The insulin-like growth factors and their regulatory proteins

Acknowledgements

Publication of this volume was made possible by the generous financial support of Pharmacia Kabi Peptide Hormones.

The insulin-like growth factors and their regulatory proteins

Proceedings of the Third International Symposium on Insulin-Like Growth Factors, Sydney, 6–10 February 1994

Editors:

R.C. Baxter

Kolling Institute of Medical Research
Royal North Shore Hospital
Sydney, NSW, Australia

P.D. Gluckman

Research Centre for Developmental Medicine and Biology
University of Auckland
Auckland, New Zealand

R.G. Rosenfeld

Department of Pediatrics
School of Medicine, Oregon Health Sciences University
Portland, Oregon, U.S.A.

 1994

Excerpta Medica

Amsterdam, Lausanne, New York, Oxford, Shannon, Tokyo

International Congress Series No. 1056
ISBN 0-444-81756-5

This book is printed on acid-free paper.

Published by:
Elsevier Science B.V.
P.O. Box 211
1000 AE Amsterdam
The Netherlands

Library of Congress Cataloging in Publication Data:

```
International Symposium on Insulin-Like Growth Factors (3rd : 1994 :
  Sydney, N.S.W.)
   The insulin-like growth factors and their regulatory proteins :
  proceedings of the Third International Symposium on Insulin-Like
  Growth Factors, Sydney, 6-10 February 1994 / editors, R.C. Baxter,
  P.D. Gluckman, R.G. Rosenfeld.
       p.    cm. -- (International congress series ; no. 1056)
   Includes bibliographical references and index.
   ISBN 0-444-81756-5 (alk. paper)
   1. Somatomedin--Congresses.  2. Insulin-like growth factor-binding
  proteins--Congresses.  3. Somatomedin--Receptors--Congresses.
  I. Baxter, R. C. (Robert C.)  II. Gluckman, Peter D.
  III. Rosenfeld, Ron G.  IV. Title.  V. Series.
   [DNLM: 1. Somatomedins--congresses.  2. Carrier Proteins-
  -congresses.  3. Gene Expression Regulation--congresses.   W3 EX89
  no.1056 1994 / QU 107 I612 1994]
  QP552.S65I578   1994
  612'.015756--dc20
  DNLM/DLC
  for Library of Congress                                   94-15908
                                                                CIP
```

In order to ensure rapid publication this volume was prepared using a method of electronic text processing known as Optical Character Recognition (OCR). Scientific accuracy and consistency of style were handled by the author. Time did not allow for the usual extensive editing process of the Publisher.

Printed in the Netherlands

Preface

In the three years since the Second International Symposium on Insulin-like Growth Factors was held in San Francisco, many exciting advances have been made. That meeting occurred at a turning point in the evolution of IGF research, when the structures of the six binding proteins (IGFBPs) had recently been elucidated, a novel signalling pathway for the type II IGF receptor had just been identified and reports of therapeutic trials of IGF-I were beginning to appear. Since then, there have been major developments in many areas, from investigations of posttranslational processing of IGFBPs to novel clinical applications. As a result of increased availability of the growth factors and their binding proteins, and of newly developed analytical techniques, the door to IGF research has been opened to many investigators who previously would have found it inaccessible.

The Third International Symposium aimed to provide a forum both for researchers with a long-standing commitment to IGF research and those who had entered the area more recently, to present their latest data to an audience of similar enthusiasts. Fourteen sessions of invited presentations, supplemented by papers selected from submitted abstracts, addressed a range of topics from growth hormone signalling pathways, IGF gene regulation and IGF receptors, IGFBP regulation and actions, metabolic studies and clinical applications of IGFs. In addition, a number of specific body system including bone, muscle, brain, kidney and reproduction were covered. To provide delegates with up-to-date technical information on molecular biology approaches, immunoassay methods, analysis of IGFBPs and IGF receptors, four interactive workshops were integrated into the program of research presentations. Finally, some 300 posters, presented over two major sessions, provided a lively forum for detailed discussion of recent advances over the complete range of IGF research. Methodological papers based on the workshop topics, and abstracts of all oral and poster presentations, were published at the time of the meeting[*].

This volume presents over 40 papers by acknowledged leaders in current IGF research, the invited symposium speakers. Since the book is not subject to the programming constraints of the meeting, the order of papers has been rearranged to allow grouping into the following eight thematic sections, with papers relating to specific organ systems integrated into these topics:
— Regulation of IGF expression
— Structural and functional relationships
— Receptors
— IGF binding proteins

---

[*]Growth Regulation 1994;4(suppl. 1):1—140.

— Growth, development and differentiation
— Reproduction
— In vivo actions
— Clinical applications.

Together these papers provide a detailed insight into important areas of IGF investigation. Each paper is self-contained, to be of maximum benefit both to the casual reader and the active researcher. Thus, the book aims not only to provide a record of major recent advances, but also to point the way to future studies.

Special thanks are due to Pharmacia Kabi for their generous sponsorship of this Symposium.

Editors
Robert C. Baxter
Peter D. Gluckman
Ron G. Rosenfeld

Sydney, February 1994

Contents

Regulation of IGF expression

Structural and functional relationships

Receptors

viii

Binding proteins

Growth, development and differentiation

Reproduction

x

In vivo actions

Clinical studies

Regulation of IGF expression

©1994 Elsevier Science B.V. All rights reserved
The insulin-like growth factors and their regulatory proteins
R.C. Baxter, P.D. Gluckman and R.G. Rosenfeld, editors

Growth hormone signalling between the receptor and the nucleus

Jessica Schwartz, Christin Carter-Su, Debra Meyer, Elaine Stephenson, Lawrence Argetsinger and George Campbell
Department of Physiology, University of Michigan, Ann Arbor, MI 48109-0622, USA

Growth hormone (GH) was among the first regulators of IGFs identified [1]. Thus, in considering IGF expression it is appropriate to discuss the signalling mechanisms by which GH regulates gene expression.

Signal transduction by GH can be viewed as short-term changes that are initiated when GH interacts with target cells. These short-term events are believed to culminate in long-term changes recognized as growth, evident in some cells as proliferation and in others as differentiation [2,3]. IGF-I is implicated in many of these growth responses [1,3]. GH also elicits metabolic changes, among them induction of insulin resistance [4]. One of the most sensitive in vitro targets for GH is the 3T3-F442A cell line which requires GH for differentiation of fibroblasts to adipocytes [2]. These cells have been useful in analysis of several aspects of GH signal transduction.

The binding of GH to its receptor is the initial event in GH action. It had been hypothesized [5] that the GH receptor (GHR), like receptors for a variety of growth promoting factors, including IGF-I, acts by stimulating a tyrosine kinase [6–8]. Evidence in support of this hypothesis included observations that highly purified GH-GHR complexes contain tyrosine kinase activity [9,10] and that GH promotes the tyrosyl phosphorylation of multiple proteins, including the GHR [5,9,11].

However, the cloned liver GHR was found to be a single membrane-spanning polypeptide that showed no homology to known tyrosine kinases [12]. Two alternatives could reconcile these observations. There might be two different GHRs, one that had been cloned without a kinase and another hypothetical GHR with tyrosine kinase activity. Alternatively, a single GHR might be able to associate with a cellular tyrosine kinase. This was supported by the observation that the cloned GHR (which lacks homology to known tyrosine kinase), when expressed in a variety of different cell types, coprecipitated with a tyrosine kinase [13]. The putative kinase appeared on gels to be similar in size to GHR, approximately 120,000 Da.

In searching for such a kinase the Janus kinase (JAK) family of kinases, presently consisting of JAK1, JAK2 and tyk2, was of greatest interest. These kinases migrate with a molecular weight appropriate for the GHR-associated kinase. All three kinases lack a membrane spanning domain and are expressed fairly ubiquitously [14,15]. tyk2 had recently been identified as a signaling molecule for interferon α [16] and JAK1, and JAK2 were kinases of unknown function [14,15]. Recent studies have established

4

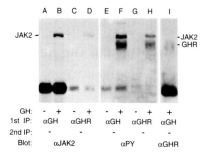

Fig. 1.

JAK2 as a GHR-associated tyrosine kinase [17].

Since autophosphorylation is often the earliest manifestation of an activated kinase, the tyrosyl phosphorylation of JAK2 in response to GH was investigated [17]. JAK2 immunoprecipitates from GH-treated 3T3-F442A fibroblasts were electrophoresed and probed on a western blot with antiphosphotyrosine antibody. A single band migrating with Mr 130,000 was present within 30 sec of GH treatment. JAK2 phosphorylation was evident at physiological concentrations of GH, as low as 0.5 ng/ml. Phosphorylation of JAK2 was specific for GH. Responses with other growth factors, including PDGF, EGF and IGF-I, were no different from control [17].

The kinase activity of JAK2 was examined directly by addition of ^{32}P-ATP to αJAK2 immunoprecipitates from GH-treated 3T3-F442A cells. ^{32}P was incorporated into a protein migrating at about 130,000, appropriate for JAK2, but only when cells had been incubated with GH. Phospho-amino acid analysis of the labelled band indicated that ^{32}P was incorporated into tyrosine indicating that JAK2 is tyrosyl phosphorylated [17].

For JAK2 to be the GHR-associated tyrosine kinase, it was necessary to show that JAK2 associates with the GHR (Fig. 1). Purified GHR was obtained from 3T3-F442A fibroblasts by immunoprecipitating with αGH or αGHR and blotted with αJAK2. In Fig. 1, lanes B and D show the presence of JAK2 in GHR preparations from GH-treated cells. Since αGHR precipitates GHR whether or not GH is bound to receptor, the absence of JAK2 in lane C indicates that GH promotes the association of JAK2 with GHR. When antiphosphotyrosine antibody was used for blotting instead of αJAK2, as shown in lanes E—H (Fig. 1), two bands were observed. One corresponds to JAK2 and the other is most likely to be GHR since it is the right size and since a similar protein is recognized in western blots using αGHR (lane 1). Overall, the results of the experiments depicted in Fig. 1 suggest that GH promotes the association of JAK2 with GHR, activates JAK2 and stimulates the tyrosyl phosphorylation of both JAK2 and GHR. The identification of JAK2 as a signalling molecule for the GHR is important, since JAK2 is the first signalling molecule identified that interacts with GHR.

The finding that JAK2 is a signalling molecule for GHR has a broad impact because recent findings indicate that JAK2 is also utilized by other members of the

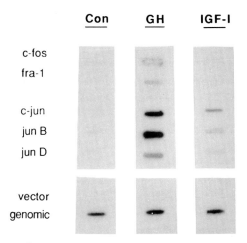

Con	GH	IGF-I

c-fos
fra-1

c-jun
jun B
jun D

vector
genomic

Fig. 2.

cytokine/hematopoietin receptor family. This association has now been demonstrated for a variety of these receptors including receptors for prolactin, erythropoietin and other cytokines, and the more distinctly related receptor for IFNγ [18–21]. The fact that all of these receptors can activate JAK2 makes it seem likely that these receptors share signalling pathways and possibly elicit some of the same responses.

Among the short-term consequences of the GH-GHR interaction are rapid changes in the nucleus. GH induces early-response genes such as c-*fos* and c-*jun*, which encode transcription factors that regulate target genes implicated in growth and differentiation pathways [22]. The rapid induction of c-*fos* by GH has been shown in 3T3-F442A fibroblasts [23] and in a variety of other cell types [24–26].

Nuclear run-off experiments show that the GH induced increase in expression of c-*fos* reflects stimulation of transcription (Fig. 2). GH also stimulates, within 15 min, the transcription of other genes in the Fos family and several genes in the Jun family (Fig. 2, middle lane), whose products can work in coordination with c-*fos* [22]. IGF-I, at an equimolar concentration to GH (22nM), was consistently less effective than GH in inducing c-*fos* and c-*jun* transcription (Fig. 2, right lane). Since the induction of these genes by GH occurs so rapidly, and is consistently greater than the effect of

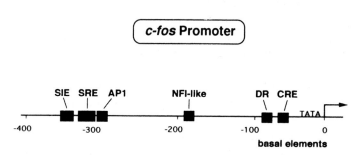

Fig. 3.

6

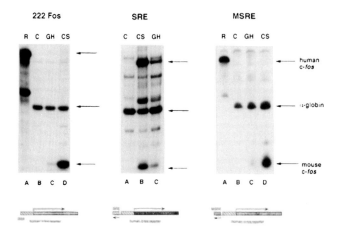

Fig. 4.

IGF-I, it is unlikely to be mediated by IGF-I.

Once it was established that GH stimulated the transcription of c-*fos*, it was logical to look for GH-responsive DNA sequences in the c-*fos* promoter (Fig. 3). A fragment of the well-studied c-*fos* promoter, containing growth factor sensitive regions known as the serum response element (SRE), the c-*sis* inducible element (SIE), and an AP-1 site were found to contain a GH-responsive DNA sequence which could mediate expression of a reporter [27].

To identify a GH responsive DNA sequence in this fragment with more refinement, the ability of the SRE to mediate stimulation of reporter expression by GH was examined (Fig. 4). An oligonucleotide based on the sequence of the SRE, upstream of a human c-*fos* reporter [28] was transfected transiently into NIH-3T3 mouse fibroblasts. Human α globin was cotransfected to assess transfection efficiency. Cells were treated with or without GH and RNA was prepared. RNAse protection assays using a c-*fos* riboprobe distinguished between endogenous mouse c-*fos* and the transfected human c-*fos*, which would only be detected if the promoter was stimulated by treatment of the cells with GH. A riboprobe for α-globin was used to detect expression of the control plasmid.

The middle panel of Fig. 4 shows that the SRE can mediate induction of c-*fos* by GH. The top bands (H) indicate that in GH treated cells (lane C) expression of the transfected human c-*fos* reporter was stimulated relative to untreated controls (lane A) that exhibited the same transfection efficiency (α, middle bands). Not surprisingly serum also stimulated expression through the SRE (lane B). In the same cells, GH and serum also stimulated expression of the endogenous mouse c-*fos*, as expected (M, bottom bands). Controls are shown using the reporter without a SRE (panel A) and with a mutated SRE (panel C) [29] which cannot mediate reporter expression. Thus, the SRE is a GH-responsive DNA sequence in the c-*fos* promoter.

These results raise several interesting questions. First, since a number of nuclear proteins have been identified which are transcription factors which bind to or associate with the SRE [30], it will be of interest to determine whether any of these factors are regulated by GH. Second, the present results with the SRE do not preclude that other DNA sequences in the c-*fos* gene might also respond to GH. In this regard, our recent experiments show that the SIE sequence in the c-*fos* promoter, which lies just upstream of the SRE, is also regulated by GH.

To determine whether GH might induce the binding of nuclear proteins to the SIE sequence, electrophoretic mobility shift assays (EMSA) were used. Nuclear extracts from 3T3-F442A cells treated with or without GH were incubated with ^{32}P-labelled oligonucleotide representing a high-affinity SIE sequence [28]. GH stimulated the binding of nuclear proteins to the SIE (Fig. 5). The GH-induced binding was specific, since it was competed by unlabelled probe but was poorly competed by a mutated SIE sequence [31]. We have named this GH-inducible DNA binding factor GHIF. Since GHIF runs as multiple bands, it may contain a complex of multiple proteins or contain proteins in multiple phosphorylation states. Induction of GHIF binding is specific for GH (Fig. 5). It is not evident in cells treated with IGF-I (22 nM). It is induced to a lesser extent by PDGF (25 ng/ml), although PDGF is a potent stimulator of binding to SIE in other cell types [29].

To identify components of GHIF, analogy to interferon signalling pathways were considered for several reasons. IFNα and IFNγ receptors, like the GHR, utilize JAK family kinases as signalling molecules. It is now known that IFNα uses JAK1 and tyk2 [16,32] and that IFNγ utilizes JAK2 in signalling [21]. IFNα and IFNγ stimulate the tyrosyl phosphorylation of DNA binding proteins [33]. In response to IFNα, a 91 kDa cytoplasmic protein undergoes tyrosyl phosphorylation and forms a complex (ISGFα) with two other tyrosyl phosphorylated proteins (p84 and p113) and with a DNA binding subunit (p48) to form a DNA binding complex that initiates transcription of IFNα stimulated genes [34–36]. With IFNγ treatment, p91 appears to be tyrosyl phosphorylated, to translocate to the nucleus and to bind directly to IFNγ

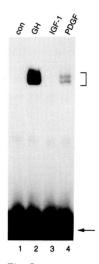

Fig. 5.

8

responsive DNA sequences [37–39]. Interestingly, the sequences of the interferon responsive DNA sequences share striking homologies with the sequence of the c-*fos* SIE [40]. Thus, it seemed possible that GHIF might contain p91 or a related protein. This idea was supported by observations that GH stimulated tyrosyl phosphorylation of p91 or a related protein in 3T3-F442A cells. When proteins from GH or IFNγ treated cells were immunoprecipitated using αp91 and blotted with antiphosphotyrosine antibodies, both GH and IFNγ stimulated tyrosyl phosphorylation of proteins immunoprecipitated by αp91 [31]. One band in GH-treated cells appeared to be p91, since it was blotted with p91 antibody. Antibodies that recognize p84 or p113 did not recognize protein in the αp91 immunoprecipitate.

To test whether p91 might be a component of the GHIF complex, nuclear extracts were prepared from GH treated cells and tested in the EMSA (Fig. 6). The GHIF complex was clearly seen (lane 2). Addition of αp91 to nuclear extract, prior to its interaction with the SIE probe, resulted in a supershift of the GHIF-SIE complex (lane 3), suggesting the presence of p91 or an antigenically related protein. This supershift was specific for αp91, since αp113 and two unrelated antibodies did not cause the supershift in this experiment (lanes 4,5,7). Incubation of the nuclear extract with antiphosphotyrosine reduced the formation of the GHIF-SIE complex, consistent with the presence of tyrosyl phosphorylated proteins in GHIF (lane 6). These results provide evidence that GH induces the binding of the GHIF DNA binding complex to the c-*fos* SIE. The complex contains p91 or p91-related proteins and phosphotyrosine. GHIF activity was found to appear in the cytoplasm earlier (5 min) and in the nucleus (15 min) (not shown), consistent with translocation. These findings also

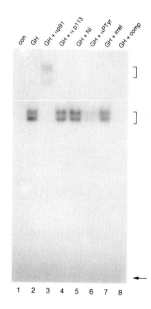

Fig. 6.

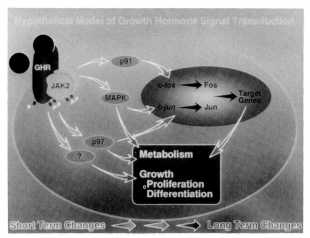

Fig. 7. Hypothetical model of growth hormone signal transduction.

have broad impact since p91 has recently been implicated in signalling pathways of a variety of receptors that utilize JAK2 [18–21].

A model of GH signal transduction can now be hypothesized which links GH-induced changes in the nucleus to events at the receptor (Fig. 7). Beginning at the membrane, the binding of GH to the GH receptor causes JAK2 to bind to GHR and become activated. Once bound, JAK2 phosphorylates itself and GHR, and presumably other proteins. This appears to initiate a cascade of events involving phosphorylation. Among the phosphorylated intermediates are MAP kinases, which are stimulated by GH [41–43] and which participate in regulation of transcription factors associated with SRE [44,45]. Obviously of interest are p91 and related proteins, which participate in binding to the c-*fos* SIE and appear to play a similar role in other signaling pathways utilizing JAK2 [20,37].

We believe that c-*fos* and other Fos and Jun family genes in turn regulate expression of target genes implicated in long term physiological changes associated with growth and metabolic regulation. In some systems, we can speculate that genes encoding IGF-I, or other GH-dependent components associated with IGF-I, may also be dependent on these pathways of GH signaling. Identification of these signaling pathways represents a major advance in understanding how GH signals between the receptor and nucleus. These findings should enable us to make substantial progress in the future in understanding how GH acts and interacts with other growth factors to regulate body growth and metabolism.

Acknowledgements

These studies were supported by grants DCB8918289 from NSF, 9202770 from USDA (to JS) and DK34171 from NIH (to CCS and IS). Figures are reprinted by permission as follows; Fig. 1 [Ref. 17], Fig. 4 [Ref. 27] and Fig. 6 [Ref. 31].

10

References

1. Isaksson OGP, Eden S, Jansson, JO. Ann Rev Physiol 1985;47:483–499.
2. Morikawa M, Nixon T, Green H. Cell 1982;29:783–789.
3. Billestrup N, Nielsen JH. Endocrinology 1991;129:883–888.
4. Davidson MB. Endocrine Rev 1987;8:115–131.
5. Foster CM, Shafer JA, Rozsa FWW, Wang X, Lewis SD, Renken DA, Natale JE, Schwartz J, Carter-Su C. Biochemistry 1988;27:326–334.
6. Jacobs S, Kull FC, Earp HS, Suoboda M, VanWyk JJ, Cuatrecasas P. J Biol Chem 1983;258:951–9584.
7. Rubin JB, Shia MA, Pilch PF. Nature 1983;305:438–440.
8. Ullrich A, Schlessinger J. Cell 1990;61:203–212.
9. Carter-Su C, Stubbart JR, Wang X, Stred SE, Argetsinger LS, Shafer JA. J Biol Chem 1989;264: 18654–18661.
10. Stred SE, Stubbart JR, Argetsinger LS, Smith WC, Shafer JA, Talamantes F, Carter-Su C. Endocrinology 1992;130:1626–1636.
11. Campbell GS, Christan LJ, Carter-Su C. J Biol Chem 1993;268:7427–7434.
12. Leung DW, Spencer SA, Cachianes G, Hammonds RG, Colling C, Henzel WJ, Barnard R, Waters MJ, Wood WI. Nature 1987;330:537–543.
13. Stred SE, Stubbart JR, Argetsinger LS, Shafer JA, Carter-Su C. Endocrinology 1990;127:2506–2516.
14. Silvennoinen O, Witthuhn B, Quelle FW, Cleveland JL, Yi T, Ihle JN. Proc Natl Acad Sci USA 1993;90:8429–8433.
15. Wilks AF, Harpur AG, Kurban RR, Ralph SI, Zurcher G, Ziemiecki A. Mol Cell Biol 1991;11: 2057–2065.
16. Velazquez L, Fellous M, Stark GR, Pellegrini S. Cell 1992;70:313–322.
17. Argetsinger L, Campbell GS, Yang X, Witthuhn BA, Silvennoinen O, Ihle JN, Carter-Su C. Cell 1993;74:237–244.
18. Campbell GS, Argetsinger LS, Ihle JN, Kelly PA, Rillema JA, Carter-Su C. Activation of JAK2 tyrosine kinase by prolactin receptors in Nb$_2$ cells and mouse mammary gland explants. Proc Natl Acad Sci USA 1994 (in press).
19. Witthuhn BA, Quelle FW, Silvennoinen O, Yi T, Tang B, Miura O, Ihle JN. Cell 1993;74:227–236.
20. Stahl N, Boulton TG, Fartuggella T, Ip NY, Davis S, Witthuhn BA, Quelle FW, Silvennoinen O, Barbieri G, Pellegrine S, Ihle JN, Yancopoulos GD. Science 1994;263:92–95.
21. Watling D, Guschin D, Muller M, Silvennoinen O, Witthuhn BA, Quelle FW, Rogers NC, Schindler C, Stark GR, Ihle JN, Kerr IM. Nature 1993;366:166–170.
22. Cuttan T, Franza BR Jr. Cell 1988;55:395–397.
23. Gurland G, Ashcom G, Cochran BH, Schwartz J. Endocrinology 1990;127:3187–3195.
24. Doglio A, Dani C, Grimaldi P, Ailhaud G. Proc Nat Acad Sci USA 1989;86:1148–1152.
25. Slootweg MC, deGroot RP, Herrmann-Erlee MPM, Koornneef I, Kruijer W, Kramer YM. J Mol Endocrinol 1991;6:179–188.
26. Tollet P, Legraverend C, Gustafsson J, Mode A. Mol Endocrinol 1991;5:1351–1358.
27. Meyer DJ, Stephenson EW, Johnson L, Cochran BH, Schwartz J. Proc Nat Acad Sci USA 1993;90: 6721–6725.
28. Wagner BJ, Hayes TH, Hoban CJ, Cochran BH EMBO J 1990;9:4477–4484.
29. Hayes TE, Kitchen AM, Cochran BH. Proc Nat Acad Sci USA 1987;84:1272–1276.
30. Treisman R. Trends Biochem Sci 1992;17:423–426.
31. Meyer DJ, Campbell GS, Cochran BH, Argetsinger LS, Larner AC, Finbloom DS, Carter-Su C, Schwartz J. J Biol Chem 1994;269:4701–4704.
32. Muller M, Briscoe J, Laxton C, Guschin D, Ziemiecki A, Silvennoinen O, Harpur AG, Barbieri G, Witthuhn BA, Schindler C, Pellegrini S, Wilks AF, Ihle JN, Stark GR, Kerr IM. Nature 1993;366: 129–135.
33. Shuai K, Stark GR, Kerr IM, Darnell JE Jr. Science 1993;261:1744–1746.

34. Schindler C, Shuai K, Presioso VR, Darnell JE Jr. Science 1992;257:809–813.
35. Fu XY, Schindler C, Improta T, Aebersold R, Darnell JE. Proc Natl Acad Sci USA 1992;89:7840–7843.
36. Kessler DS, Veals SA, Fu XY, Levy DE. Genes Devel 1990;4:1753–1765.
37. Shuai K, Schindler C, Prezioso VR, Darnell JE Jr. Science 1992;258:1808–1812.
38. Pearse RN, Feinman R, Shuai K, Darnell JE Jr, Ravetch JV. Proc Natl Acad Sci USA 1993;90:4314–4318.
39. Wilson KC, Finbloom DS. Proc Natl Acad Sci USA 1992:89:11964–11968.
40. Fu XY, Zhang J-J. Cell 1993;74:1135–1145.
41. Campbell GS, Miyasaka T, Pang L, Saltiel AR, Carter-Su C. J Biol Chem 1992;267:6074–6080.
42. Winston LA, Bertics PJ. J Biol Chem 1992;267:4747–4751.
43. Moller C, Hansson A, Enberg B, Lobie PE, Norstedt G. J Biol Chem 1992;267:23403–23407.
44. Marais R, Wynne J, Treisman R. Cell 1993;73:381–393.
45. Janknecht R, Ernst WH, Pingoud V, Nordheim A. EMBO J 1993;12:5097–5104.

©1994 Elsevier Science B.V. All rights reserved
The insulin-like growth factors and their regulatory proteins
R.C. Baxter, P.D. Gluckman and R.G. Rosenfeld, editors

The somatomedin hypothesis revisited: early events in growth hormone action

Peter Rotwein[1,2], Michael J. Thomas[1,2], Ann M. Gronowski[1,2], David P. Bichell[3] and Kiyoshi Kikuchi[1,2]
Departments of [1]Medicine, [2]Biochemistry and Molecular Biophysics and [3]Surgery, Washington University School of Medicine, St. Louis, MO 63110, USA

Introduction

In mammals, somatic growth is regulated by the interplay of hormonal, genetic, developmental, nutritional and metabolic factors [1,2]. The growth-promoting effects of many of these agents are secondary to the actions of IGF-I a highly-conserved, 70 amino acid secreted protein that is produced in many tissues [3,4]. The critical role of one of these factors, growth hormone (GH), in regulating postnatal growth through IGF-I has been appreciated since the original formulation of the somatomedin hypothesis by Salmon and Daughaday in 1957 [5], although progress has been slow in understanding the biochemical mechanisms of GH action. In this report we review recent research on this topic, focusing on early events in GH-mediated signal transduction. The results presented outline a physiologically-significant pathway of growth control, in which signals initiated by the binding of GH to its cell-surface receptor are rapidly propagated to the nucleus to stimulate transcription of the IGF-I gene.

Early events in GH action

The GH receptor

Since the initial cloning of the 620 amino acid human and rabbit growth hormone (GH) receptors in 1987 [6], much progress has been made in defining the biochemistry of this glycoprotein. Receptor homologues have been characterized from several mammalian species and from the chicken [7,8]. The human GH receptor is a transmembrane protein consisting of an extracellular domain of 246 amino acids, a single membrane-spanning segment of 24 residues, and a cytoplasmic region of 350

Address for correspondence: Peter Rotwein, Washington University School of Medicine, Box 8231, 660 South Euclid Avenue, St. Louis, MO 63110, USA. Tel.: +1-314-362-2703. Fax: +1-314-362-7183.

amino acids that both lack typical protein tyrosine kinase motifs and domains that are involved in receptor G-protein coupling (reviewed in [7,9]). The extracellular part of the receptor has also been characterized as the serum GH-binding protein [6]. The GH receptor was the first member identified in an expanding group of related proteins that are known collectively as the cytokine receptors [9–11] and include receptors for prolactin, erythropoietin, granulocyte and granulocyte-macrophage colony stimulating factors, leukemia inhibitory factor, ciliary neurotrophic factor, interleukins 3–7 and others [9,11–13]. These proteins share limited amino acid identity in their extracellular domains, including pairs of cysteine residues that are involved in ligand binding [7], and a signature motif, WSxWS (W-tryptophan, S-serine, x-any residue), that is located in the juxtamembrane region [10]. This latter motif is absent in the GH receptor [6–8].

First steps in GH action

A series of studies published in the past few years have defined the initial events in GH action [14–24]. Experiments performed in vitro have indicated that the binding of GH to the extracellular portion of the receptor induces receptor dimerization [14] and the sites that are necessary for ligand-receptor binding have been identified [22,25]. Based on studies using chimeric receptors, it has been suggested that hormone-induced dimerization is a critical first step in GH receptor activation [15,26].

Studies using cultured cells have shown additionally that GH binding stimulates the interaction of the GH receptor with an intracellular protein kinase termed JAK2 [17], a member of the Janus kinase family [27]. This interaction occurs within minutes of addition of GH to 3T3F442A cells and leads to the autophosphorylation on tyrosine residues of JAK2 and to the tyrosine phosphorylation of the GH receptor itself [17]. The role of JAK2 as a protein kinase toward exogenous substrates and its function in GH-mediated signal transduction remain to be defined.

Rapid changes in cellular protein tyrosine phosphorylation are induced by GH

Recent studies have demonstrated that activation of the GH receptor by ligand binding leads to the rapid tyrosine phosphorylation of multiple intracellular proteins [16,17,21,22,28,29]. Experiments using cultured cells have shown that GH treatment stimulates both the phosphorylation and activation of MAP (or ERK) kinases [21,22]. Both the 44 kDa (ERK1) and 42 kDa (ERK2) isoforms are regulated by GH [21,22]. Our laboratory has demonstrated that in vivo GH treatment also leads to the rapid tyrosine phosphorylation of MAP kinases in the liver of hypophysectomized (hypox) male rats [30]. We also have evidence that translocation of both isoforms to the nucleus is another early event in GH action [30]. MAP kinases are ubiquitous intracellular enzymes that are induced by many extracellular signals through activation of the protein kinase MEK [31–34]. The pathway of stimulation of MAP kinases by GH and their roles in GH action are currently unknown; however, since these proteins phosphorylate other intracellular enzymes, such as ribosomal S6

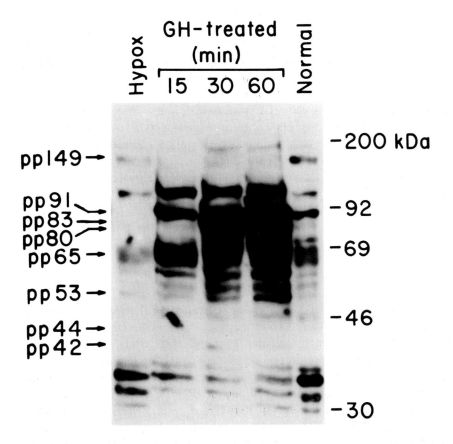

Fig. 1. GH treatment induces rapid changes in hepatic nuclear protein tyrosine phosphorylation. Liver nuclear proteins were extracted from normally growing male rats and from hypox male rats before or after a single intraperitoneal injection of human recombinant GH. Proteins were separated by SDS-polyacrylamide gel electrophoresis, transferred to PVDF membranes and were detected using a monoclonal antibody to phosphotyrosine [30]. Molecular weight markers are indicated.

kinases and transcription factors, including c-*jun*, c-*myc* and others [32,34,35], MAP kinases may mediate GH-regulated activation of early response genes [36,37].

In related experiments we have examined other early steps in GH action in vivo by investigating changes in hepatic protein phosphorylation that follow a single GH injection to hypox male rats. Since our major interest is in the mechanisms by which GH induces target gene transcription, we have focused on alterations within the nucleus. GH rapidly stimulated the tyrosine phosphorylation of several nuclear proteins, ranging in mass from 42 to ~205 kDa and caused the dephosphorylation of a single ~150 kDa protein (Fig. 1). Using specific antibodies we have identified two of these proteins as 42 and 44 kDa MAP kinases, as noted above, and have shown that the prominent 91 kDa phosphoprotein is STAT91, a component of the interferon α-stimulated gene factor 3 complex [38]. In addition to its role in mediating the immediate transcriptional response to interferon α, STAT91 is also activated by interferon γ [39] and is induced by treatment of cells with a variety of growth factors and cytokines [40–44]. One consequence of the activation of STAT91 by GH is the appearance of GH-stimulated nuclear DNA binding activity, as shown by gel-mobility shift assay with an oligonucleotide probe derived from the c-*sis* inducible element (SIE) of the c-*fos* promoter [30]. GH appears to be as potent as epidermal growth factor in inducing DNA-binding activity toward the SIE in liver nuclear extracts [40]. In aggregate our results show that nuclear tyrosine phosphorylation is another early event in GH action, occurring within minutes of hormone administration [30], and identify a biochemical link between GH-stimulated signal transduction pathways and target gene expression. The identities of the other nuclear tyrosine-phosphorylated proteins that are modified by GH are unknown.

Regulation of IGF-I gene expression by GH

IGF-I gene and mRNA structure

The IGF-I gene is composed of 5 or 6 exons depending on the species [45,46]. In mammals the large 6 exon gene (80 kb in the rat, >70 kb in the human) consists of 2 overlapping transcription units. Exons 1 and 2 each contain 5′ noncoding sequences and the beginning portions of signal peptide coding regions and are each preceded by a distinct promoter [46–48]. Exons 3 and 4 encode the mature 70 residue IGF-I protein, as well as part of the signal peptide on exon 3 and the beginning of the E domain on exon 4. In the human IGF-I gene exon 5 encodes the COOH-terminal portion of the E_B peptide, 3′ untranslated sequences, and a polyadenylation signal, exon 6 contains the distal part of the E_A domain, a 3′ untranslated region (UTR) and multiple polyadenylation signals [45,46]. Because of alternative RNA splicing these two exons are uniquely present in different classes of IGF-I mRNAs. In the rat gene several nucleotide changes have occurred within exon 5 during speciation and have created a splice donor site for RNA processing [49], so that IGF-I_B mRNAs contain exons 5 and 6 and IGF-I_A transcripts contain exon 6 [48].

As evidenced by the complicated anatomy of IGF-I genes and mRNAs summarized above, multiple mechanisms are potentially important in the regulation of IGF-I gene expression. The diversity and relative concentration of different IGF-I transcripts is the consequence of the interplay among several processes, including transcription from 2 promoters, heterogeneous transcription initiation within each promoter, alternative RNA splicing, differential RNA polyadenylation and variable mRNA stability [45,50]. Although each of these mechanisms are involved in determining the steady-state levels of IGF-I mRNAs under different physiological conditions, as indicated below the most potent acute effect of GH is to stimulate IGF-I gene transcription [51].

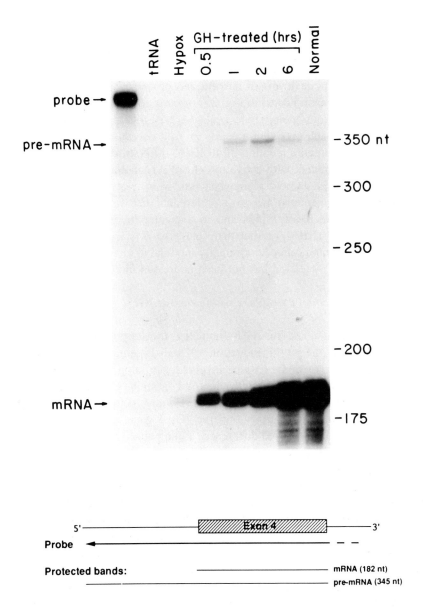

Fig. 2. Rapid stimulation of nuclear IGF-I mRNA after GH treatment. Hypox male rats were given a single intraperitoneal injection of human GH, hepatic nuclei and nuclear RNA were isolated [51]. The autoradiograph shows results of a ribonuclease protection experiment using a ^{32}P-labeled antisense RNA probe derived from rat IGF-I exon 4 and its 5′ intron, as illustrated. An increase in unspliced and processed IGF-I mRNA is apparent within 30 min of GH treatment (the former is seen more clearly on a longer radiographic exposure (data not shown)). The locations of the full-length probe and protected fragments are indicated. Calibration was performed using the DNA sequencing ladder visible in the two rightmost lanes.

Rapid activation of IGF-I gene transcription by GH treatment

As assessed by "run-on" assays with isolated liver nuclei, IGF-I gene transcription increased within 30 min of intraperitoneal injection of GH into hypox juvenile male rats [51]. By this early time point levels of nascent and processed IGF-I RNA had also increased in the nucleus, as indicated in Fig. 2. Transcriptional activation, which affects both IGF-I promoters equivalently [51], peaked at >10-fold above baseline by 2 hr after GH administration and preceded a nearly 20-fold rise in all IGF-I mRNA species [51]. The rapid, coordinate induction of all IGF-I mRNAs after a single GH injection was temporally coincident with activation of Spi 2.1, another GH-regulated gene [52], and contrasted with effects seen when rats were treated with GH for several days. Multiple GH injections led to a preferential rise in IGF-I mRNAs containing exon 2 rather than exon 1 [53] and to a greater increase in mRNAs encoding both exons 5 and 6 (IGF-I$_B$) rather than just exon 6 (IGF-I$_A$) [49]. These more chronic effects of GH may reflect hormonally-modulated alterations in IGF-I mRNA stability, although this question has not been addressed directly.

GH regulates changes in chromatin structure within the rat IGF-I gene

Recently we have begun to look for GH-stimulated transcriptional regulatory proteins that might mediate the rapid induction of IGF-I gene expression described above. Our approach to this problem involved assuming that interaction of GH-regulated DNA binding proteins with their recognition sites would alter chromatin organization somewhere within the IGF-I locus. We therefore first developed a map of chromatin structure within the IGF-I gene, using the nuclease DNase I as a probe, and then analyzed differences among normal, hypox and GH-treated rats. We mapped 15 DNase I hypersensitive (HS) sites within the 120 kb IGF-I gene and flanking regions [54]. A single site, HS7, located in the second intron, was present in normal rats but absent after hypophysectomy. By 30 min after GH injection HS7 reappeared, only to disappear by 6 hr [51]. This time course coincided with the onset and decline in IGF-I transcription described above. More recently we have used in vivo DNase I footprinting to map this hormonally-responsive chromatin domain to a ~350 nucleotide region and have identified DNA-protein interactions within HS7 by in vitro gel-mobility shift assays and in vitro DNase I footprinting studies [55]. DNA-protein binding was localized to two adjacent segments of 32 and 48 nucleotides. DNA binding activity was present in hypox rats and was not modified by GH treatment, as determined by gel-shift assay, although acute hormonally-regulated changes were evident after analysis by DNase I footprinting [55]. These results define a rapid and reversible genomic alteration in response to GH in a GH-regulated gene and delineate a target within chromatin for GH action.

Table 1. Timetable of early events in GH action

1. GH-induced receptor dimerization.
2. Interaction of the activated GH receptor with JAK2.
3. Tyrosine phosphorylation of JAK2 and the GH receptor.
4. Changes in cytoplasmic and nuclear protein phosphorylation.
5. Stimulation of target gene transcription.

Summary and perspectives on future studies

In this chapter we have presented recent information from our laboratory and from other groups on the acute actions of GH. Our principal focus has been on signal transduction from the cell surface to the nucleus and on the mechanisms by which GH activates a key target gene, IGF-I. Based on the preliminary evidence described in this report we propose a multi-step pathway from the GH receptor in the cell membrane to stimulation of target gene expression within the nucleus (Table 1). Goals for the future will be to understand each of these steps in detail, to establish the links among them and to characterize the signaling molecules. Then the somatomedin hypothesis will be elucidated at a molecular level.

Acknowledgements

The studies from our laboratory were supported by U.S. National Institutes of Health Grant 5RO1-DK37449 (to P.R.). M.J.T. and A.M.G. are postdoctoral trainees in Endocrinology and Metabolism (NIH Training Grant 5T32DK07120) and D.P.B. is a postdoctoral trainee in Surgical Oncology (NIH Training Grant 5T32CA09621) at Washington University School of Medicine. K.K. was supported by the Washington University-Searle-Monsanto Research Program.

References

1. Daughaday WH. Trends Genet 1985;2:194–195.
2. Rudd BT. Ann Clin Biochem 1991;28:542–555.
3. Daughaday WH, Rotwein P. Endocrine Rev 1989;10:68–91.
4. Humbel RE. Eur J Biochem 1990;190:445–462.
5. Salmon WD, Daughaday WH. J Lab Clin Med 1957;49:825–836.
6. Leung DW, Spencer SA, Cachianes G, Hammonds RG, Collins C, Henzel WJ, Barnard R, Waters MJ, Wood WI. Nature 1987;330:537–543.
7. Kelly PA, Ali S, Rozakis M, Goujon L, Nagano M, Pellegrini I, Gould D, Djiane J, Edery M, Finidori J, Postel-Vinay MC. Recent Prog Horm Res 1993;48:123–165.
8. Burnside J, Shuenn SL, Cogburn LA. Endocrinol 1991;128:3183–3192.
9. Kelly PA, Djiane J, Postel-Vinay M-C, Ederly M. Endocrine Rev 1991;12:235–251.

10. Cosman D, Lyman S, Idzerda RL, Beckmann MP, Goodwin RG, March CJ. Trends Biochem Sci 1990;15:265–270.

11. Miyajima A, Hara T, Kitamura T. Trends Biochem Sci 1992;17:378–382.

12. Gearing DP, Comeau MR, Friend DJ, Gimpel SD, Thut CJ, McGourty J, Brasher KK, King JA, Gillis S, Mosley B, Ziegler SF, Cosman D. Science 1992;255:1434–1437.

13. Davis S, Aldrich TH, Valenzuela D, Wong V, Furth ME, Squinto S, Yancopoulos GD. Science 1991; 253:59–63.

14. Cunningham BC, Ultsch M, De Vos AM, Mulkerrin MG, Clauser KR, Wells JA. Science 1991;253: 821–825.

15. Fuh G, Cunningham BC, Fukunaga R, Nagata S, Goeddel DV, Wells JA. Science 1992;256:1677–1680.

16. Campbell GS, Christian LJ, Carter-Su C. J Biol Chem 1993;268:7427–7434.

17. Argetsinger LS, Campbell GS, Yang X, Witthuhn BA, Silvennoinen O, Ihle JN, Carter-Su C. Cell 1993;74:237–244.

18. Foster CM, Shafer JA, Rozsa FW, Wang X, Lewis SD, Renken DA, Natale JE, Schwartz J, Carter-Su C. Biochem 1988;27:326–334.

19. Stred SE, Stubbart JR, Argentsinger LS, Shafer JA, Carter-Su C. Endocrinol 1990;127:2506–2516.

20. Stred SE, Stubbart JR, Argentsinger LS, Smith WC, Shafer JA, Talamantes F, Carter-Su C. Endocrinol 1992;130:1626–1636.

21. Winston LA, Bertics PJ. J Biol Chem 1992;267:4747–4751.

22. Moller C, Hansson A, Enberg B, Lobie PE, Norsted G. J Biol Chem 1992;267:23403–23408.

23. Ishizaka-Ikeda E, Fukunaga R, Wood WI, Goeddel DV, Nagata S. Proc Natl Acad Sci USA 1993; 90:123–127.

24. Colosi P, Wong K, Leong S, Wood WI. J Biol Chem 1993;268:12617–12623.

25. deVos AM, Ultsch M, Kossiakof AA. Science 1992;255:306–312.

26. Wells JA, Cunningham BC, Fuh G, Lowman HB, Bass SH, Mulkerrin MG, Ultsch M, deVos AM. Recent Prog Horm Res 1993;48:253–275.

27. Harpur AG, Andres A-C, Ziemiecki A, Aston RR, Wilks AF. Oncogene 1992;7:1347–1353.

28. Silva CM, Weber MJ, Thorner MO. Endocrinol 1993;132:101–108.

29. Campbell GS, Pang L, Miyasaka T, Saltiel AR, Carter-Su C. J Biol Chem 1992;267:6074–6080.

30. Gronowski AM, Rotwein P. J Biol Chem 1994;269 (in press).

31. Lange-Carter CA, Pleiman CM, Gardner AM, Blumer KJ, Johnson GL. Science 1993;260:315–319.

32. Davis RJ. J Biol Chem 1993;268:14553–14556.

33. Crews CM, Erikson RL. Cell 1993;74:215–217.

34. Egan SE, Weinberg RA. Nature 1993;365:781–783.

35. Janknecht R, Ernst WH, Pingoud V, Nordheim A. EMBO J 1993;12:5097–5104.

36. Gurland G, Ashcom G, Cochran BH, Schwartz J. Endocrinol 1990;127:3187–3195.

37. Slootweg MC, de Groot RP, Herrmann-Erlee MPM, Koornneef I, Kruijer W, Kramer YM. J Mol Endocrinol 1991;6:179–188.

38. Schindler C, Shuai K, Prezioso VR, Darnell JE Jr. Science 1992;257:809–813.

39. Shaui K, Schlindler C, Prezioso VR, Darnell JE Jr. Science 1992;258:1808–1812.

40. Ruff-Jamison S, Chen K, Cohen S. Science 1993;261:1733–1736.

41. Sadowski HB, Shaui K, Darnell JE Jr, Gilman MZ. Science 1993;261:1739–1744.

42. Larner AC, David M, Feldman GM, Igarashi K-i, Hackett RH, Webb DSA, Sweitzer SM, Petricoin F III, Finbloom DS. Science 1993;261:1730–1733.

43. Silvennoinen O, Schindler C, Schlessinger J, Levy DE. Science 1993;261:1736–1739.

44. Bonni A, Frank DA, Schindler C, Greenberg ME. Science 1993;262:1575–1579.

45. Rotwein P. Growth Factors 1991;5:3–18.

46. Sussenbach JS, Steenbergh PH, Holthuizen P. Growth Reg 1992;2:1–9.

47. Kim SW, Lajara R, Rotwein P. Mol Endocrinol 1991;5:1964–1972.

48. Hall LJ, Kajimoto Y, Bichell DP, Kim SW, James PL, Counts D, Nixon L, Tobin G, Rotwein P. DNA Cell Biol 1992;11:301–313.

49. Lowe WL Jr, Laskey SR, LeRoith D, Roberts CT Jr. Mol Endocrinol 1988;2:528–535.
50. Hepler JE, Van Wyck JJ, Lund PK. Endocrinol 1990;127:1550–1552.
51. Bichell DP, Kikuchi K, Rotwein P. Mol Endocrinol 1992;6:1899–1908.
52. Yoon JB, Berry SA, Seelig S, Towle HC. J Biol Chem 1990;265:19947–19954.
53. Lowe WL Jr, Roberts CT Jr, Laskey SR, LeRoith D. Proc Natl Acad Sci USA 1987;84:8946–8950.
54. Kikuchi K, Bichell DP, Rotwein P. J Biol Chem 1992;267:21505–21511.
55. Thomas MJ, Kikuchi K, Bichell DP, Rotwein P. J Biol Chem 1994;269 (in press).

©1994 Elsevier Science B.V. All rights reserved
The insulin-like growth factors and their regulatory proteins
R.C. Baxter, P.D. Gluckman and R.G. Rosenfeld, editors

Posttranscriptional regulation of IGF-I gene expression

Martin L. Adamo, Anatoly Koval, Derek LeRoith and Charles T. Roberts Jr

Diabetes Branch, NIH, Bethesda, MD 20892, USA

Abstract. Expression of the insulin-like growth factor-I (IGF-I) gene involves the use of leader exons whose transcription may be regulated by multiple promoters, alternative splicing of leader and coding exons, and the use of multiple polyadenylation sites. As a result, IGF-I mRNAs vary with respect to the length and sequence of their 5'-and 3'-untranslated regions (UTRs) and the signal and E-peptide coding regions. These variations raise the possibility that IGF-I gene expression may be regulated at the levels of mRNA translation and degradation and, due to the potential synthesis of multiple forms of the IGF-I prepro and prohormones, at the posttranslational level as well.

Introduction

Insulin-like growth factor-I (IGF-I) is a 70-amino acid growth factor containing B, C, and A domains analogous to the B and A chains and the C peptide of insulin and is a member of the insulin family of peptides that contains, in addition to IGF-I and insulin, IGF-II and relaxin. IGF-I plays important roles in the growth and development of many tissues, as evidenced by the widespread expression of the IGF-I gene, which is detectable in all tissues examined, particularly during postnatal development [1]. Additional proof of the importance of IGF-I function in growth and development has come from analyses of mice in which the IGF-I gene has been inactivated by gene targeting [2–4]. Homozygous IGF-I-deficient animals exhibit a 30% reduction in growth during prenatal development and die immediately after birth.

While the liver is the main source of IGF-I mRNA and accounts for the majority of circulating peptide [5], extensive local production of IGF-I is consistent with its functioning in an autocrine or paracrine mode in addition to a more classical endocrine mode, each involving activation of the IGF-I receptor that is also widely expressed both prenatally and postnatally. Given the numerous sources of IGF-I, the variety of target tissues and its multiple modes of action, it is clear that IGF-I biosynthesis would be likely to be tightly controlled, perhaps at a number of different levels. In the sections that follow, we shall discuss the structure of the IGF-I gene and the possible levels at which regulation could occur. We will focus on posttranscriptional mechanisms, since transcription of the IGF-I gene and its regulation at this level are described in an accompanying chapter.

24

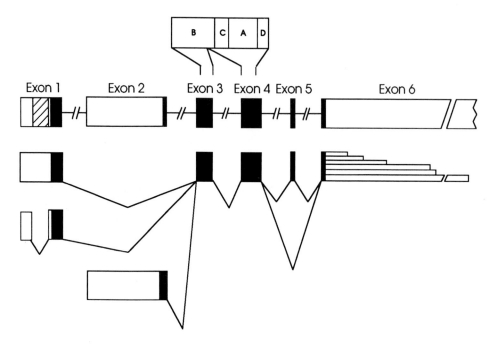

Fig. 1. Schematic representation of the structure of the rat IGF-I gene (above) and the variations in mRNA structure resulting from multiple leader exons and transcription start sites, alternative splicing in exon 1 and of exon 5, and alternative polyadenylation site usage in exon 6 (below). Open boxes represent 5′ and 3′-UTRs. Translated regions are represented by filled-in boxes. Exons are shown to scale, introns are not.

IGF-I gene structure

The human and rat IGF-I genes consist of six exons spanning ~100 kb of genomic DNA [6–9]. As illustrated in Fig. 1, exons 1 and 2 encode distinct 5′-untranslated regions (UTRs) and some signal peptide sequences. Exon 3 encodes the remainder of the signal peptide and the first part of the B domain. Exon 4 encodes the remainder of the B, C, A, and D domains (the latter representing a sequence of the mature IGF-I peptide that does not have an analogue in the insulin molecule) and the initial part of the E peptide moiety of the prohormone. In the mouse [10] and rat [11] IGF-I genes, exon 5 is an alternatively spliced "cassette" exon of 52 nt whose inclusion in the IGF-I mRNA sequence changes the reading frame and the remainder of the E peptide sequence from that encoded by IGF-I mRNAs in which exon 4 is spliced directly to exon 6. Exon 6 encodes the carboxy-terminus of the E peptide and a long (>6-kb) 3′-UTR and contains multiple polyadenylation sites. In the human IGF-I gene, exon 5 is much longer than in the rodent genes and encodes an extended version of the E peptide and a different 3′-UTR sequence [6].

The patterns of transcription and processing seen in the IGF-I gene are complex and derive from the architecture just described. Transcription initiation in exon 1 occurs from multiple sites dispersed over several hundred base pairs [12—15], whereas transcription initiation in exon 2 occurs from a more restricted region ~60 bp upstream of the 3' end of exon 2 [12,13]. A 186-base sequence in exon 1 itself is spliced out of some exon 1 mRNAs initiated at the upstream start sites in the rat gene [16], but this sequence does not appear to function as a "part-time" intron in the human gene (J.S. Sussenbach, pers. comm.). In primary transcripts initiated in exon 1 and, therefore, containing both exon 1 and exon 2 sequences, exon 1 always appears to be spliced to exon 3. There is no evidence of IGF-I mRNAs containing exon 1 sequences spliced to exon 2 sequences, presumably because the requisite splice acceptor site does not occur in the region flanking exon 2. Thus, IGF-I mRNAs contain different lengths of exon 1 sequences or exon 2 sequences due to the obligate splicing of exon 1 sequences (whenever present) on exon 2 sequences to exon 3 rather than to alternative splicing per se. The exon 5 cassettes seen in the rodent IGF-I genes represent true alternative splicing in that they can be differentially retained in mRNAs containing both flanking exon sequences. The presence or absence of human exon 5 sequences, however, depends upon which splice acceptor site (at the 5' end of exon 5 or of exon 6) is used in processing of a particular primary transcript. Finally, the choice of polyadenylation site in the exon 6 sequence determines the length of the 3'-UTR. Thus, a combination of multiple leader exons and transcription start sites, differential splicing involving exon 5 sequences, and the presence of multiple polyadenylation sites in exon 6, produces an array of IGF-I mRNAs that differ with respect to the length and sequence of the 5'-UTR, the sequences encoding the signal and E peptides, and the length of the 3'-UTR.

Potential levels of regulation of IGF biosynthesis

There are many levels at which production of a specific gene product can be controlled. These include changes in active gene number (through amplification or imprinting), alteration of chromatin structure, initiation, elongation or termination of transcription, splicing, 3' end formation and polyadenylation of the primary transcript, nucleocytoplasmic transport, translation (including initiation, elongation and termination) and degradation of the mature mRNA and the processing, intracellular trafficking and secretion of the primary translation product. The complex architecture of the IGF-I gene and the fact that it encodes a preprohormone that is eventually secreted, clearly provide opportunities for regulation of IGF-I production at all of the levels just described.

For a number of years, the majority of studies on the regulation of gene expression have focussed on transcriptional control, particularly transcription initiation. This has also tended to be the case in the area of IGF-I gene expression. Transcriptional control is obviously extremely important in regulation of IGF-I biosynthesis, given that leader exons 1 and 2 of the rat and human genes appear to be flanked by distinct promoter regions [14,15,17—19]. Furthermore, chromatin alterations accompany changes in IGF-I gene expression during development [20] and growth hormone (GH)

[21–25], PGE_2 [26], estradiol [27], experimental diabetes [28] and angiotensin II [29], affect the rate of IGF-I gene transcription. As the transcriptional aspects of IGF-I gene transcription are discussed in an accompanying chapter, this brief review will emphasize the importance of posttranscriptional mechanisms that may affect IGF-I biosynthesis.

In view of the size of the mammalian IGF-I gene and the estimated transcription site of RNA polymerase II, generation of the primary transcript and its processing to a mature, translationally competent cytoplasmic mRNA could conceivably take several hours. Thus, changes in the rate of transcription may underlie much of the developmental and tissue-specific differences in IGF-I mRNA levels, but such a mechanism would appear to be somewhat unwieldy in engendering rapid changes in IGF-I production. Posttranscriptional control, therefore, may provide the possibility for more acutely modulating IGF-I biosynthesis.

Translational control of IGF-I gene expression

In the case of the IGF-I gene, there are two aspects of potential control of mRNA translation. One is intimately tied to transcription itself and involves the production of IGF-I mRNAs that have inherent differences in their translatability. The other involves the differential translatability of a given species of IGF-I mRNA under various conditions due to the action of specific factors that regulate the translation process itself. As shown in Fig. 2, multiple transcription initiation sites and alternative splicing in the leader exons of the rat IGF-I gene produce a collection of IGF-I mRNAs that have different 5'-UTR sequences (some of which would also encode

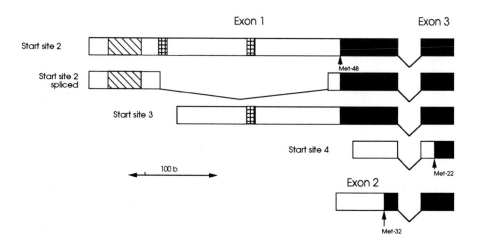

Fig. 2. Structure of 5'-UTRs in the major transcripts of the rat IGF-I gene. Translated regions are in black and the location of the various AUG codons initiating the prepro IGF-I ORF are shown. The singly and doubly cross-hatched boxes in the 5'-UTR represent the upstream ORF and the AUGUGA motifs, respectively, described in the text.

different signal peptide sequences, as described in a subsequent section). In addition to differences in the length of the various 5′-UTRs, there are several specific motifs in the exon 1 sequence that are differentially retained in exon 1-derived mRNAs, depending upon the particular start site used and the alternative splicing of the 186-base "part-time intron". Thus, transcripts initiated at the major upstream start site (#2) in exon 1 of the rat gene, would contain a short open reading frame (ORF) and two pairs of potential translation initiation and termination codons (5′-AUGUGA-3′) prior to the ORF encoding preproIGF-I itself; each of these motifs would be expected to impair translation of the preproIGF-I ORF by impeding transit of the scanning 40S ribosomal subunit to the AUG codon initiating the latter ORF. Transcripts that are initiated from this site and that have been completely spliced to remove the 186-base intronic sequence, described previously, would retain the upstream ORF, but would lack both AUGUGA motifs, whereas transcripts initiated at the major downstream start site in exon 1 (#3) would only contain the more downstream of the AUGUGA motifs. Finally, transcripts initiated at the most downstream site in exon 1 (#4) or at the major site in exon 2 would have short 5′-UTRs lacking any of these elements, but would, of course, differ in sequence.

Given this arrangement, the first type of translational control described above, i.e., that resulting indirectly from differential transcriptional start site usage and splicing, would be achieved by expressing different 5′-UTR versions of the IGF-I mRNA under various conditions. The potential basis for such a mechanism is supported by the finding that those exon 1 IGF-I mRNAs predicted to be more translatable by virtue of their lack of interfering sequence motifs, are, in fact, enriched in polysomal RNA fractions from liver, a tissue that expresses all the various IGF-I mRNA variants [30,31].

In fact the relative abundance of human and rat IGF-I mRNAs with different 5′-UTR sequences (both exon 1-derived and exon 2-derived) does vary in a tissue and developmental stage-specific fashion [13,32—35] and as a function of GH status [31]. Specifically, all of the IGF-I mRNA variants are present in liver, whereas this heterogeneity is more limited in extrahepatic tissues with exon 1 transcripts initiated at the major downstream start site (#3) predominating. In liver, the various exon 1 transcripts are seen throughout development and these levels increase at a constant rate, with their relative proportions remaining constant. Exon 2 transcripts, however, appear postnatally at the time of acquisition of GH responsiveness, where they rapidly come to represent ~30% of total IGF-I mRNA. Additionally, exon 2 transcripts are preferentially decreased by hypophysectomy and restored by GH treatment. Thus, to the extent that different IGF-I mRNAs are translated differently, indirect translational control by differential transcriptional initiation and splicing may be one level at which IGF-I biosynthesis is regulated. There are a number of conditions such as experimental diabetes and nutritional deprivation, however, in which overall IGF-I mRNA levels change without any significant variation in the proportions of the various IGF-I mRNA species [33]. The possibility of more direct translational control of IGF-I biosynthesis follows from the observations mentioned above, that the majority of IGF-I mRNAs in extrahepatic tissues (as well as a significant fraction of those in

28

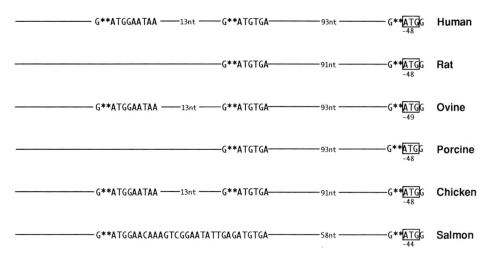

Fig. 3. Sequence motifs in the 5'-UTR of the major extrahepatic exon 1-derived transcript of the mammalian, chicken and fish IGF-I genes.

liver) are derived from transcription initiation at the major downstream start site in exon 1. As shown in Fig. 3, certain aspects of the structure of the 5'-UTR of this IGF-I mRNA species are highly conserved. The mammalian and chicken sequences each contain an AUGUGA motif 91–93 nt upstream of the Met-48 codon of the preproIGF-I ORF. In each case these motifs are preceded by a G residue 3 nt upstream, thus placing the AUG sequences in an appropriate context for translation initiation [36]. In the human, ovine and chicken sequences, the AUGUGA motif is preceded, 16 nt upstream, by a two-amino acid ORF whose AUG codon is preceded by a G residue 3 nt further upstream, thus placing this sequence in an appropriate context for translation initiation also. In the salmon IGF-I gene, these motifs bracket a 9-amino acid ORF that occurs 58 nt upstream of the preproIGF-I ORF; the AUG at the beginning of this upstream ORF is also in an appropriate context for translation initiation.

The existence of these conserved sequence elements in the 5'-UTR of the predominant extrahepatic IGF-I mRNA species, would be predicted to impair the translatability of the mRNA by interfering with the ability of 40S ribosomal subunits to scan past these ORFs and to effect efficient translation of the downstream ORF encoding preproIGF-I. The production of IGF-I would then depend upon the frequency of reinitiation of protein synthesis following translation termination at upstream ORFs. A potential mediator of this process is eukaryotic initiation factor 2 (eIF-2), which is responsible for the association of charged methionyl tRNAs with the 40S ribosomal subunit. eIF-2 functions as a GTP-binding protein and both it and its guanine nucleotide exchange factor, eIF-2B, are subject to phosphorylation events that modulate their activity and, hence, the rate of translation of certain mRNA species [37,38]. The phosphorylation of eIF-2B by glycogen synthase kinase-3, for example, is regulated by insulin [39].

Control of IGF-I mRNA stability

In addition to variability of at their 5′ ends, IGF-I mRNAs can differ in the length and (in humans) sequence of the 3′-UTR due to the presence of alternative splicing of exons 5 and 6 and the existence of multiple polyadenylation sites in exon 6 itself. As human exon 5-containing mRNAs are rare [34], we will focus on the heterogeneity due to the inclusion of different lengths of exon 6 sequences.

The existence of alternative polyadenylation sites in exon 6 results in IGF-I mRNA species that range in size from <1 kb to ~7.5 kb in length. Although variations at the 5′ end of IGF-I mRNAs make some contribution to length heterogeneity, RNase H mapping experiments have established that differential polyadenylation site usage is primarily responsible for variation in the size of IGF-I mRNAs [40]. The exon 6 sequence has been determined for the human [41] and rat [42] genes and predicts the existence of A-U-rich, potentially destabilizing sequences in the more distal region of this exon. Thus, the high-molecular-weight IGF-I mRNAs produced as a result of 3′ end formation at the end of exon 6 would be expected to contain such sequences, whereas the lower-molecular weight species, generated by use of the more proximal polyadenylation sites, would be relatively deficient in these motifs.

Based upon this data, it would be predicted that the longer IGF-I mRNA species would be less stable than the shorter transcripts. In fact, the recovery of the high-molecular weight IGF-I mRNA in polysomal RNA fractions varies from tissue to tissue (Foyt, H.L., unpublished observations) and as a function of experimental procedures [30,43] and the levels of this transcript in liver decrease more rapidly than those of the smaller IGF-I mRNAs after administration of a bolus of GH to hypophysectomized rats [44]. These findings are consistent with the differential stability of the high molecular weight IGF-I mRNA both in vitro and in vivo.

A significant fraction of hepatic IGF-I mRNA occurs on the 7.5-kb form and most, in some cases all, IGF-I mRNA in extrahepatic tissues [45] is in this form. This widespread occurrence of a potentially unstable mRNA strongly suggests that control of mRNA stability, potentially through RNA binding proteins, may be an important level of regulation of IGF-I biosynthesis. Pertinent in this regard is the fact that most techniques commonly employed to determine mRNA levels, including Northern blot analyses, solution hybridization/RNase protection assays and reverse transcription-polymerase chain reaction (RT-PCR) approaches, do not distinguish between changes in transcription vs. changes in stability.

Posttranslational control of IGF-I biosynthesis

The possibility that IGF-I production may be regulated at a posttranslational level is suggested by the existence of IGF-I mRNAs that encode multiple signal and E peptides and, thus, variant forms of prepro- and proIGF-I. Thus, as shown in Fig. 2, translation of different exon 1 and exon 2-derived mRNAs may generate prepro-IGF-I proteins with N-terminally divergent signal peptides 48, 32, or 22 (25 in the human) amino acids in length, depending upon whether AUG codons encoded by exon 1, 2 or 3 are employed. These different forms of preproIGF-I can be produced by in vitro translation of synthetic IGF-I mRNAs [46,47] and, if also produced in vivo, may be subject to differential processing, intracellular trafficking or secretion.

With respect to divergent E-peptide sequences, differential inclusion of exon 5 sequences results in the synthesis of proIGF-I peptides containing E-peptide moieties that differ in the length and sequence of their C termini. In the rat gene the change in the E-peptide sequence, due to the inclusion of the exon 5 sequence in the mRNA, causes the loss of two N-linked glycosylation sites that have been shown to be functional in vitro [48]. The in vivo significance of different E-peptides is unclear, however, since exon 5-containing IGF-I mRNAs are rare in all the rat [49] and human [34] tissues examined. Additionally, their proportions do not appear to significantly change under conditions in which overall IGF-I mRNA levels vary, except in liver of GH-treated hypophysectomized rats [49].

Conclusions

Mammalian IGF-I genes are complex structures whose expression, from alteration of chromatin structure at sites of transcription initiation through secretion of the fully processed mature peptide, involves numerous steps. While a great deal of attention and research effort has, quite reasonably, focussed on transcriptional regulation, many of these steps represent potential levels at which control of IGF-I gene expression and IGF-I biosynthesis could be exerted. In this brief review we have attempted to highlight some of the more obvious posttranscriptional control mechanisms that may be relevant to overall regulation of the IGF-I gene. Given the widespread expression of this gene and the fundamental biological importance of the gene product, it perhaps should not be surprising that nature has exploited many avenues of control to finely modulate its production.

References

1. Daughaday WH, Rotwein PS. Endocrine Rev 1989;10:68–91.
2. Liu J-P, Baker J, Perkins AS, Robertson EJ, Efstratiadis A. Cell 1993;75:59–72.
3. Baker J, Liu J-P, Robertson EJ, Efstratiadis A. Cell 1993;75:73–82.
4. Powell-Braxton L, Hollingshead P, Warbuton C, Dowd M, Pitts-Meek S, Dalton D, Gillett N, Stewart TA. Genes Devel 1993;7:2609–2617.
5. Schwander H, Hauri C, Zapf J, Froesch E. Endocrinology 1983;113:297–305.
6. Rotwein PS, Pollock K, Didier D, Krivi G. J Biol Chem 1986;261:4828–4832.
7. Shimatsu A, Rotwein PS. J Biol Chem 1987;262:7894–7900.
8. Bucci C, Malluci P, Roberts CT Jr, Frunzio R, Bruni CB. Nucl Acid Res 1989;9:3596.
9. Tobin G, Yee D, Brunner N, Rotwein PS. Mol Endocrinol 199;4:1914–1920.
10. Bell GI, Stempien MM, Fong NM, Rall LB. Nucl Acid Res 1986;14:7873–7882.
11. Roberts CT Jr, Lasky SR, Lowe WL Jr, Seaman WT, LeRoith D. Mol Endocrinol 1987;1:243–248.

12. Adamo ML, Ben-Hur H, LeRoith D, Roberts CT Jr. Biochem Biophys Res Commun 1991;176:887–893.
13. Jansen E, Steenbergh PH, LeRoith D, Roberts CT Jr, Sussenbach JS. Mol Cell Endocrinol 1991;78:115–125.
14. Kim S-W, Lajara R, Rotwein PS. Mol Endocrinol 1991;5:1964–1972.
15. Hall IK, Kajimoto Y, Bichell D, Kim S-J, James PL, Counts D, Nixon LJ, Tobin G, Rotwein PS. DNA Cell Biol 1992;11:301–313.
16. Shimatsu A, Rotwein PS. Nucl Acid Res 1988;15:719.
17. Lowe WL Jr, Teasdale RM. Biochem Biophys Res Commun 1992;189:972–978.
18. Jansen E, Steenbergh PH, van Schaik FMA, Sussenbach JS. Biochem Biophys Res Commun 1992;187:1213–1226.
19. Adamo ML, Lanau F, Neuenschwander S, Werner H, LeRoith D, Roberts CT Jr. Endocrinology 1993;132:935–937.
20. Kikuchi K, Bichell DP, Rotwein PS. J Biol Chem 1992;267:21505–21511.
21. Mathews LS, Norstedt G, Palmiter RD. Proc Natl Acad Sci USA 1986;83:9343–9347.
22. Doglio A, Dani C, Fredrikson G, Grimaldi R, Ailhaud G. EMBO J 1987;6:4011–4016.
23. Tollet P, Enberg B, Mode A. Mol Endocrinol 1990;4:1934–1942.
24. Johnson TR, Rudin SD, Blossey BK, Ilan J, Ilan J, Proc Natl Acad Sci USA 1991;88:5287–5291.
25. Bichell DP, Kikuchi K, Rotwein PS. Mol Endocrinol 1992;6:1899–1908.
26. Bichell DP, Rotwein PS, McCarthy TL. Endocrinology 1993;133:1020–1028.
27. Ernst M, Rodan GA. Mol Endocrinol 1991;5:1081–1089.
28. Pao C-I, Farmer PK, Begovic S, Goldstein S, Wu G-J, Phillips LS. Mol Endocrinol 1992;6:969–977.
29. Delafontaine P, Lou H. J Biol Chem 1993;35:16866–16870.
30. Foyt HL, LeRoith D, Roberts CT Jr. J Biol Chem 1991;266:7300–7305.
31. Foyt HL, Lanau F, Woloschak M, LeRoith D, Roberts CT Jr. Mol Endocrinol 1992;6:1881–1888.
32. Adamo ML, Lowe WL Jr, LeRoith D, Roberts CT Jr. Endocrinology 1989;124:2737–2744.
33. Adamo ML, Ben-Hur H, Roberts CT Jr, LeRoith D. Mol Endocrinol 1991;5:1677–1686.
34. Hernandez E, Hurwitz A, Pellicer A, Adashi EY, LeRoith D, Roberts CT Jr. J Clin Endocrinol 1992;74:419–425.
35. Shemer J, Adamo ML, Roberts CT Jr, LeRoith D. Endocrinology 1992;131:2793–2799.
36. Kozak M. J Cell Biol 1991;115:887–903.
37. Hershey JWB. J Biol Chem 1989;264:20823–20826.
38. Samuel CE. J Biol Chem 1993;268:7603–7607.
39. Welsh GI, Proud CG. Biochem J 1993;294:625–629.
40. Lund PK, Hoyt E, Van Wyk JJ. Mol Endocrinol 1989;3:2054–2061.
41. Steenbergh PH, Koonen-Reemst AMCB, Cleutiens CBJM, Sussenbach JS. Biochem Biophys Res Commun 199;175:507–514.
42. Hoyt EC, Hepler JC, Van Wyk JJ, Lund PK. DNA Cell Biol 1992;11:433–442.
43. Thissen JP, Underwood LE. J Endocrinol 1992;132:141–147.
44. Heppler JE, Van Wyk JJ, Lund PK. Endocrinology 1990;127:1550–1552.
45. Peter MA, Winterhalter KH, Böni-Schnetzler M, Froesch ER, Zapf J. Endocrinology 1993;133:2624–2631.
46. Rotwein PS, Folz RJ, Gordon JI. J Biol Chem 1987;262:11807–11812.
47. Simmons JG, Van Wyk JJ, Hoyt EC, Lund PK. Growth Factors 1993;9:205–221.
48. Bach MA, Roberts CT Jr, Smith EP, LeRoith D. Mol Endocrinol 1990;4:899–904.
49. Lowe WL Jr, Lasky SR, LeRoith D, Roberts CT Jr. Mol Endocrinol 1988;2:528–535.

Molecular mechanisms for nutritional regulation of genes for IGF-I, IGF-binding proteins and other plasma proteins

Daniel S. Straus, John M. Hayden and Norman W. Marten

Biomedical Sciences Division and Biology Department, University of California, Riverside, CA 92521, USA

Abstract. Insulin-like growth factor-I (IGF-I) mRNA abundance is consistently decreased in animals whose growth is arrested due to nutritional restriction. In fasting animals this decrease is caused primarily by a decrease in IGF-I gene transcription, whereas in protein-restricted animals it appears to be caused by a posttranscriptional mechanism such as decreased IGF-I mRNA stability. In addition to the reduction of IGF-I mRNA that occurs in protein-restricted rats, the abundance of serum albumin, transthyretin, carbamyl phosphate synthetase-I and class I alcohol dehydrogenase mRNA is also decreased. Finally, expression of the IGFBP-1 and -2 genes is increased in nutritionally restricted rats, due primarily to increased gene transcription.

Juvenile animals stop growing if they are fed a diet containing an inadequate amount of energy or protein. The molecular basis for this growth arrest is not completely understood [1]. In general, the decreased growth velocity observed in nutritionally-restricted animals is not accounted for by a decrease in circulating pituitary growth hormone (GH). In most species, nutritional restriction leads to an increase rather than a decrease in plasma GH levels [2]. In contrast, circulating levels of insulin-like growth factor-I (IGF-I) are consistently decreased in animals that are growing slowly because of inadequate nutrient intake [1]. This suggests that the synthesis of IGF-I is a key control point for nutritional regulation of growth [1]. The molecular mechanism(s) by which nutrition regulates IGF-I synthesis remain to be fully elucidated. Current findings regarding the regulation of IGF-I, IGF-binding proteins and other plasma proteins are summarized below.

Nutritional regulation of IGF-I

Early studies indicated that circulating levels of IGF-I peptide were consistently decreased in animals consuming inadequate amounts of protein or energy [1]. Subsequently, it was demonstrated that the steady-state abundance of IGF-I mRNA in liver was decreased in fasting [3–5], protein-restricted [6–8] and energy-restricted animals [9]. IGF-I mRNA abundance was also decreased in fetal animals under conditions of intrauterine growth retardation caused by maternal fasting [10]. These results indicated that nutritional regulation of IGF-I occurs at least partly at the level of IGF-I gene expression. Interestingly, although IGF-I mRNA abundance is consistently decreased by nutritional restriction, there is a difference in the way in which IGF-I mRNA decreases in response to various types of nutritional insufficiency. In particular, in fasting and energy-restricted animals there is a coordinate decrease in the three major size species of IGF-I mRNA (8 kb, 1.7 kb and 1.0 kb) [5,9]. In contrast, in protein-restricted animals there is a greater decrease in the abundance of the 8 kb IGF-I mRNA species as compared with the shorter species [6–8]. The 8 kb IGF-I mRNA differs from the shorter mRNA species primarily in having a very long 3'-untranslated region (UTR) and is less stable than the shorter species, perhaps due to a greater number of sites for endonucleolytic cleavage in the very long 3'-UTR [11,12]. The observation that the 8 kb IGF-I mRNA species is preferentially regulated by protein restriction, is consistent with the possibility that the regulation of IGF-I mRNA abundance in protein restricted animals occurs at least partly at the posttranscriptional level (see below).

In early experiments aimed at determining whether the decrease in IGF-I mRNA, that occurs in fasting animals, is caused by a decrease in IGF-I gene transcription, IGF-I transcription was quantified by nuclear transcription run-on assay [5]. Initial measurements of IGF-I gene transcription in control ad libitum fed animals indicated that the level of IGF-I gene transcription varied considerably from animal to animal [5,6]. This variation in IGF-I gene transcription was specific for IGF-I, since it was detected with two different IGF-I gene targets in transcription run-on assays and a similar variation was not observed in the level of β-actin or serum albumin gene transcription [5,6]. The level of IGF-I gene transcription exhibited a downward trend in fasting animals; however, this decrease was not usually statistically significant within a single experiment because of the animal-to-animal variation in IGF-I gene transcription in the control animals [5].

An alternative method to the run-on assay for estimating gene transcription, involves quantifying the steady-state abundance of nuclear transcripts by Northern blot analysis [13] or RNase protection assay [14,15] using probes specific for intron sequences. Since nuclear transcripts are rapidly processed to mRNA, measurement of the steady-state abundance of nuclear transcripts provides an estimate of transcriptional activity. We have recently used this method for estimating transcriptional activity of the IGFBP-1 gene [13] and IGF-I gene [14]. The intron probe used for quantifying IGF-I transcripts was provided to us by Peter Rotwein, Washington University, St. Louis [15]. We have constructed intron-specific probes for several other transcripts either by PCR amplification or direct subcloning of genomic sequences (Table 1). The advantages of the Northern blot or RNase protection assay for nuclear transcripts over the run-on assay as a means for estimating transcription have been discussed in detail [13,14].

We have recently used the RNase protection assay for quantifying IGF-I nuclear transcripts in control and fasting animals [14]. Bichell et al. [15] demonstrated that the kinetics of induction by GH of IGF-I nuclear transcripts measured by the RNase protection assay and IGF-I transcriptional activity measured by run-on assay were very similar. In addition, when transcription run-on assays and RNase protection assays of nuclear transcripts were performed with liver samples from the same

Table 1. Probes used for quantifying nuclear transcripts

Gene	Region of gene	Source	Type of assay
IGF-I	Intron 3-exon 4	P. Rotwein	RNase protection
IGFBP-1	Intron 3	PCR	Northern blot
	Intron 1	PCR	Northern blot
Serum albumin	Intron 13	Genomic subclone	Northern blot
	Intron 13-exon 14	Genomic subclone	RNase protection
Transthyretin	Intron 1	PCR	RNase protection
Carbamyl phosphate synthetase-I	Intron 1	PCR	RNase protection
H-Ferritin	Intron 1	PCR	Northern blot
Ribosomal RNA	5'-Leader	Genomic subclone	Northern blot

animals, the results of the assays were strongly correlated (r >0.90, p <0.001). In particular, animals that exhibited a high signal in the IGF-I run-on assay also had a high level of IGF-I nuclear transcripts measured by RNase protection assay [14]. These results indicate that the RNase protection assay provides an accurate estimate of IGF-I gene transcription.

An example of such an RNase protection assay performed with six control and six fasting rats is shown in Fig. 1. The RNase protection assay for IGF-I nuclear transcripts uses a riboprobe containing the last 163 base pairs of intron 3 and all 182 base pairs of exon 4 of the rat IGF-I gene [14,15]. Hybridization of the probe with nuclear transcripts containing intron 3 and exon 4, protects a 345 base portion of the probe; hybridization of the probe with fully processed IGF-I mRNA protects a 182 base portion. Therefore, the steady-state level of IGF-I nuclear transcripts and IGF-I mRNA are measured simultaneously in the same assay. The results of the RNase protection assay were very similar to results of earlier transcription run-on assays: a uniformly low IGF-I transcript level was observed in the fasting animals (Fig. 1B, lanes 1—6) whereas the level of IGF-I transcripts in the fed animals varied considerably from animal to animal (lanes 7—12). For example, in the experiment shown in Fig. 1, the expression of IGF-I nuclear transcripts was high in the fed control animals in lanes 8, 10 and 11, moderate in the animal in lane 9 and low in the animals in lanes 7 and 12 (Fig. 1B). Very similar results were obtained in three other fasting experiments. The overall results of the four experiments (n = 18 and 19 for ad libitum fed and fasted treatments, respectively) indicated that fasting produced a 78% reduction (p < 0.001) in hepatic IGF-I nuclear transcripts (range 71—84%) which paralleled a 70% decrease (p < 0.001) in IGF-I mRNA abundance. The repression of IGF-I transcription observed in fasting animals was specific, as the abundance of serum albumin, H-ferritin and ribosomal RNA nuclear transcripts were not decreased

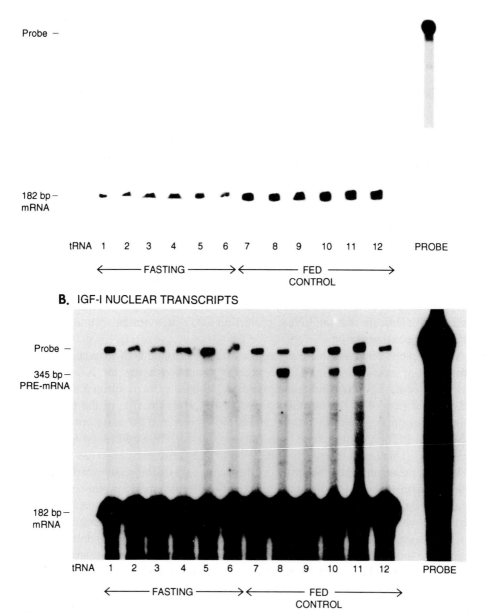

Fig. 1. RNase protection assay showing the effect of fasting on hepatic IGF-I mRNA (A) and nuclear transcript (B) abundance. Assays were performed with 10 μg portions of whole cellular RNA isolated from six animals fasted for 72 h (lanes 1–6) or fed ad libitum (lanes 7–12). The figure shows two autoradiograms of the same gel exposed for different times: A, 1-h exposure; and B, 96-h exposure. Reproduced from Ref. [14] with permission of the Endocrine Society.

by fasting. The overall results of these experiments indicate that the decrease in IGF-I mRNA abundance in fasting animals is caused primarily by a decrease in IGF-I gene transcription.

The animal-to-animal variability in IGF-I gene transcription is of interest. As noted above, this variability is specific for IGF-I and is observed both in transcription run-on assays and in RNase protection assays of IGF-I nuclear transcripts. One explanation for this variability is that transcription of the IGF-I gene is controlled in a pulsatile manner, with surges of IGF-I gene transcription occurring in response to pulses of GH released by the pituitary. In support of this hypothesis, GH levels vary in a pulsatile manner in male rats [16] and GH is known to stimulate transcription of the IGF-I gene [15]. According to this interpretation, IGF-I mRNA levels do not exhibit the same moment-to-moment variability as IGF-I nuclear transcript levels, because the mRNA has a longer turnover time than the nuclear transcripts which damps the variation.

The molecular basis for the decreased IGF-I gene transcription in fasting rats remains to be elucidated. However, previous studies have indicated that GH secretion is severely impaired in fasting rats [17]. (This decrease in GH secretion contrasts with the increased GH secretion that occurs during fasting in other species [1].) In addition, fasting produces a state of GH resistance, possibly related to decreased expression of GH receptors on target tissues [5,18,19]. Therefore, the decreased IGF-I gene transcription in fasting animals may be caused in part by the reduction in circulating GH levels and resistance to GH action. The severe decrease in plasma insulin that occurs during fasting may also contribute to the decline in IGF-I gene transcription, since insulin positively regulates transcription of the IGF-I gene [20].

We have recently examined the effect of dietary protein restriction on the abundance of IGF-I nuclear transcripts. This study involved the measurement of IGF-I mRNA and nuclear transcript abundance in two different experiments in which rats were fed a diet containing 20% protein (control) or 4% protein (restricted) [Hayden JM and Straus DS, manuscript in preparation]. In each of the experiments there were six animals per treatment group. In this study, protein restriction caused a consistent 64–65% decrease in IGF-I mRNA abundance in rats on the 4% protein diet as compared with rats on the 20% protein diet. In contrast, no significant effect of protein restriction was observed on IGF-I nuclear transcript abundance in either of the two experiments, despite the fact that we were able to detect a decrease in nuclear transcripts for two other nutritionally sensitive genes (serum albumin and transthyretin, see below). These results differ from those obtained with fasting animals and suggest that in protein-restricted rats IGF-I mRNA abundance is decreased primarily by a posttranscriptional mechanism. The observation that IGF-I gene transcription is not diminished in protein-restricted rats is curious in view of a recent report indicating that GH secretion in rats is severely impaired by protein restriction [21]. Evidently, the plasma GH concentration in the protein-restricted animals, although diminished, is nevertheless adequate to stimulate IGF-I gene transcription. Protein restriction differs from fasting in that fasting decreases the expression of GH receptors in liver whereas protein restriction does not [1,6,7 and references therein].

Apparently, the repression of IGF-I gene transcription that occurs in fasting rats results from both lowered plasma GH and GH resistance resulting from a decrease in GH receptors.

Nutritional regulation of IGF-binding proteins

In tissues and in serum, IGF-I and -II are complexed with binding proteins that are thought to modulate their actions. Two of the binding proteins, IGFBP-1 and IGFBP-2, are very sensitive to regulation by nutrition. In general, the regulation of these two binding proteins is opposite to the regulation of IGF-I: they are induced under conditions of nutritional restriction and repressed by refeeding. Early studies of IGFBP-1 in humans indicated that its levels in serum were increased during a short-term (overnight) fast [22]. Subsequent studies performed with rats demonstrated that fasting caused an increase in IGFBP-1 mRNA abundance in the liver, indicating that the induction of serum IGFBP-1 occurs at least partly at the level of synthesis [23]. Chronic dietary protein restriction also leads to an induction of hepatic IGFBP-1 mRNA [13]. In this case, Northern blot analysis of IGFBP-1 nuclear transcripts [13] and nuclear transcription run-on assays [24] have shown that the induction of IGFBP-1 mRNA is caused largely by an increase in IGFBP-1 gene transcription.

The metabolic signal(s) leading to the induction of IGFBP-1 expression under conditions of nutritional restriction remain to be fully elucidated. Recent studies have demonstrated that transcription of the IGFBP-1 gene is induced by glucocorticoids and cAMP, and repressed by insulin, with the repressive effect of insulin being dominant over the inductive effect of the other two agents [22]. Elements responsible for the positive response to cAMP [25] and negative response to insulin [26], have recently been identified in the human IGFBP-1 gene promoter. The reduction in serum insulin that occurs during fasting and protein restriction is very likely a major factor leading to induction of IGFBP-1 gene transcription. It is also possible that limitation for substrate (i.e., glucose or essential amino acids) plays a direct role in IGFBP-1 induction in nutritionally restricted animals. Some studies have suggested that intracellular glucose directly represses the synthesis or secretion of IGFBP-1 [27]. In addition, limitation of rat hepatoma cells for essential amino acids causes an increase of IGFBP-1 mRNA abundance [13]. In the amino acid-limited rat hepatoma cells, the induction of IGFBP-1 gene expression appears to be caused partly by an increase in IGFBP-1 transcription and partly by a posttranscriptional mechanism [13].

In the rat, hepatic IGFBP-2 gene expression is also increased by fasting [28], protein-restriction [6] and energy restriction [9]. In fasting rats, the increase in IGFBP-2 mRNA abundance is caused largely by an increase in IGFBP-2 gene transcription [28]. Interestingly, the induction of IGFBP-2 gene expression in nutritionally restricted animals is tissue-specific: it occurs in the liver but not in the brain or kidney [6,9,28]. Recent studies have shown that transcription of the IGFBP-2 gene is driven at least partly by the binding of the ubiquitous transcription factor Sp1 to three sites contained in a single large footprint spanning nucleotide −125 to −189 of the IGFBP-2 promoter [29]. It remains to be determined whether the nutritional regulation of IGFBP-2 transcription involves modulation of Sp1 binding to these three sites, or perhaps the regulated binding of a yet to be identified liver-enriched transcription factor such as C/EBP, HNF-1, HNF-3 or HNF-4. It should also be noted that changes in IGFBP-2 gene expression may not always be accompanied by similar changes in IGFBP-2 protein levels in serum. For example, fasting of neonatal pigs increases the level of immunoreactive IGFBP-2 in serum. However, the increase in IGFBP-2 is accounted for by an increase in proteolyzed IGFBP-2 fragments that do not bind IGF-I or -II, so that the amount of IGFBP-2 detected by ligand blotting is actually decreased in serum of the fasting animals [30].

Nutritional regulation of other plasma proteins

In addition to the reduction of IGF-I levels that occurs in the serum of protein-restricted animals, levels of several other plasma proteins including serum albumin, transthyretin and transferrin, are also decreased [31]. The decrease in serum albumin is a hallmark of protein malnutrition and serum albumin concentration is used routinely for evaluating the nutritional status of hospital patients [31]. In multivariate analysis of children admitted to the hospital with severe protein-energy malnutrition, a low serum albumin concentration (<16 g/l) was the best single predictor of subsequent risk of dying [32].

Previous studies have indicated that the abundance of serum albumin mRNA is decreased in the liver of protein-restricted rats, indicating that, as with IGF-I, the decreased circulating albumin concentration is caused at least partly by a decrease in albumin gene expression [6,33]. In order to define the specificity of this phenomenon, we have recently surveyed the effect of protein restriction on the abundance in rat liver of mRNAs for a number of genes. The results of these experiments have indicated that the genes can be divided into three groups based on their response to protein restriction: the expression of group 1, 2 and 3 genes is decreased, unchanged or increased in response to protein restriction (Table 2). The results presented in Table 2 indicate that the negative response to protein restriction is highly specific and is restricted to a limited number of genes. In addition to IGF-I and serum albumin, other genes exhibiting decreased expression in response to protein restriction included the genes encoding the thyroid hormone-binding plasma protein transthyretin, the urea cycle enzyme carbamyl phosphate synthetase-I and class I alcohol dehydrogenase, which is the rate-limiting enzyme in the metabolism of ingested ethanol and is also involved in the metabolism of retinol and a variety of other endogenous and xenobiotic alcohols.

As noted above, the decrease in IGF-I mRNA that occurs in protein-restricted animals appears to be caused primarily by a posttranscriptional mechanism such as a decrease in IGF-I mRNA stability. To determine whether this is also true of the other group 1 genes, nuclear transcripts for the serum albumin and transthyretin genes were quantified by Northern blot analysis and RNase protection assay using the

Table 2. Effect of dietary protein restriction on mRNA abundance for 12 genes in rat liver

---

Group 1: Expression decreased in protein-restricted animals
  IGF-I
  Serum albumin
  Transthyretin (TTR)
  Carbamyl phosphate synthetase-I (CPS-I)
  Alcohol dehydrogenase (class I)

Group 2: Expression not changed in protein-restricted animals
  Hypoxanthine-guanine phosphoribosyl transferase (HPRT)
  Ubiquitin (*UbB* and *UbC* genes)

Group 3: Expression increased in protein-restricted animals
  IGFBP-1
  IGFBP-2
  IGFBP-4
  H-ferritin

---

probes described in Table 1. The results of these experiments indicated that protein restriction significantly decreased the abundance of serum albumin and transthyretin nuclear transcripts [Straus DS, Marten NW, Hayden JM and Burke EJ, manuscript submitted]. Therefore, in contrast to the posttranscriptional regulation of IGF-I mRNA abundance that occurs in protein-restricted rats, the decrease in albumin and transthyretin mRNA appears to be caused at least partly by a decrease in albumin and transthyretin gene transcription. Transcriptional control of the albumin and transthyretin genes has been studied extensively [34–36]. For both genes, the high level of transcription observed in liver is caused by binding of liver-enriched as well as ubiquitous transcription factors to promoter and enhancer elements. A comparison of the factors involved in regulating albumin and transthyretin transcription indicates that both genes use hepatocyte nuclear factor-1 (HNF-1), HNF-3 and proteins of the CCAAT/enhancer binding protein (C/EBP) family. It is possible that the coordinate repression of albumin and transthyretin transcription in protein-restricted animals results from a decrease in activity of HNF-1, HNF-3 and/or C/EBP. HNF-1 seems to be a less likely candidate for this than the other two factors, since HNF-1 also positively controls IGFBP-1 transcription [37], which increases rather than decreases in the liver of protein-restricted rats [13]. Further studies are underway to fully elucidate the molecular mechanisms for the posttranscriptional down-regulation of IGF-I mRNA and the repression of albumin and transthyretin gene transcription, that occurs in protein-restricted rats.

Acknowlededgments

This research was supported by NIH grants R01-DK39739 and T32-DK07310.

References

1. Straus DS. FASEB J 1994;8:6–12.
2. Vance ML, Hartman ML, Thorner MO. Horm Res 1992;38(suppl 1):85–88.
3. Emler CA, Schalch DS. Endocrinology 1987;120:832–834.
4. Lowe WL Jr, Adamo M, Werner H, Roberts CT Jr, LeRoith D. J Clin Invest 1989;84:619–626.
5. Straus DS, Takemoto CD. Mol Endocrinol 1990;4:91–100.
6. Straus DS, Takemoto CD. Endocrinology 1990;127:1849–1860.
7. VandeHaar MJ, Moats-Staats BM, Davenport ML, Walker JL, Ketelslegers JM, Sharma BK, Underwood LE. J Endocrinol 1991;130:305–312.
8. Miura Y, Kato H, Noguchi T. Br J Nutr 1992;67:257–265.
9. Straus DS, Takemoto CD. J Nutr 1991;121:1279–1286.
10. Straus DS, Ooi GT, Orlowski CC, Rechler MM. Endocrinology 1991;128:518–525.
11. Hepler JE, Van Wyk JJ, Lund PK. Endocrinology 1990;127:1550–1552.
12. Hoyt EC, Hepler JE, Van Wyk JJ, Lund PK. DNA Cell Biol 1992;11:433–441.
13. Straus DS, Burke EJ, Marten NW. Endocrinology 1993;132:1090–1100.
14. Hayden JM, Marten NW, Burke EJ, Straus DS. Endocrinology 1994;134:760–768.
15. Bichell DP, Kikuchi K, Rotwein P. Mol Endocrinol 1992;6:1899–1908.
16. Tannenbaum GS, Martin JB. Endocrinology 1976;98:562–570.
17. Tannenbaum GS, Rorstad, O, Brazeau P. Endocrinology 1979;104:1733–1738.
18. Baxter RC, Bryson JM, Turtle JR. Metabolism 1981;30:1086–1090.
19. Maes M, Underwood LE, Ketelslegers J-M. J Endocrinol 1983;97:243–252.
20. Pao C-I, Farmer PK, Begovic S, Goldstein S, Wu GJ, Phillips LS. Mol Endocrinol 1992;6:969–977.
21. Harel Z, Tannenbaum GS. Endocrinology 1993;133:1035–1043.
22. Lee PDK, Conover CA, Powell DR. Proc Soc Exp Biol Med 1993;204:4–29.
23. Murphy LJ, Seneviratne C, Ballejo G, Croze F, Kennedy TG. Mol Endocrinol 1990;4:329–336.
24. Miura Y, Uchijima Y, Takahashi S-I, Noguchi T. Biosci Biotechnol Biochem 1993;57:358–359.
25. Suwanichkul A, DePaolis LA, Lee PDK, Powell DR. J Biol Chem 1993;268:9730–9736.
26. Suwanichkul A, Morris SL, Powell DR. J Biol Chem 1993;268:17063–17068.
27. Lewitt MS, Baxter RC. Endocrinology 1990;126:1527–1533.
28. Tseng LHY, Ooi GT, Brown AL, Straus DS, Rechler MM. Mol Endocrinol 1992;6:1195–1201.
29. Boisclair YR, Brown AL, Casola S, Rechler MM. J Biol Chem 1993;268:24892–24901.
30. McCusker RH, Cohick WS, Busby WH, Clemmons DR. Endocrinology 1991;129:2631–2638.
31. Spiekerman AM. Clin Lab Med 1993;13:353–369
32. Dramaix M, Hennart P, Brasseur D, Bahwere P, Mudjene O, Tonglet R, Donnen P, Smets R. Br Med J 1993;307:710–713.
33. Sakuma K, Ohyama T, Sogawa K, Fujii-Kuriyama Y, Matsumura Y. J Nutr 1987;117:1141–1148.
34. Maire P, Wuarin J, Schibler U. Science 1989;244:343–346.
35. McPherson CE, Shim E-Y, Friedman DS, Zaret KS. Cell 1993;75:387–398.
36. Mirkovitch J, Darnell JE Jr. Genes Devel 1991;5:83–93.
37. Powell DR, Suwanichkul A. DNA Cell Biol 1993;12:283–289.

Regulation of IGF-II gene expression and posttranscriptional processing of IGF-II mRNAs

P. Elly Holthuizen, Richard J.T. Rodenburg, Wiep Scheper and John S. Sussenbach
Laboratory for Physiological Chemistry, Utrecht University, Stratenum, Postbus 80042, 3508 TA Utrecht, The Netherlands

Abstract. The human insulin-like growth factor-II (IGF-II) gene constitutes a complex transcription unit that is controlled by four promoters. Expression of the IGF-II gene is development- and tissue-specific. This study aims to establish the molecular basis of the regulation of expression of the human IGF-II gene and characterize the nucleotide sequences and factors involved in transcriptional activation of the adult liver-specific promoter P1 and the major fetal promoter P3. In addition, regulation at the posttranscriptional level occurs. IGF-II mRNAs are subject to site-specific endonucleolytic cleavage, directed by two widely separated elements in the 3′ untranslated region (UTR) of the IGF-II RNAs.

Introduction

Proliferation in a multicellular eukaryotic organism is a complex process strictly regulated by specific proteins such as growth factors. The insulin-like growth factors (IGFs) are important regulators of growth, which exert their functions through endocrine, paracrine and autocrine mechanisms of action in a variety of cell types. IGFs have also been detected in a variety of tumors, where they can stimulate growth and cell division in an autocrine or paracrine manner.

IGF-II plays a central role in regulating mammalian growth and fetal development [1]. In addition to the stimulation of cellular proliferation, IGF-II can induce differentiation [2]. The involvement of IGF-II in fetal growth control has elegantly been demonstrated by DeChiara and colleagues, who showed that marked growth retardation occurs in mice bearing a disrupted IGF-II allele [3]. IGF-II is also involved in the generation of several types of tumors and may have autocrine effects on tumor progression [4].

The human IGF-II gene is a complex transcription unit. Its regulation of expression is governed by an intricate mechanism, which enables synthesis of IGF-II under various conditions. Multiple transcripts that all encode the same IGF-II precursor, are synthesized as a result of alternate promoter usage [5]. Several functional poly(A) addition signals in the last exon contribute further to the heterogeneity of the IGF-II mRNAs. Transcription from the various IGF-II promoters leads to the formation of IGF-II mRNAs, that are translated with varying efficiencies. In addition, regulation at the posttranscriptional level occurs, since IGF-II mRNAs are subject to site-specific endonucleolytic cleavage. Cleavage of IGF-II mRNAs yields

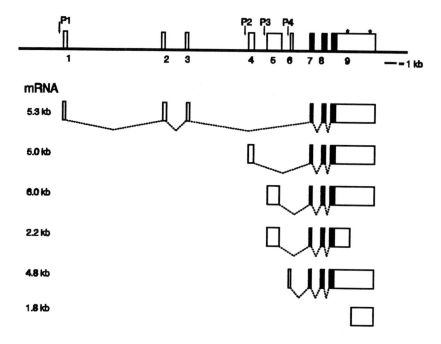

Fig. 1. Schematic representation of the human IGF-II gene and corresponding mRNAs. The numbered boxes indicate the nine exons of the IGF-II gene (1–9). The four promoters (P1–P4) and the two poly(A) addition signals (*) are indicated. Solid boxes represent exon sequences encoding preproIGF-II, open boxes denote 5' and 3' untranslated sequences [9].

a capped, but not polyadenylated 5'-specific fragment, which is subject to rapid degradation and a stable polyadenylated uncapped 3'-specific cleavage product of 1.8 kb.

Studying the molecular mechanisms underlying the differential regulation of the IGF-II genes will help to understand the complex roles of IGF-II in growth and development.

IGF-II gene structure

The human gene encoding IGF-II is located on chromosome 11 and spans 30 kb of chromosomal DNA. It consists of nine exons, 1–9, of which exons 7, 8 and the first part of 9 code for the IGF-II precursor protein. The 5' part of the gene consists of noncoding leader exons 1–6, of which exons 1, 4, 5 and 6 are each preceded by a distinct promoter (P1–P4) (Fig. 1). The IGF-II promoters (P1–P4) are activated in a development-dependent and tissue-specific manner [5–8].

The human promoter P1 is exclusively active in adult liver tissue, whereas activity of promoter P2 has only been detected in certain human tumor cell lines [10]. The major promoters in fetal and nonhepatic adult tissues are P3 and P4 [11]. The degree

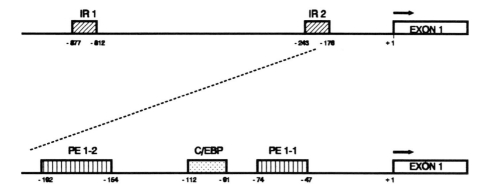

Fig. 2. Schematic representation of the human IGF-II P1 region. The distal promoter P1 region contains an inverted repeat of 67 nucleotides long, separated by 568 nucleotides. As shown by transient transfection experiments this distal region of P1 exerts a 3-fold repressing effect. Three domains of the proximal promoter are protected by specific nuclear proteins as was shown by DNaseI footprint analysis. Binding of C/EBP was also shown by oligonucleotide competition experiments [14].

of differential activation of each of these promoters depends on the cell type of origin [12], and the state of development.

Characterization of the adult liver specific IGF-II promoter P1

A distinct example of differential regulation of the IGF-II promoters is found in the liver. In the fetal stage of liver development promoter P3 is the major IGF-II promoter, whereas P2 and P4 are moderately active. After birth, these three promoters are switched off and P1 is activated (Fig. 1). Promoter P1 can be subdivided into two regions: a proximal region which contains sequence information required for basal transcription, and a distal region, which has a negative effect on transcription [13] (Fig. 2).

We have shown that the adult liver-specific IGF-II promoter P1, contains a functional binding site at positions −112 to −91 relative to the site of transcription initiation for CCAAT/Enhancer Binding Protein (C/EBP) [14], which is a member of the bZIP-type transcription factor family [15]. Several other promoters of genes which are transcribed at high levels in adult liver tissue contain one or more binding sites for C/EBP, e.g., albumin, alcohol dehydrogenase and PEP carboxykinase.

Binding sites for C/EBP are also recognized by several factors that are closely related to C/EBP. One of these is the liver-enriched activating protein (LAP) [16], which is expressed at high levels in adult liver. The LAP gene further encodes the liver-enriched inhibiting protein (LIP), that lacks the LAP transactivation domain, but contains a functional DNA-binding domain. C/EBP, LAP and LIP contain a leucine-zipper dimerization domain through which they can form both homo- and heterodimers [17]. LIP is coexpressed with LAP albeit at a much lower level and the ratio

LAP/LIP changes during development in favor of LAP. The capability of C/EBP and LAP to activate transcription can be inhibited by LIP, probably through the formation of inactive heterodimers. The expression patterns of C/EBP and LAP during the development of the liver are very similar. Little or no expression of these transcription factors is detected in fetal rat liver, whereas adult liver contains high levels of C/EBP and LAP [18]. However, hepatoma cells contain less than 5% of the C/EBP level as found in adult liver, while C/EBP is also downregulated in regenerating liver.

In order to study the binding of C/EBP, LAP and LIP to P1, we made a synthetic double-stranded (ds) oligonucleotide CBS (P1 C/EBP Binding Site) which was used as a probe in electrophoretic mobility shift assays (EMSAs). Bacterially expressed C/EBP, LAP and LIP are able to bind to the P1 CBS oligonucleotide both as homodimers and as heterodimers. To analyze the effect of C/EBP, LAP and LIP on P1 promoter activity, a 200 bp P1 fragment, which shows maximal promoter activity and contains the C/EBP binding sequence, was coupled to the firefly luciferase reporter gene and cotransfected together with expression plasmids encoding either C/EBP, LAP or LIP into Hep3B human hepatoma cells. Expression of C/EBP results in a 3–6-fold increase in P1 activity, whereas LAP gives rise to a 5–15-fold increase. LIP, which hardly influences P1 activity directly, is able to inhibit the P1 activation of both C/EBP and LAP. When C/EBP and LAP are coexpressed no additional stimulation of P1 activity is observed, suggesting that C/EBP-LAP heterodimers activate transcription equally well as LAP homodimers (Fig. 3).

In order to investigate the importance of the C/EBP binding site in IGF-II P1 activation, we further compared this site to the strong liver-specific enhancer of the rat albumin gene (Alb. D) and a weak C/EBP site also found in the rat albumin

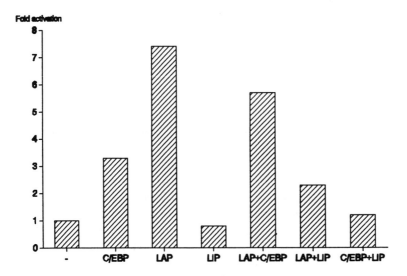

Fig. 3. Transactivation of IGF-II promoter P1 by C/EBP and LAP in transient transfected Hep3B cells. Cotransfections of P1 (–207 to +52) luciferase reporter constructs with C/EBP, LAP and LIP expression plasmids. Hep3B cells were transfected in 25 cm^2 flasks and transfected with 2 µg P1-luc construct, 1 µg of transcription factor(s) and 0.5 µg of RSV lacZ, which served as an internal standard.

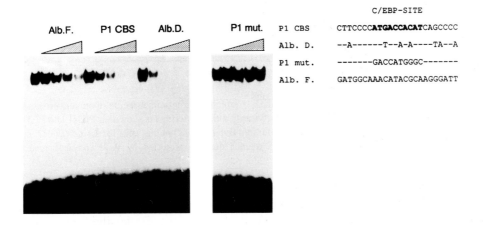

C/EBP-SITE

P1 CBS	CTTCCCC**ATGACCACAT**CAGCCCC
Alb. D.	--A------T--A-A----TA--A
P1 mut.	-------GACCATGGGC-------
Alb. F.	GATGGCAAACATACGCAAGGGATT

Fig. 4. Comparison of the binding of C/EBP to P1 CBS, Alb. D. and Alb. F., using EMSA. Approximately 10 ng of recombinant C/EBP protein was incubated with 0.5 ng of radiolabeled ds P1 CBS oligonucleotide. Binding of C/EBP was competed for by the addition of increasing amounts of unlabelled P1 CBS, Alb. D., Alb. F. or P1 mut. oligonucleotides, respectively.

promoter (Alb. F) [19]. Electrophoretic mobility shift assays show that the Alb. D. site binds C/EBP, LAP and LIP with a higher affinity, and the Alb. F. site with a lower affinity than the P1 CBS site (Fig. 4). Additional quantitative electrophoretic mobility shift competition assays revealed that the P1 CBS site has a 2-fold lower binding activity than the Alb. D. site and approximately 13-fold higher binding activity than the Alb. F. site for C/EBP, LAP and LIP.

Summarizing, we conclude that C/EBP and LAP play a major role in the liver-specific activation of the human IGF-II promoter P1.

Characterization of the most active IGF-II promoter, P3

The human IGF-II promoter P3 is expressed in many fetal and nonhepatic adult tissues and in most IGF-II expressing cell lines. P3 contains a TATA- and a CCAAT-box and approximately 75% of the promoter consists of GC basepairs. Transfections with various P3-reporter gene constructs indicated that P3 consists of a proximal region that supports transcription in most cell types and an upstream region that enhances P3 activity in endogenously IGF-II expressing cells [13]. DNase footprint analysis, electrophoretic mobility shift assays and in vitro transcription have revealed that the proximal promoter region contains a number of elements that are recognized by nuclear proteins (PE3-1 to PE3-4) [22]. Element PE3-4 is bound by a still unidentified transcription factor, which has a strong activating effect on P3 transcription. Using in vitro transcription it was shown that element PE3-3 alone has no effect on transcription, suggesting that it can only act in concert with adjacent transcription factors (Fig. 5). In addition, five binding sites are present for the early

48

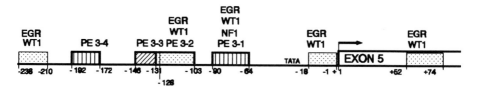

Fig. 5. Schematic representation of the human IGF-II promoter P3 proximal region. Domains protected by specific nuclear proteins are indicated. In vitro transcription experiments show that PE3-1 and PE3-4 are involved in activation of transcription. In addition, five putative binding sites for krox20/EGR2 and krox24/EGR1 (activators) are present. The P3 regions that are protected by WT1 (repressor) were identified by Drummond et al. [20,21].

growth response (EGR/krox) zinc-finger proteins, which act as transcriptional activators [23,24]. In order to study the putative binding of these factors to the IGF-II P3 promoter, we constructed five ds oligonucleotides, specific for the five putative EGR/krox binding sites. After incubation of these ds oligonucleotides with nuclear extracts prepared from recombinant vaccinia virus infected cells expressing krox20/EGR2 or krox24/EGR1, respectively, we could show that both proteins do indeed recognize and bind to these five sites, albeit with different affinities. Furthermore, we could show that binding of krox20/EGR2 and krox24/EGR1 to the P3 region is competed for by oligos specific for krox/EGR, suggesting an activating role for krox/EGR in P3 directed IGF-II expression.

To further investigate the role of the krox/EGR elements in P3, we cotransfected Hep3B cells with a construct bearing a P3 fragment (–138 to +140) coupled to the luciferase gene and a krox20/EGR2 expression plasmid. We could show that P3 is activated 8-fold by this factor (Fig. 6).

Interestingly, the same binding sites are also recognized by the Wilms' tumor locus zinc finger protein WT1 [20,21], which can also bind to the P3 promoter [25]. The WT1 protein is found in vivo to be present in four different isoforms, due to alternative splicing of WT1 mRNAs. It was shown that one of these isoforms, the -KTS form, can act as a transcriptional repressor of P3 activity [21]. From these and other results it is postulated that the krox/EGR proteins may play a role in overexpression of the IGF-II gene resulting in autocrine growth stimulation of various tumors, whereas WT1 may act as a repressor of P3 activity. Given the complexity of the structure of promoter P3, however, the in vivo effect may be quite different.

Site-specific endonucleolytic cleavage of IGF-II mRNAS

Regulation of mRNA stability is a common mechanism of controlling gene expression in eukaryotic cells. In general, degradation of mRNAs proceeds through the action of exo- and endonucleases in cooperation with regulatory factors. Cis-acting sequences involved in stability regulation are often found in the 3′ untranslated regions (UTRs) [26].

We have reported previously the existence of an unusually stable intermediate in

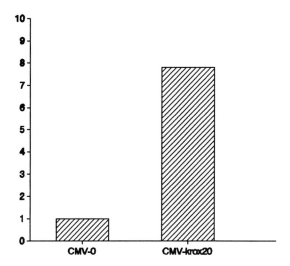

Fig. 6. Cotransfection of IGF-II P3-luc construct (−138 to +140) and the expression vector CMV-krox20. The luciferase activity of P3 cotransfected with the empty expression vector pCMV-0 was arbitrarily set to 1. Hep3B cells were transfected in 25 cm² flasks with 2 μg P3-luc construct, 2 μg of transcription factor(s) expression plasmid and 1 μg of RSV lacZ DNA, which served as an internal standard.

degradation of human IGF-II mRNAs [7,27,28]. This 1.8 kb RNA is the uncapped polyadenylated 3′-cleavage product of endonucleolytic cleavage in the 3′-UTR of IGF-II mRNAs. The capped 5′-cleavage product, which contains the entire IGF-II coding region, can be detected, but it is usually very unstable, probably because it lacks a poly(A)-tail. Although the precise function of this cleavage reaction is not known, there are indications that it is the initial step in degradation of IGF-II mRNAs that can be influenced by the growth conditions of the cells [27].

In search for cis-acting stability determinants we have shown that cleavage of IGF-II mRNAs in vivo requires two widely separated sequence elements (elements I and II) of about 300 nt located in the 3′-UTR of exon 9 (Fig. 7). Element II exhibits two conserved features: a) two stable stem-loop structures upstream of the cleavage site and b) a G-rich domain encompassing the cleavage site. Element I is located 1786 nt upstream of element II and does not display any obvious structural domains. Interestingly, computer-aided folding of elements I and II reveals the possibility that these two elements form a very stable secondary structure of considerable length (Fig. 7). That this interaction between elements I and II is of physiological relevance is further suggested by the fact that a similar interaction can be found for rat and mouse IGF-II mRNAs that undergo endonucleolytic cleavage like their human analogues. Moreover, comparison of the sequences of the three species reveals that base changes in element I are usually compensated for by an additional mutation in element II leading to maintenance of the double-stranded stem structure. This further provides evidence that the RNA/RNA interaction plays a major role in the cleavage reaction.

The identification of a putative stem structure between elements I and II raises the question what role this structure plays in endonucleolytic cleavage of IGF-II mRNAs.

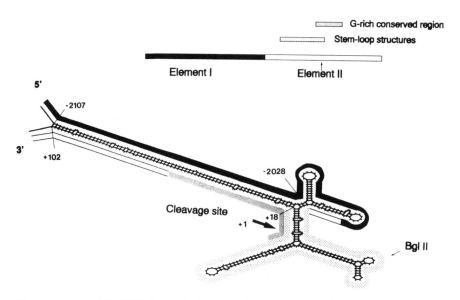

Fig. 7. A putative RNA/RNA interaction between elements I and II in human IGF-II mRNAs. Computer prediction of the secondary structure of elements I and II was performed according to the Zuker and Stiegler algorithm [29]. On top, the positions of the elements, starting with +1 as the cleavage site, the stem-loop structures and G-rich region are depicted in a linear format. For clarity, 5′ and 3′ flanking sequences are omitted.

To investigate the mechanism of cleavage in vivo we performed compensatory mutagenesis in the interacting regions. For this purpose we constructed three plasmids. The first construct Sense/Sense (S/S) contains a minimal element I (−2114/−2012). In the resulting mRNAs of 2.8 kb the stem structure can be formed, because both regions involved in stem formation are present in the wild-type configuration. A second construct Antisense/Sense (AS/S) was prepared by inverting element I. Transcripts derived from AS/S (2.8) kb are not able to form the stem structure, because the regions can no longer basepair. It is expected that this abolishes cleavage of the mRNA. When the interaction between elements I and II acts merely by providing a nonspecific stretch of ds RNA, cleavage should be retained when the basepairing is restored by compensatory mutations in the interacting region of element II. When not only the secondary structure, but also the primary sequence is involved in recognition of the RNA by trans-acting factors, no cleavage will take place after restoration of the stem structure. Therefore, in the third construct Antisense/Antisense (AS/AS) we restored the interaction, by also inverting the interacting region in element II so that the primary sequence of the interacting regions is different, but the secondary structure is maintained. Both the upstream stem-loop structures and the cleavage site are unchanged.

After transient transfection of the constructs into 293 cells, total RNA was analyzed on a Northern blot. Transcripts derived from S/S are cleaved very efficiently, but mRNAs derived from AS/S (2.8 kb) are not cleaved, probably because

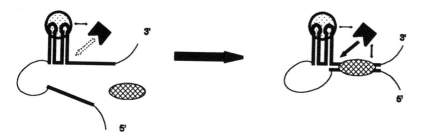

Fig. 8. Putative model for site-specific endonucleolytic cleavage of IGF-II mRNAs. Once the interaction between elements I and II forms, it is recognized by a sequence-specific trans-acting factor (depicted by the shaded ellipse). The stem structure provides specificity for RNA-protein complex formation, possibly in conjunction with other RNA regions and protein factors, for the endonucleolytic cleavage of the IGF-II mRNA.

no basepairing between the antisense element I and the sense element II can occur. Surprisingly, for AS/AS mRNAs, a full length transcript of 2.8 kb could be detected, but no cleavage products were present. Therefore, restoration of the secondary structure does not suffice to render the mRNA substrate for the cleavage reaction. This result indicates that the long-range RNA/RNA interaction between elements I and II functions probably as a sequence-specific double-stranded structure. We currently favor the following model for site-specific endonucleolytic cleavage of IGF-II mRNAs (Fig. 8). It involves specific recognition by one or more transacting factors of at least the interaction between elements I and II and possibly also of some other structure/sequence elements where the long-range interaction is recognized in a sequence-specific manner.

Cleavage of IGF-II mRNAs represents an up to now unique and unusual mRNA processing event. Although the function of the cleavage reaction is still elusive, it is tempting to speculate that this endonucleolytic cleavage is the first step in the degradation of IGF-II mRNAs. After cleavage the 5′ product containing the IGF-II coding region is very unstable, supporting a model of rapid change in IGF-II mRNA availability. Another interesting possibility is that a product of the cleavage reaction has a (yet unknown) function itself. Rastinejad and Blau [30] recently showed that 3′-UTRs can induce myogenic differentiation in a differentiation-deficient cell line. In this respect, it is interesting that IGF-II has been implicated in myogenic differentiation [31], opening new perspectives for an unconventional role of the 1.8 kb RNA cleavage product.

In conclusion, we have shown that the human IGF-II gene expression is controlled at different levels. First, at the transcriptional level, various promoters can be activated, depending on the availability of different transcription factors that are expressed in a development-specific manner or that are cell type-specific. Secondly, regulation takes place at the posttranscriptional level by means of site-specific endonucleolytic cleavage of the IGF-II mRNAs.

52

Acknowledgements

The authors wish to thank Mrs. A.M.C.B. Koonen Reemst and Mrs. W.R. Teertstra for excellent technical assistance.

References

1. Daughaday WH. In: Spencer EM (ed) Modern Concepts of Insuline-like Growth Factors. New York: Elsevier Science Publishing Co., 1991;557–565.
2. D'Ercole AJ. J Dev Physiol 1987;9:481–495.
3. DeChiara TM, Efstratiadis A, Robertson EJ. Nature 1990;345:78–80.
4. Sussenbach JS. Prog Growth Factor Res 1989;1:33–48.
5. De Pagter-Holthuizen P, Jansen M, Van Schaik FMA, Van der Kammen RA, Oosterwijk C, Van den Brande JL, Sussenbach JS. FEBS Lett 1987;214:259–264.
6. Jansen M, Van Schaik FMA, Van Tol H, Van den Brande JL, Sussenbach JS. FEBS Lett 1985;179:243–246.
7. De Pagter-Holthuizen P, Jansen M, Van der Kammen RA, Van Schaik FMA, Sussenbach JS. Biochim Biophys Acta 1988;950:282–295.
8. Holthuizen P, Van der Lee FM, Ikejiri K, Yamamoto M, Sussenbach JS. Biochim Biophys Acta 1990;1087:341–343.
9. Gloudemans T, Prinsen I, Van Unnik JAM, Lips CJM, Den Otter W, Sussenbach JS. Cancer Res 1990;50:6689–6695.
10. Sussenbach JS, Holthuizen P, Steenbergh PH. Growth Reg 1992;2:1–9.
11. Holthuizen P, LeRoith D, Lund PK, Roberts CT Jr, Rotwein P, Spencer EM, Sussenbach JS. In: Spencer EM (ed) Modern Concepts of Insulin-like Growth Factors. New York: Elsevier Science Publishing Co., 1991;733–736.
12. Schneid H, Holthuizen PE, Sussenbach JS. Endocrinology 1993;132:1145–1150.
13. Van Dijk MA, Van Schaik FMA, Bootsma HJ, Holthuizen P, Sussenbach JS. Mol Cell Endocrinol 1991;81:81–94.
14. Van Dijk MA, Rodenburg RJT, Holthuizen P, Sussenbach JS. Nucl Acids Res 1992;20:3099–3104.
15. Johnson PF, Landschulz WH, Graves BJ, McKnight SL. Genes Devel 1987;1:133–146.
16. Descombes P, Chojkier M, Lichtsteiner S, Falvey E, Schibler U. Genes Devel 1990;4:1541–1551.
17. Descombes P, Schibler U. Cell 1991;67:569–579.
18. Birkenmeier EH, Gwynn B, Howard S, Jerry J, Gordon JI, Landschulz WH, McKnight SL. Genes Devel 1989;3:1146–1156.
19. Maire P, Wuarin J, Schibler U. Science 1989;244:343–346.
20. Rauscher-III FJ, Morris JF, Tournay OE, Cook DM, Curren T. Science 1990;250:1259–1262.
21. Drummond IA, Madden SL, Rohwer-Nutter P, Bell GI, Sukhatme VP, Rauscher-III FJ. Science 1992;257:674–678.
22. Van Dijk MA, Holthuizen P, Sussenbach JS. Mol Cell Endocrinol 1992;88:175–185.
23. Lemaire P, Relevant O, Bravo R, Charnay P. Proc Natl Acad Sci USA 1988;85:4691–4695.
24. Lemaire P, Vesque C, Schnitt J, Stunnenberg H, Frank R, Charnay P. Mol Cell Biol 1990;10:3456–3467.
25. Madden SL, Cook DM, Morris JF, Gashler A, Subhatme VP, Rauscher-III FJ. Science 1991;253:1550–1553.
26. Peltz SW, Brewer G, Bernstein P, Hart PA, Ross J. Crit Rev Euk Gene Exp 1991;1:99–126.
27 Meinsma D, Holthuizen P, Van den Brande JL, Sussenbach JS. Biochem Biophys Res Commun 1991;179:1509–1516.
28. Meinsma D, Scheper W, Holthuizen P, Van den Brande JL, Sussenbach JS. Nucl Acids Res 1992;20:5003–5009.

29. Zuker M, Stiegler P. Nucl Acids Res 1981;9:133—148.
30. Rastinejad F, Blau HM. Cell 1993;72:903—917.
31. Tollefsen SE, Sadow JL, Rotwein PS. Proc Natl Acad Sci USA 1989;86:1543—1547.

Structural and functional relationships

Molecular interactions of IGF-I and IGF-II with their binding proteins and receptors

Geoffrey L. Francis, Sally E. Aplin, Kerrie A. McNeil, Steven J. Milner, Briony E. Forbes, Marina Ross, F. John Ballard and John C. Wallace
Cooperative Research Centre for Tissue Growth and Repair, CSIRO Division of Human Nutrition and Department of Biochemistry, University of Adelaide, Adelaide, SA 5000, Australia

Abstract. IGF-I and IGF-II binding to the type 1 and type 2 IGF receptors and the IGF-binding proteins (IGFBPs) have been extensively studied. We have defined the role of the N-terminal region of the B-domain, in particular the equivalent Glu^3 and Glu^6 residues in IGF-I and IGF-II respectively, as being important in the binding to IGFBPs. We previously established that the reduced association of IGF-I analogs with IGFBPs results in increased anabolic potency in cultured cells. Investigation of the relative biological potency of IGF-I and IGF-II and their B-domain analogs, reinforces the conclusion that IGFBPs play an important role in determining IGF actions. However, the observed biological potency in different cell types indicates that all binding sites in the IGF system, the signalling type 1 receptor, the potentially inhibitory type 2 IGF receptor and IGFBPs, must be taken into account.

Introduction

Insulin-like growth factors-I, IGF-I and IGF-II, are potent growth factors in many cell types, where they stimulate a number of anabolic processes. The pleiotropic response to IGFs, which includes the stimulation of DNA and protein synthesis and inhibition of intracellular protein breakdown, is believed to be mediated through the type 1 IGF receptor in most cell types [1]. The type 1 IGF receptor is a homolog of the insulin receptor as they share extensive structural homology, both having a heterotetrameric structure incorporating a cytoplasmic tyrosine kinase, presumably involved in transmembrane signalling [2]. IGFs bind to the insulin receptor with much lower affinity than insulin, but have the potential to interact with the insulin receptor in insulin-responsive tissues or cells. Characterisation of insulin and IGF-I receptor structure and function, has revealed the existence of insulin/IGF-I hybrid receptors. At the present time it is not clear whether such hybrid receptors are formed in living cells and modulate the actions of IGF-I and IGF-II. Another receptor that binds IGF-II with high affinity is the type 2 IGF receptor which has been shown to be identical to the cation-independent mannose 6-phosphate receptor [3]. The role of the type 2 IGF receptor in IGF-II signalling remains to be established for specific growth and

Address for correspondence: G.L. Francis, CSIRO Division of Human Nutrition, P.O. Box 10041, Gouger Street, Adelaide, SA 5000, Australia.

differentiation related functions.

In addition to their receptor binding, the actions of the IGFs are controlled by their association with a group of binding proteins that are unrelated to the IGF cell-surface receptors. This third component of the IGF system, the IGF-binding proteins (IGFBPs), are made up of six different classes. Most cells in culture secrete one or more types of IGFBPs into the extracellular medium where they are able to bind the IGFs and modify their interactions with the cell-surface IGF receptors. In certain situations IGFBPs are associated with the cell surface, where they may have a different role in IGF function [4]. Clearly, the nature of the interaction of the IGFs with their binding proteins is important in defining the role of the IGFs in vivo as well as in vitro. In this paper we will focus our work to evaluate the importance of the N-terminal region of the B-domain in the binding of IGF-I and IGF-II to the IGFBPs. Moreover, we will discuss the impact of altered IGFBP binding on the observed growth factor actions of IGF-I and IGF-II in cultured cells.

Characterisation of a potent analog of IGF-I with reduced binding to IGFBPs

Several years ago an IGF purified from bovine colostrum, was found to more potent in stimulating DNA and protein synthesis and the inhibiting intracellular protein breakdown in rat L6 myoblasts [5]. The sequence of this IGF with enhanced biological activity was found to lack the first three amino acids from the N-terminus of IGF-I and referred to as des(1—3)IGF-I. All three elements of the IGF system were evaluated for their role in the enhanced anabolic actions of the truncated analog. Competitive binding radioreceptor assays and affinity cross-linking experiments, using radiolabelled IGF-I and des(1-3)IGF-I, supported the conclusion that both growth factors bound to the signalling type 1 IGF receptor with similar affinity [6]. IGF-I and des(1-3)IGF-I both bound the type 2 IGF receptor with very low apparent affinity. Consequently, it did not appear as if differences in binding to the cell surface receptors were responsible for the increased biological potency in rat L6 myoblasts.

During the mid 1980s it became apparent that the family of IGFBPs secreted by many cell types had the potential to modulate the biological actions of the IGFs [4]. Binding of des(1-3)IGF-I to bIGFBP-2 purified from culture medium conditioned by bovine kidney (MDBK) cells was markedly reduced compared to the parent IGF-I molecule [7]. Thus, the increased bioactivity of des(1-3)IGF-I appeared to be the result of reduced affinity for IGFBPs secreted into the extracellular medium. We tested this hypothesis directly by employing chicken embryo fibroblasts, a cell that does not secrete detectable amounts of IGFBPs [8]. In these experiments we were able to evaluate the effect of adding two different IGFBPs, bIGFBP-2 and hIGFBP-1 on the inhibition of protein breakdown in chicken embryo fibroblasts. All three IGFs tested, IGF-I, des(1-3)IGF-I and IGF-II, were equally potent in this cell line, unlike in the rat L6 myoblasts. Addition of bIGFBP-2 or hIGFBP-1 had no effect on the dose-response curve for des(1-3)IGF-I. However, the response to IGF-I and IGF-II was changed so that much higher concentrations were required to reach the same level of inhibition of protein breakdown. The different response to addition of the two IGFBPs reflects the known relative affinity of the IGFs for these binding proteins [9]. The poor binding of des(1-3)IGF-I to the IGFBPs would result in higher concentrations of free growth factor to bind to the signalling type 1 IGF receptor.

From these experiments we concluded that the inhibitory effects of IGFBPs on IGF actions depends first on the ratio of IGF peptide and secondly on IGFBP present and the relative affinity of the IGFBPs for the IGF.

Defining the N-terminal amino acid residues important for reduced IGFBP binding

IGF-I and IGF-II are single chain polypeptides that share significant amino acid homology with insulin [1]. The IGF molecules are organised into four structural domains designated as B, C, A and D from the N-terminal. The B- and A-domains correspond to the B and A chains of insulin. To further define the role of the N-terminal region of the B-domain in the biological actions of IGF-I, we chemically synthesised a library of analogs lacking from 1 to 5 amino acids from the N-terminus [10]. Ability to stimulate protein synthesis in rat L6 myoblasts was not affected by removal of 1 or 2 amino acids from the N-terminus, but as expected, loss of Glu^3 in des(1—3)IGF-I resulted in an 8-fold increase in potency relative to IGF-I. The further removal of Tar^4 in des(1—4)IGF-I, resulted in a growth factor with activity intermediate between that of IGF-I and des(1—3)IGF-I. Des(1—5) possessed very low activity that may reflect the presence of incorrectly folded forms of the molecule.

The pattern of binding for the IGF-I deletion analogs to IGFBPs present in rat L6 myoblast conditioned medium supported the role of IGFBPs in modulating the actions of IGFs. Moreover, the critical role of Glu^3 in the N-terminal tripeptide for binding to IGFBPs was established. The essential role of the signalling type 1 IGF receptor was apparent from the reduced biological activity of des(1—4)IGF-I compared with des(1—3)IGF-I, despite the lower affinity of the former for the IGFBPs present. Des(1—4)IGF-I binds 2-fold less well to the type 1 IGF receptor compared with des(1—3)IGF-I. Hence the observed biological potency is a function of binding to the IGFBP and type 1 IGF receptor.

Modification of the N-terminal region of the B-domain in IGF-I affects both IGFBP binding and its anabolic actions

To further define the structure and function relationships of residues at the N-terminus of IGF-I, we produced three classes of recombinant IGF-I analogs: 1. The truncated analog, des(1—3)IGF-I; 2. Substitution of Glu^3 by a neutral Gly or oppositely charged Arg to give [Gly^3]-IGF-I and [Arg^3]-IGF-I respectively [11]; 3. Addition of a 13-amino acid extension derived from porcine growth hormone to the IGF-I sequence. These IGFs referred to as Long IGF-I, Long [Gly^3]-IGF-I and Long [Arg^3]-IGF-I were fusion proteins expressed directly in *Escherichia coli* [12]. We found these IGF-I fusion proteins could be refolded successfully and were biologically active, provided the N-terminal fusion partner linked to the IGF-I sequence was kept short (e.g., 13 amino acids).

The biological activities of the IGF-I fusion proteins were compared with authentic IGF-I and the truncated analog, des(1–3)IGF-I. In rat L6 myoblasts all of the analogs were more potent than IGF-I in their abilities to stimulate DNA and protein synthesis and inhibit protein breakdown. The order of biological potency was Long [Arg^3]-IGF-I ≥ des(1-3)IGF-I > Long [Gly^3]-IGF-I > Long IGF-I > IGF-I. This was almost the inverse order of their apparent affinity for the IGFBPs secreted by rat L6 rat myoblasts. Surprisingly, the only analog that displayed significantly reduced binding to the type 1 IGF receptor was the most biologically active analog, Long [Arg^3]-IGF-I.

To evaluate the ability of rat L6 myoblast derived IGFBPs to modulate the biological activity of these IGF-I fusion proteins, we once again utilised the chicken embryo fibroblasts. In the absence of added IGFBPs des(1–3)IGF-I and IGF-I were equipotent in inhibiting protein breakdown while Long [Arg^3]-IGF-I was about 3-fold less potent. The observed biological potency exactly reflected the type 1 IGF receptor binding pattern in these cells, which was similar to that in rat L6 myoblasts. Addition of L6 myoblast conditioned medium IGFBPs had a negligible effect on the activity of des(1–3)IGF-I and Long [Arg^3]-IGF-I, but reduced the activity of IGF-I by 20-fold.

From these studies we concluded that the addition of a hydrophobic 13-amino acid extension to the N-terminus interferes with binding to IGFBPs either directly by steric hindrance or indirectly by masking an essential residue on either IGF-I or IGFBP required for formation of an IGF-IGFBP complex. Further modification of the IGF-I sequence by substitution of Glu^3 with a neutral Gly or oppositely charged Arg results in an incremental reduction of IGFBP binding. The effect of these changes in structure at the N-terminus indicated that IGFBP binding was the most important factor in determining biological potency, provided binding to the type 1 IGF receptor was not reduced more than 5-fold.

Role of the N-terminal region of the B-domain in IGF-II binding to IGFBPs

The function of IGF-II has been the subject of much speculation and experimentation recently [1,13]. Our aim was to address two major questions: 1. In IGF-II is the N-terminal region of the B-domain of similar importance for IGFBP binding as observed for the corresponding region in IGF-I? 2. Do changes in IGF-II binding to IGFBPs result in altered growth factor potency in cultured cells?

The solution structure of IGF-I and insulin has been determined, but not for IGF-II [14]. However, the strong amino acid homology between IGF-II, IGF-I and insulin suggests that the same structural features will be shared between the three polypeptides. Thus it would be expected that modification of the corresponding N-terminal residues in IGF-II and IGF-I would lead to equivalent changes in biological

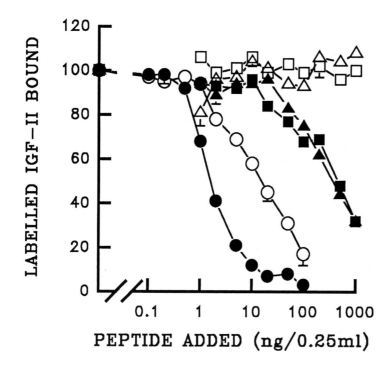

Fig. 1. Competition for binding of ^{125}I-labelled IGF-II to purified rat IGFBP-2 by IGF-I(O), [Arg³]-IGF-I (□), des(1—3)IGF-I (Δ), IGF-II (●), [Arg⁶]-IGF-II (■) and des(1—6)IGF-II (▲). Values are the means of triplicate determinations at each peptide concentration. S.E.M. are shown by the descending symbols.

properties. We constructed two analogs of IGF-II, [Arg⁶]-IGF-II and des(1—6)IGF-II, and compared their biological properties with the corresponding structural analogs of IGF-I, [Arg³]-IGF-I and des(1—3)IGF-I. To answer the first question about the impact of these modifications on the binding of IGF-II to IGFBPs, we tested the binding of both sets of IGFs to purified rIGFBP-2, pIGFBP-3 and oIGFNP-4. The binding of these B-domain analogs to rIGFBP-2 are compared in a competition binding assay in Fig. 1.

IGF-II binds to rIGFBP-2 with 9-fold greater apparent affinity than IGF-I. There is a clear difference in binding between the B-domain analogs of IGF-I and IGF-II, with both IGF-I analogs showing very little competition for labelled IGF-II binding. The IGF-II analogs, [Arg⁶]-IGF-II and des(1—6)IGF-II bind with approximately 200-fold reduced potency compared with the parent IGF-II. Different patterns of reduced binding were found for the B-domain mutants of IGF-I and IGF-II with pIGFBP-3 and oIGFBP-4 (data not shown).

What was the effect of the alterations in IGFBP binding on the biological potency of these B-domain analogs? In L6 myoblast protein synthesis bioassay, the IGF-II analogs, des(1—6)IGF-II and [Arg⁶]-IGF-II were slightly more potent than IGF-II, but about 10-fold less potent than IGF-I and 100-fold less potent than the corresponding IGF-I analogs, des(1—3)IGF-I and [Arg³]-IGF-I (Table 1). Reduced binding to the

Table. 1. Biological potencies of the insulin-like growth factors (IGFs) in rat L6 myoblasts and H35 hepatoma cells are expressed relative to IGF-II. The values have been calculated from the ED_{50} in the assays

Assay	IGF-I	[Arg³]-IGF-I	des(1–3)IGF-I	IGF-II	[ARG⁶]-IGF-II	des(1–6)IGF-II
L6 myoblast:						
Protein synthesis	11	150	160	1.0	1.5	1.3
Type 1 IGF receptor	4.7	1.9	5.4	1.0	0.56	0.56
Type 2 IGF receptor	<0.001	<0.001	<0.001	1.0	2.9	0.42
IGFBP	0.065	<0.001	<0.001	1.0	0.008	0.003
H35 hepatoma:						
Protein breakdown	2.2	8.6	6.0	1.0	4.3	2.7
Insulin receptor	0.17	0.12	0.26	1.0	0.58	0.14
Type 2 IGF receptor	<0.001	<0.001	<0.001	1.0	1.9	0.26
IGFBP	1.7	0.005	0.007	1.0	0.015	0.006

Reproduced with permission from [21].

type 1 IGF receptor by the IGF-II peptides can partly explain their lower potency compared with the IGF-I peptides. Furthermore, the IGF-II peptides bind with a more than a 100-fold higher apparent affinity to the type 2 IGF receptor compared to IGF-I and its analogs. Thus the type 2 IGF receptor could act as an inert "sink" for the IGF-II peptides decreasing the concentration of free peptide to bind to the signalling type 1 IGF receptor. The expected positive effect of the reduced binding to the IGFBPs on biological potency of the IGF-II analogs is apparently attenuated by the combined effects of binding to the type 2 receptor and reduced binding to the type 1 IGF receptor.

As a result of the differences in receptor binding and the biological potencies in L6 myoblasts for the different analogs, we investigated their biological potency in H35 hepatoma cells. These cells do not possess a type 1 IGF receptor and the actions of IGF-I and IGF-II are mediated through the related insulin receptor [15]. The hepatoma cells also possess a large number of type 2 IGF receptors, which are not involved in mediating the anabolic responses to IGF-II [16]. Intracellular protein breakdown in these cells was inhibited by $[Arg^6]$-IGF-II and des(1—6)IGF-II with a 4.4-fold and 2.4-fold greater potency than IGF-II respectively (Table 1). The corresponding IGF-I analogs, $[Arg^3]$-IGF-I and des(1—3)IGF-I, showed very similar changes to this in their biological potency relative to IGF-I in the hepatoma cells, in strong contrast to the situation in L6 myoblasts. There are two main differences between the two cell types that could explain the different relative potency of IGF-II. First, in H35 hepatoma cells the IGF-II peptides bind as well or better than the IGF-I peptides to the signalling receptor. Secondly, the binding to the secreted IGFBPs in the hepatoma cells is very similar for IGF-I and IGF-II and their corresponding analogs. Thus in hepatoma cells the basis exists for IGF-II analogs to display enhanced activity in a similar fashion to the IGF-I analogs.

In both the hepatoma and myoblast cells the greater potency of IGF-I over IGF-II may be explained by the type 2 IGF receptor acting as an inert "sink" for IGF-II. Selective binding of IGF-II over IGF-I would reduce the free concentration of IGF-II peptides able to bind to the signalling receptor. The concept of the type 2 receptor acting as a "sink" to reduce IGF-II binding to the type 1 IGF receptor, was proposed previously to explain the opposite genomic imprinting of IGF-II and the type 2 receptor [13].

A simpler picture is presented by the activity of these analogs in chicken embryo fibroblasts, as these cells do not secrete detectable amounts of IGFBPs and lack the type 2 IGF receptor [17]. The anabolic response to IGFs is mediated via the signalling type 1 IGF receptor which was previously established by affinity cross-linking experiments [17]. IGF-I and IGF-II and their B-domain analogs, show similar biological potency in inhibiting intracellular protein breakdown (Fig. 2). Moreover, the biological potencies reflect the similar binding pattern of these peptides in type 1 IGF receptor binding assays (data not shown). These results support the conclusion that in the absence of type 2 IGF receptor binding the IGF-II peptides are free to bind the type 1 IGF receptor as well as IGF-I and stimulate an anabolic response.

64

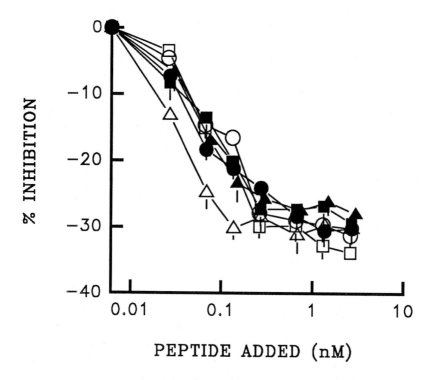

Fig. 2. Inhibition of intracellular protein breakdown in chicken embryo fibroblasts by IGF-I (O), [Arg³]-IGF-I (□), des(1—3)IGF-I (Δ), IGF-II (●), [Arg⁶]-IGF-II (■) and des(1—6)IGF-II (▲). Values are the means of triplicate determinations on three cultures at each peptide concentration. S.E.M. are shown by the descending symbols.

Conclusions and Speculations

The biological actions of the IGFs are dependent on the role of two other components making up the IGF system, the cell surface receptors and the family of IGFBPs [4]. Understanding the nature of the interaction between IGF-I and IGF-II and these binding sites at the molecular level has been facilitated by the production of analogs of the IGFs, where one or more residues have been altered [10—12,18—21]. Substitutions or deletions of amino acids based on insulin and other strategies in these studies have identified key residues in the interaction of IGF-I and IGF-II with both the type 1 and type 2 IGF receptors and members of the IGFBP family. The evaluation of critical residues for binding to IGFBPs has taken advantage of the availability of analogs designed primarily to probe receptor binding. Residues in the IGFs important for the binding of IGFBPs have been identified in the A-domain and B-domain employing these analogs [22,23]. The A-domain mutants of particular interest involve the substitution of [Phe⁴⁹, Arg⁵⁰, Ser⁵¹] in IGF-I and [Phe⁴⁸, Arg⁴⁹, Ser⁵⁰] in IGF-II by the equivalent residues from insulin, [Thr, Ser, Ile]. These substitutions were found to markedly reduce binding to the type 2 IGF receptor [19,24]. More recently these mutants have helped identify the relative importance of IGF residues that occupy the IGFBP binding pocket. For example, the identification of the A-domain residues as important for binding of IGFBP-1 and -2 compared with IGFBP-3 is noted [22,23]. IGFBP-4 and IGFBP-5 are affected by all mutations in either the A- or B-domains of IGF-I and IGF-II. The B-domain residue at position 3 in IGF-I and the corresponding residue at 6 in IGF-II, appear to have a large influence on binding to all the classes of IGFBPs [20,21,25]. Moreover, our studies on the N-terminal B-domain analogs of both IGF-I and IGF-II, suggest that the nature of the substitution can have a significant effect on the apparent affinity for different IGFBPs. Hence caution should be shown in assigning importance for particular residues in the binding reaction.

Our studies in cultured cells relating affinity for IGFBPs and the potency of IGFs to stimulate an anabolic response, substantiates the involvement of the various components of the IGF system. In rat L6 myoblasts a relatively straightforward relationship between reduced binding to the IGFBPs secreted into the culture medium and increased biological potency exists. Thus it appears that binding to IGFBPs decreases the concentration of free IGF available to bind to the type 1 IGF receptor and hence reduces its biological potency compared with IGFs that possess lower affinity for the IGFBPs. Reduction of receptor binding can reduce biological potency to a lesser value than might be expected, as in the case of the truncated analog des(1—4)IGF-I compared with the more potent des(1—3)IGF-I [10]. This is to be compared with the properties of Long [Arg³]-IGF-I which has 4-fold lower apparent affinity for the type 1 receptor compared with des(1—3)IGF-I (and IGF-I). In this case the approximately 20-fold reduced binding to L6 myoblast IGFBPs displayed by Long [Arg³]-IGF-I compared with des(1—3)IGF-I presumably explains the slightly greater biological potency of the former analog. Thus, in L6 myoblasts the observed biological potency of IGF-I appears to be largely a function of the competing type 1 IGF and IGFBP binding sites.

In L6 myoblasts the IGF-II analogs, des(1—6)IGF-II and [Arg⁶]-IGF-I, fail to show the expected increase in biological potency resulting from reduced affinity for IGFBPs, as observed with the corresponding IGF-I analogs. One explanation for this is the reduced affinity of the IGF-II peptides for the signalling type 1 IGF receptor. This contrasts with the situation in H35 hepatoma cells where binding to the signalling insulin receptor by the IGF-II peptides is greater than observed for the IGF-I peptides. Here the IGF-II analogs display the expected increase in biological potency compared with IGF-II.

The situation with the IGF-II analogs, des(1—6)IGF-II and [Arg⁶]-IGF-I, is complicated by the presence of the anabolically inert type 2 IGF receptor. In both the L6 myoblasts and H35 hepatoma cells this receptor appears to act as an inert "sink" that reduces the concentration of free IGF-II peptides available to bind to the signalling type 1 receptors. This was clearly shown in chicken embryo fibroblasts, a cell that does not possess this receptor type. Moreover the chicken embryo fibroblasts do not secrete IGFBPs. The net effect of these properties results in IGF-I, IGF-II and

66

their respective B-domain analogs having similar biological potencies in this cell type.

From our cell culture studies it is clear that caution must be exercised in extrapolating the in vitro properties of IGF analogs to the more complex situation in vivo. However, the library of IGF analogs available from different laboratories should provide useful probes for dissecting the role of the various elements of the IGF system in physiological processes.

References

1. Humbel RE. Eur J Biochem 1990;190:445—462.
2. Frattali AL, Pessin JE. Ann NY Acad Sci 1993;687:77—89.
3. MacDonald RG, Pfeffer SR, Coussens L, Tepper MA, Brocklebank CM, Mole JE, Anderson JK, Chen E, Czech MP, Ullrich A. Science 1988;239:1134—1137.
4. Rechler MM. Vit Horm 1993;47:1—114.
5. Francis GL, Upton FM, Ballard FJ, McNeil KA, Wallace JC. Biochem J 1988;251:95—103.
6. Ballard FJ, Ross M, Upton FM, Francis GL. Biochem J 1988;249:721—726.
7. Szabo L, Mottershead DG, Ballard FJ, Wallace JC. Biochem Biophys Res Commun 1988;151:207—214.
8. Ross M, Francis GL, Szabo L, Wallace JC, Ballard FJ. Biochem J 1989;258:267—272.
9. Forbes B, Szabo L, Baxter RC, Ballard FJ, Wallace JC. Biochem Biophys Res Commun 1988;157:196—202.
10. Bagley CJ, May BL, Szabo L, McNamara PJ, Ross M, Francis GL, Ballard FJ, Wallace JC. Biochem J 1989;259:665—671.
11. King R, Wells JRE, Krieg P, Snoswell M, Brazier J, Bagley CJ, Ballard FJ, Ross M, Francis GL. J Mol Endo 1992;8:29—41.
12. Francis GL, Ross M, Ballard FJ, Milner SJ, Senn C, McNeil KA, Wallace JC, King R, Wells JRE. J Mol Endo 1992;8:213—223.
13. Haig D, Graham C. Cell 1991;64:1045—1046.
14. Cooke RM, Harvey TS, Campbell ID. Biochemistry 1991;30:5484—5489.
15. Mottola C, Czech MP. J Biol Chem 1984;259:12705—12713.
16. Massague J, Blinderman LA, Czech MP. J Biol Chem 1982;257:13958—13963.
17. Kallincos NC, Wallace JC, Francis GL, Ballard FJ. J Mol Endo 1990;124:89—97.
18. Cascieri MA, Bayne ML. In: LeRoith D, Raizada MK (eds) Molecular and Cellular Biology of Insulin-like Growth Factors and their Receptors. New York: Plenum, 1989;225—229.
19. Sokano K, Enjoh T, Numata F, Fujiwara H, Marumoto Y, Higashihashi N, Sato Y, Perdue JF, Fujita-Yamaguchi Y. J Biol Chem 1991;266:20626—20635.
20. Luthi C, Roth BV, Humbel RE. Eur J Biochem 1992;205:483—490.
21. Francis GL, Aplin SE, Milner SJ, McNeil KA, Ballard FJ, Wallace JC. Biochem J 1993;293:713—719.
22. Clemmons DR, Dehoff ML, Busby WH, Bayne ML, Cascieri MA. Endocrinology 1992;131:890—895.
23. Bach LA, Hsieh S, Sokano K, Fujiwara H, Perdue JF, Rechler MM. J Biol Chem 1993;268:9246—9254.
24. Bayne ML, Applebaum J, Chicchi GG, Hayes NS, Green BG, Cascieri MA. J Biol Chem 1988;263:6233—6239.
25. Oh Y, Muller HL, Lee DY, Feilder PJ, Rosenfeld RG. Endocrinology 1993;132:1337—1344.

Structural determinants for the binding of insulin-like growth factor-II to IGF and insulin receptors and IGF binding proteins

J.F. Perdue[1], L.A. Bach[2], R. Hashimoto[3], K. Sakano[3], Y. Fujita-Yamaguchi[4], H. Fujiwara[3] and M.M. Rechler[2]

[1]*American Red Cross, Department of Molecular Biology, 15601 Crabbs Branch Way, Rockville, MD 20855, USA;* [2]*NIDDK, National Institutes of Health, Bethesda, MD 20892, USA;* [3]*Molecular Biology Research Laboratory of Daiichi Pharmaceutical Co., Ltd., Tokyo 134, Japan; and* [4]*Beckman Research Institute of the City of Hope, Duarte, CA 91010, USA*

Abstract. Nineteen deletion and amino acid substitution mutants of rIGF-II were prepared and characterized for their apparent relative affinity for IGF and insulin receptors and binding proteins. The results of these studies indicated that Phe^{26}, Tyr^{27} in the B-domain and Val^{43} in the A-domain, specified IGF-II's affinity for IGF-I and insulin receptors while Phe^{48}, Arg^{49}, Ser^{50}, Ala^{54} and Leu^{55} defined it for IGF-II/CIM6-P receptors. Phe^{48}, Arg^{49} and Ser^{50} also interacted with IGFBP 1–6. In studies with N-terminal mutants of IGF-II, Leu^8 was identified as a probable three dimensional determinant of structure that is essential for IGF and insulin binding to receptors and binding proteins.

Introduction

Structure function characterization of natural mutants of insulin that have been isolated from diabetic patients and of mutants and have been synthesized with amino acid substitutions in the B and A chains of insulin [1] or the B to D domains of IGF-I [2], have provided a frame work for understanding the role the different amino acids serve in forming the molecules three-dimensional structures and in facilitating high affinity protein-protein interactions. In the case of insulin, these interactions are with additional insulin molecules to form dimers and hexamers and with insulin receptors [1]. For IGF-I they are with IGF receptors and binding proteins [2].

Present in human serum, to the extent of about 10% of total IGF-II (Perdue, unpublished), is a natural mutant of IGF-II called IGF-II variant, that arose as a consequence of an error in mRNA splicing. This error resulted in the substitution of Arg, Leu, Pro, Gly for Ser^{29} at the carboxy-terminal end of the B-domain and decreased the affinity this IGF-II had for IGF-I receptors and its mitogenic activity on MCF-7 cells by 50% [3]. Recently several laboratories, including our own, used site-directed mutagenesis procedures and expression in bacteria and *Bombyx mori* to produce mutants of IGF-II that have deletions or specific amino acid substitutions in the B-, C-, A- or D-domains. These mutants have been used to identify the residues that are required for IGF-II binding to IGF-I, IGF-II/CIM6-P and insulin receptors [4–6] and IGFBP 1–6 [7]. For example, Phe^{26} and Tyr^{27} in the B-domain [4–6] and

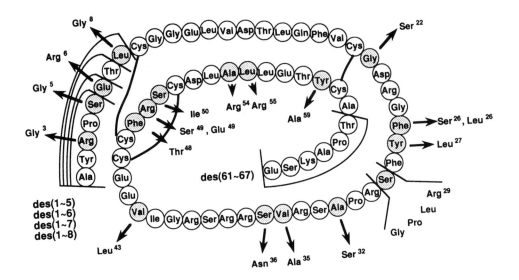

Fig. 1. Schematic representation of the amino acid substitution and deletion mutants that were used in earlier [6,7] and the present studies.

Val[43] in the A-domain are essential for its binding to IGF-I and insulin receptors and Phe[48], Arg[49], Ser[50], Ala[54] and Leu[55] in the A-domain for its binding to IGF-II/CIM6-P receptors [6]. More recently, we determined that Phe[48], Arg[49], Ser[50] and Phe[26] are critical residues for IGF-II binding to IGFBP 1—6 [7]. In this paper we review these past results and describe new experiments that point to additional residues in the B- and A-domains that are involved in the interactions of IGF-II with its receptors and binding proteins.

Materials and Methods

Materials

Enzymes, isotopes and radioactivity-labeled and unlabeled insulin, IGF-I and IGF-II that were used to construct, express, purify and characterize IGF-II mutants were purchased from previously described sources [6].

IGF-II mutants

The rIGF-II deletion and substitution mutants that were employed in this and previous studies [6] are shown in Fig. 1. [Ser[26]] rIGF-II, [Leu[27]] rIGF-II, [Leu[43]] rIGF-II, des [62—68] rIGF-II and the disulfide-bonded isomer of rIGF-II were expressed and purified from *B. mori* larvae as previously described [6]. [Thr[48], Ser[49], Ile[50]] rIGF-II,

[Arg^{54}, Arg^{55}] rIGF-II, [Leu^{26}] rIGF-II, [Ser^{22}] rIGF-II, [Ser^{32}, Ala^{35}, Asn^{36}] rIGF-II, [Glu^{49}] rIGF-II, [Ala^{59}] rIGF-II, [Gly^3, Gly^5] rIGF-II, [des (1—5)] rIGF-II, [Gly^8] rIGF-II and [des (1—8)] rIGF-II were expressed and purified from *Escherichia coli* as previously described [6]. [Arg^6] rIGF-II and [des (1—6)] rIGF-II were purchased from GroPep Pty. Ltd. (Adelaide, Australia). Peptide mapping confirmed proper disulfide bond pairing of the mutants [6]. Their mass and the correct substitution of amino acids was determined by compositional and N-terminal amino acid sequence analysis [6].

Characterization of the binding of rIGF-II mutants to insulin and IGF receptors and IGFBPs

The affinities of the different IGF-II mutants for enriched preparations of human placenta insulin and IGF-I receptors and rat placenta IGF-II/CIM6-P receptors was determined in competitive ligand binding assays as previously described [6]. A similar approach, using previously described procedures, [7] was used to determine the rIGF-II mutants affinities for purified preparations of human IGFBP-1, IGFBP-2, IGFBP-4 and IGFBP-6, recombinant IGFBP-3 and IGFBP-5 and rat IGFBP-2 and IGFBP-4. The affinities of the mutants relative to that of rIGF-II were estimated by comparison of concentrations that inhibited binding of ^{125}I labeled-IGF-I, -IGF-II and -insulin by 50%.

Characterization of the biological activities of rIGF-II mutants

The magnitude of incorporation of [^{3}H] thymidine into BALB/c 3T3 cells treated for 24 h with designated concentrations of rIGF-II and rIGF-II mutants was determined as previously described [6].

Results

Preparation and characterization of rIGF-II and rIGF-II mutants

Over a period of about 4 years, 19 substitution or deletion mutants of hrIGF-II have been designed by the Molecular Biology Laboratory of the Daiichi Pharmaceutical Co., Ltd. mainly on the results of structural-functional studies with natural and synthetic mutants of insulin [1] and with mutants of rIGF-I [2]. Several of them were also designed to define the epitopes specifically recognized by anti-hIGF-II monoclonal antibodies [8]. These were expressed and purified from *B. mori* larva or *E. coli* as previously described [6]. In addition, we purchased [Arg^6] rIGF-II and [des (1—6)] rIGF-II. Figure 1 illustrates the positions of the deleted or substituted amino acids. Although all the mutants were tested for their ability to compete with human or rIGF-II or rIGF-I or porcine insulin for binding to IGF-II/CIM6-P, IGF-I or insulin receptors, respectively, we will discuss the properties of only 13 of them.

IGF-I receptors

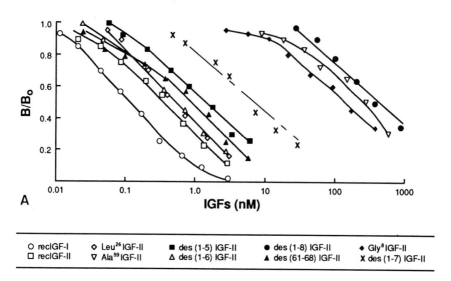

O reclGF-I	◇ Leu²⁶ IGF-II	■ des (1-5) IGF-II	● des (1-8) IGF-II	◆ Gly⁸ IGF-II
□ reclGF-II	▽ Ala⁵⁹ IGF-II	△ des (1-6) IGF-II	▲ des (61-68) IGF-II	X des (1-7) IGF-II

Insulin receptors

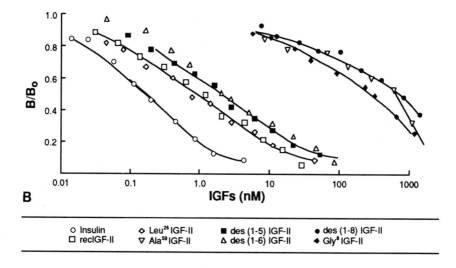

O Insulin	◇ Leu²⁶ IGF-II	■ des (1-5) IGF-II	● des (1-8) IGF-II
□ reclGF-II	▽ Ala⁵⁹ IGF-II	△ des (1-6) IGF-II	◆ Gly⁸ IGF-II

Fig. 2. Competitive ligand binding of rIGF-II mutants to IGF-I (A), insulin (B) and IGF-II/CIM6P (C) (*opposite page*) receptors.

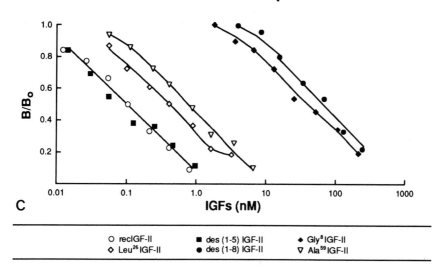

IGF-II/CIM6P receptors

O reclGF-II	■ des (1-5) IGF-II	◆ Gly^8 IGF-II
◇ Leu^{26} IGF-II	● des (1-8) IGF-II	▽ Ala^{59} IGF-II

Fig. 2C.

Isolation of rIGF-II and the mutants of rIGF-II involves SP-Toyopearl column chromatography in the presence of urea and 50 mM 2-mercaptoethanol followed by a renaturation step involving refolding of the reduced polypeptide and intrachain disulfide bond formation. The bonds are formed between Cys^9 and Cys^{47}, Cys^{21} and Cys^{60}, and Cys^{46} and Cys^{51} (Fig. 1). During renaturation, some of the rIGF-II that is formed contains disulfide-bonded isomers, i.e., Cys^9 bonds to Cys^{46} and Cys^{47} to Cys^{51}. The isomeric form has about 4% of the receptor binding affinity of rIGF-II, but can be separated from the native form of rIGF-II by rpHPLC. Since substituting certain amino acids, e.g., Leu^8, resulted in comparable losses in receptor binding activity and the elution of the mutants at different positions during rpHPLC, we determined that the disulfide bond pairs and the position of the substituted amino acid in all the IGF-II mutants were correct prior to using them in structure-function studies by peptide mapping procedures and N-terminal amino acid sequence analysis, respectively.

The specificity of binding of IGF-II and IGF-II mutants to IGF-II/CIM6-P, IGF-I and insulin receptors

rIGF-II binds to IGF-I and insulin receptors with apparent equilibrium dissociation constants ($K_d$app) of 0.3 and 0.2 nM, respectively (Fig. 2A and 2B). These values were estimated from the nM concentrations of rIGF-II that displaced 50% of specifically bound ^{125}I-labeled IGF-I or insulin and are 3 and 6 times greater than the $K_d$app of these ligands for their homologous receptors. In a previous communication

Table 1. Relative affinity of rIGF-II mutants for IGF and insulin receptors

Ligand	IGF-II/CIM6-P receptor	IGF-I receptor	Insulin receptor
	(% of IGF-II)		
rIGF-II	100	100	100
Disulfide bonded isomer of rIGF-II	4	4	2
B-domain mutants:			
[des (1—5)] rIGF-II	100	62	50
[Gly^3, Gly^5] rIGF-II	111	63	83
[des (1—6)] rIGF-II	ND[a]	73	41
[Arg^6] rIGF-II	ND[a]	73	71
[des (1—7)] rIGF-II	100	5.4	25
[des (1—8)] rIGF-II	0.3	0.1	0.1
[Gly^8] rIGF-II	0.3	0.2	0.4
[Ser^{22}] rIGF-II	12	47	50
[Ser^{26}] rIGF-II	30	20	4
[Leu^{26}] rIGF-II	26	78	143
[Leu^{27}] rIGF-II	60	0.8	11
C-domain mutants:			
[Ser^{32}, Ala^{35}, Asn^{36}] rIGF-II	53	43	50
A-domain mutants:			
[Leu^{43}] rIGF-II	50	1.3	0.5
[Thr^{48}, Ser^{49}, Ile^{50}] rIGF-II	0.7	167	200
[Glu^{49}] rIGF-II	30	29	10
[Arg^{54}, Arg^{55}] rIGF-II	No inhib.	125	200
[Ala^{59}] rIGF-II	13	0.1	0.2
D-domain mutants:			
[des (62-67)] rIGF-II	167	62	200

[a]Not determined.

[6], we identified Tyr^{27} and Val^{43}, and to a lesser extent Phe^{26}, as residues that are critical for the binding of IGF-II to IGF-I and insulin receptors. Substituting Leu for Tyr^{27} decreased IGF-II binding to IGF-I receptors more that it did to insulin receptors, while substituting Ser for Phe^{26} and Leu for Val^{43} had an opposite effect. Table 1 summarizes the earlier [6] as well as new results in a form, i.e., relative affinity, that compares rIGF-II mutants binding to the receptors to that of rIGF-II that is set at 100%. If hydrophobic Leu was substituted for Phe^{26} instead of Ser, the relative affinity of this mutant for the IGF-I and, in particular, the insulin receptors increased to values that were similar to or greater than rIGF-II.

Destabilization of the α helex in the A-domain of IGF-II between Ile^{42} and Phe^{48} by substituting Leu for Val^{43} was proposed as the explanation for this mutant's decreased affinity for IGF-I and insulin receptors [2]. Structural analysis of insulin and IGF-I and a study with synthetic mutants of insulin, suggests that this region of the molecule is stabilized by Van der Wall forces that are formed between Ile^{42} and possibly Val^{43} and Tyr^{59} [1,2]. Consistent with these interpretations, in new experiments we observed that substituting Ala for Tyr^{59} in rIGF-II dramatically decreased its affinity for the IGF-I and insulin receptors. However, this substitution had much less of an effect on the binding of the mutant to IGF-II/CIM6-P receptors (Fig. 2C and Table 1).

The $K_d$app of rIGF-II for the IGF-II/CIM6-P receptors is about 0.1 nM (Fig. 2C). In our earlier study, we observed that substituting the amino acid sequence Thr, Ser, Ile that is found in insulin for the homologous sequence of Phe^{48}, Arg^{49}, Ser^{50} of IGF-II and the Arg, Arg sequence of IGF-I for Ala^{54}, Leu^{55} in IGF-II increased the affinities of both mutants for IGF-I and insulin receptors by up to 2-fold. However, these mutants could no longer bind to IGF-II/CIM6-P receptors (Table 1). Making a single replacement of negatively charged Glu for Arg^{49} also reduced the binding of this mutant to IGF-II/CIM6-P receptors by about 70%. Unexpectedly, this substitution also decreased the affinity of the mutant for IGF-I and insulin receptors (Table 1).

Deletion of the first five or six amino acids in the N-terminal region of the B-domain or substituting Gly, Gly for Arg^3, Pro^5 as is found in mouse IGF-II or Arg for Glu^6, decreased the affinity of IGF-II for IGF-I, IGF-II/CIM6-P and insulin receptors by about 50%. Removal of Thr^7 reduced the affinity of IGF-II for IGF-I and insulin receptors, but not for that of the IGF-II/CIM6P receptor. Finally, removal of Leu^8 or the replacement of Leu^8 with Gly effectively eliminated the binding of these rIGF-II mutants to any receptor (Fig. 2A—C and Table 1).

Mutants of the D-domain

Deletion of Thr^{62}, Pro^{63}, Ala^{64}, Lys^{65}, Ser^{66} and Glu^{67} of the D-domain, i.e., [des (62—67)] rIGF-II had little effect or in some cases a stimulating effect on the relative affinity of this mutant for IGF-I, IGF-II/CIM6-P or insulin receptors (Table 1).

Mitogenic activities of rIGF-II mutants

Previously, we observed that substituting amino acids in rIGF-II that specified its binding to the IGF-II/CIM6-P receptor, i.e., Thr, Ser, Ile, for Phe^{48}, Arg^{49}, Ser^{50} and Arg, Arg for Ala^{54}, Leu^{55} made these mutants more potent as mitogens on BALB/c 3T3 cells [6]. However, rIGF-II mutants that were unable to bind to IGF-I receptors like [Leu^{27}] rIGF-II and [Val^{43}] rIGF-II were inactive on these cells [4–6]. [Ala^{59}] rIGF-II that has about one-one thousandth the affinity of rIGF-II for the IGF-I and insulin receptors also has no mitogenic activity (Fig. 3). Finally, deletion of the first five amino acids from the N-terminus of rIGF-II had no effect on its mitogenic activity. However, the additional removal of Glu^6, Thr^7 and Leu^8 or the substitution of Gly for Leu^8 decreased the mitogenic activity of the first two mutants slightly and eliminated it completely for the latter two mutants.

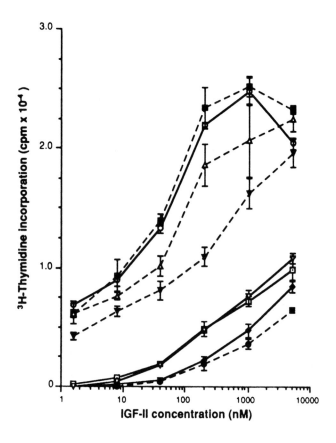

Fig. 3. Stimulation of DNA synthesis in BALB/c 3T3 cells by rIGF-II (O), [Leu^{27}] rIGF-II (□), [Ala^{59}] rIGF-II (∇), des(1–5) rIGF-II (■), des(1–6) rIGF-II (Δ), des(1–7) rIGF-II (▼), [Gly^8] rIGF-II (◆) and des(1–8) rIGF-II (●).

The specificity of binding of IGF-II and rIGF-II mutants to IGFBPs 1–6

The K_a in M^{-1} × 10^{10} of rIGF-II for human IGFBP-1 is 19 ± 8; for BP-2 it is 17 ± 0.2; for BP-3 it is 7.5 ± 1.0; for BP-4 it is 1.1 ± 0.2; for BP-5 it is 1.6 ± 0.5; and for BP-6 it is 39 ± 14 [7]. Substituting Ser for Phe^{26} in rIGF-II, but not Leu, decreased the affinity of the mutants for all the IGFBPs dramatically. This site appears to be very specific since substitution of Tyr^{27} with Leu had little effect on this mutant's binding to any of the binding proteins (Table 2). Phe^{48}, Arg^{49}, Ser^{50} in the A-domain and Leu^8 in the B-domain are even more critical residues in rIGF-II that influence the magnitude of its binding to all the binding proteins. Substituting Thr^{48}, Ser^{49} and Ile^{50} for the former eliminated binding to IGFBP-1, -4, -5 and -6 almost completely reduced its binding to IGFBP-2 and -3 to about 12% of that of rIGF-II. Replacing Arg^{49} with Glu also reduced the binding of this mutant to all the binding proteins. Of interest, replacing Ala for Tyr^{59} or Arg, Arg for Ala^{54}, Leu^{55} which dramatically

Table 2. Relative affinity of rIGF-II mutants for IGFBPs 1–6

	IGFBP-1	IGFBP-2	IGFBP-3	IGFBP-4	IGFBP-5	IGFBP-6
	(% of IGF-II)					
rIGF-II	100	100	100	100	100	100
B-domain mutants						
Ser[26]	1.3	21	19	14	6	7
Leu[26]	6	21	ND[a]	52	18	6
Leu[27]	65	71	70	105	60	37
des (1–5)	140	130		160	110	160
Gly[8]	<1	<1	<1	<1	<1	<1
A-domain mutants						
Ala[59]	25	25	ND[a]	31	32	40
Thr[48], Ser[49], Ile[50]	<1	15	12	<1	1	<1
Glu[49]	37	38	ND[a]	45	50	39
Arg[54], Arg[55]	60	100	37	25	25	21
D-domain mutants						
des (62–67)	100	230	130	150	100	150

[a]Not determined.

decreased rIGF-II binding to IGF-I or IGF-II/CIM6-P receptors, respectively, had only minor effect on the binding of these mutants to the IGFBPs. Finally, removing the D-domain sequence, i.e., [des 62–67] rIGF-II, or the first five amino acids in the B-domain, i.e., [des (1–5)] rIGF-II, enhanced the affinity of these mutants for most of the BPs marginally. Similar to what we have observed for receptor binding and mitogenic activities, however, substituting Gly for Leu[8] eliminated any significant binding of rIGF-II to the BPs (Table 2).

Discussion

During the past 4 years, 19 mutants of hrIGF-II have been characterized with respect to their proper disulfide bonds and affinities for IGF-I, IGF-II/CIM6-P and insulin receptors [6] and IGFBP 1–6 [7]. Consistent with the observations of Casciere et al. [2] using mutants of rIGF-I and the laboratories of Humbel [4] and Rosenfeld [5], we have determined that Phe[26], Tyr[27] and Val[43] are residues in rIGF-II that define its affinity, in part, for IGF-I and insulin receptors. In the case of Phe[26] and Val[43], they probably help stabilize the IGF-II's three dimensional structure. The side chain of Tyr[27] faces the external surface and most likely facilitates high affinity association between IGF-II and the IGF-I and insulin receptors. The A-domain sequences Phe[48], Arg[49], Ser[50] and Ala[54], Leu[55] also lie on the surface and define the high affinity interactions between IGF-II and the IGF-II/CIM6P receptors [6]. The former residues

76

also interact very specifically with IGFBPs [7]. This region of overlap did not extend to residues Ala^{54} Leu^{55}, however.

In studies with deletion and substitution mutants from the N-terminal region of rIGF-II (Fig. 2A–C and Tables 1 and 2), we identified Leu^8 as an essential residue of IGF-II that is required for its ability to bind to all receptors and binding proteins. A similar conclusion had been made for invariant Leu^{B6} in insulin by Nakagawa and Tager [1] based on an extensive study with chemically synthesized variants of insulin.

Recently, Cooke et al. [9], using nuclear magnetic resonance (NMR) and restrained molecular dynamic methods to study IGF-I in solution, found that its Phe^{49} Arg^{50} Ser^{51} sequence and the first three N-terminal amino acids that are analogous to Pro^4, Ser^5, Glu^6 of IGF-II formed a common patch on the growth factors surface. This near neighbor association served as the IGFBP recognition site. However, it is of interest that these residues are not essential for receptor binding. Only Leu^8 fulfilled this requirement. Its deletion or its replacement by Gly completely eliminated IGF-II receptor and binding protein interaction and this occurred even though all the N-terminal residues except Leu^8 were present in the [Gly^8] rIGF-II mutant. Thus, Leu^8 serves a function that is distinct from the other N-terminal residues. It is most likely a structural function. For example, by maintaining the local structure between Cys^9 and Cys^{47} or between the α helices of the B- and A-domains that lies within the vicinity of Leu^8's side chain. Future NMR studies of rIGF-II should clarify which of these possibilities Leu^8 serves.

Acknowledgements

We thank Ms. Kitty Wawzinski for the typing and organization of this manuscript.

References

1. Nakagawa SH, Tager HS. J Biol Chem 1991;266:11502–11509.
2. Cascieri MA, Chicchi GG, Bayne ML. In: Raizada MK, LeRoith D (eds) Molecular Biology and Physiology of Insulin and Insulin-Like Growth Factors: Advances in Experimental Medicine and Biology. New York: Plenum Press, 293;23–30.
3. Hampton B, Burgess WH, Marshak DR, Cullen KJ, Perdue JF. J Biol Chem 1989;264:19155–19160.
4. Bürgisser DM, Roth BV, Giger R, Lüthi C, Weigl S, Zarn J, Humbel RE. J Biol Chem 1991;266:1029–1033.
5. Beukers MW, Oh Y, Zhang H, Ling N, Rosenfeld RG. Endocrinology 1991;128:1201–1203.
6. Sakano K, Enjoh T, Numata F, Fujiwara H, Marumoto Y, Higashihashi N, Sato Y, Perdue JF, Yamaguchi Y. J Biol Chem 1991;266:20626–20635.
7. Bach LA, Hsieh S, Sakano K, Fujiwara H, Perdue JF, Rechler MM. J Biol Chem 1993;268:9246–9254.
8. Enjoy T, Hizuka N, Perdue JF, Takano K, Fujiwara H, Higashihashi N, Marumoto Y, Fukuda I, Sakano K. J Clin Endocrinol Metab 1993;77:510–517.
9. Cooke RM, Harvey TS, Campbell ID. Biochemistry 1991;30:5484–5491.

Unglycosylated "big" IGF-II in nonislet cell tumor hypoglycemia (NICTH) and its serum binding

W.H. Daughaday and B. Trivedi

Washington University School of Medicine, St. Louis, Missouri, USA

Abstract. Most cases of nonislet cell tumor hypoglycemia (NICTH) result from hypersecretion of "big" IGF-II. There is a small amount of "big" IGF-II in normal serum which is O-glycosylated, but the "big" IGF-II in NICTH serum is largely unglycosylated. It has been suggested by others that O-glycosylation is required for normal processing of hproIGF-II. We hypothesize that defective normal tumor glycosylation causes "big" IGF-II secretion. Another consistent abnormality of NICTH serum is the virtual absence of the 150 kDa ternary binding protein complex. This can not be attributed to "big" IGF-II, as it was found that rhproIGF-II E(1—21) forms the 150 kDa complex with normal serum but not with NICTH serum, indicating that the abnormality in NICTH serum resides in the binding proteins. As the acid labile subunit (ALS) is not limiting in most of the NICTH sera which we have examined, we conclude that IGFBP-3 has been altered so that the ternary complex fails to form. The abnormalities in the binding of "big" IGF-II, permit smaller binding protein complexes to traverse capillary membranes more readily and result in a 7-fold increase in free IGF-II related peptides in serum.

Introduction

It is now generally accepted that most cases of nonislet cell tumor hypoglycemia (NICTH) are the results of hypersecretion of IGF-II by a large tumor. The excess IGF-II suppresses growth hormone and insulin secretion. It increases peripheral utilization of glucose and decreases hepatic release of glucose (reviewed in [1]). In most, if not all, cases of NICTH there is an abnormality of the processing of proIGF-II. ProIGF-II as originally translated from its mRNA includes an 89 amino acid E domain. Zumstein et al. [2] first isolated a "big" IGF-II from human plasma protein fractions and showed that it contained the first 21 amino acids of the E domain. Subsequently, Gowan et al. [3] isolated a 15 kDa IGF-II related peptide that also contained this same 21 amino acid extension. A later publication from this same laboratory reported that normal serum "big" IGF-II was O-glycosylated on threonine 75 (the eighth position of the E domain).

A connection between defective processing of proIGF-II and neoplasia was first recognized by Haselbacher et al. [4]. They found that "big" IGF-II predominated in peptide extracts of pheochromocytomas and Wilm's tumors. We then reported that most of the IGF-II in the serum of a patient with NICTH from a fibrosarcoma was "big" IGF-II [5]. Subsequently the predominance of "big" IGF-II was present in the sera of cases of NICTH due to hepatomas, a variety of mesenchymal sarcoma and even carcinomas adrenal, stomach and prostate [6].

78

Defective glycosylation of NICTH "big" IGF-II

We were prompted by the findings of Hudgins et al. [7] that "big" IGF-II of normal serum is O-glycosylated to investigate the glycosylation of "big" IGF-II in the serum of patients with NICTH [8]. First we extracted IGFs from normal and NICTH sera with an acid Sep-Pak method. The acid alcohol eluate was vacuum dried in a Speed-Vac. The residue was taken up in a 20 mM acetic acid. Half the extract was incubated with neuraminidase and endo-N acetylgalactosaminidase (O-glycosidase) for 18 h at 37°C. The other half of the extract was incubated without enzyme. The deglycosylated and control extracts were then gel filtered through Sephadex G-50 in 0.1 M acetic acid. The E(1–21) immunoactivity of each fraction was determined by RIA [9,10]. In normal sera E(1–21) immunoactivity eluted in two major peaks (Fig. 1). The first peak eluted slightly before the cytochrome C marker and the second eluted after the ^{125}I-IGF-I marker with an estimated molecular weight of 5500. After deglycosylation of the extract from normal serum there was a shift of both peaks to a smaller size. When, however, the serum extracts of two patients with NICTH were similarly studied there was no shift of the large "big" IGF-II peak (Fig. 2). These results confirmed that the "big" IGF-II of NICTH serum lacked O-linked glycosylation.

The 5500 MW fragment with E(1–21) immunoreactivity (Fig. 3) is of current interest to us. As noted above, it appears to be glycosylated in normal serum. Partial

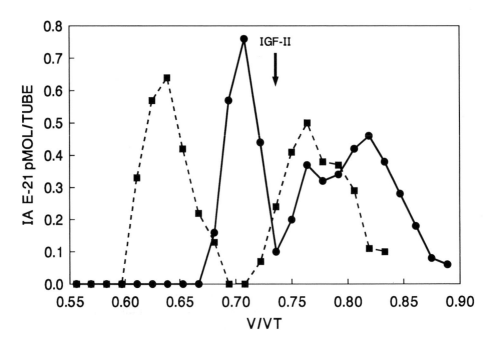

Fig. 1. IGFs extracted from normal serum were incubated with neuraminidase and O-glycosidase (●) or without enzymes (■). The extracts were then gel filtered through Sephadex in 0.1 acetic acid. E(1–21) was measured in each fraction. Reprinted with permission from Daughaday et al. [8].

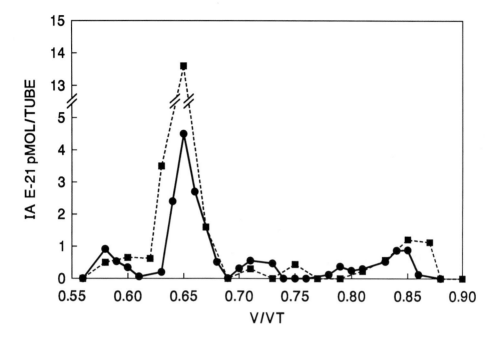

Fig. 2. IGFs extracted from a NICTH serum were similarly treated with O-glycosidase and neuraminidase as in Fig. 1. Reprinted with permission from Daughaday et al. [8].

amino acid sequencing has confirmed that it is derived from the E domain of IGF-II. Substantial quantities of this glycosylated peptide are present in the urine. We have determined that its renal clearance approaches glomerular filtration.

Because of some inconsistency of the elution position of peaks from the Sephadex G-50 column, we sought independent evidence of the glycosylation of normal and NICTH "big" IGF-II. For these studies Sep-Pak extracts of four normal and three NICTH sera were subjected to acid Sephadex G-50 chromatography. The "big" IGF-II peak was identified by E(1–21)RIA and the fractions were pooled and lyophilized. The residue was taken up in 150 mM Tris pH 7.4 buffer and passed through a 0.7 × 4 cm jacalin-agarose bead column. Jacalin is a lectin from jack beans with a selective affinity for O-linked glycopeptides [11]. When the extracts of the four normal sera were passed through these columns only 0.8 ± 0.4 pmol of E(1–21) immunoactivity was unabsorbed (therefore lacking O-linked sugars). The O-linked glycosylated peptides were retained on the column and were eluted with 8 ml of 20 mM α methylgalactopyranoside. This fraction contained 3.7 ± 0.5 pMol of E(1-21) immunoactivity. When extracts of three NICTH sera were similarly passed through the jacalin lectin column we found that 15.1 ± 1.7 pmol passed through unabsorbed. Only 1.0 ± 0.8 pmol was absorbed on the column and eluted with α methylgalacto-pyranoside. These results provide strong evidence that "big" IGF-II of the serum of patients with NICTH is grossly deficient in O-linked glycosylation.

There may be a link between the O-linked glycosylation of proIGF-II and its

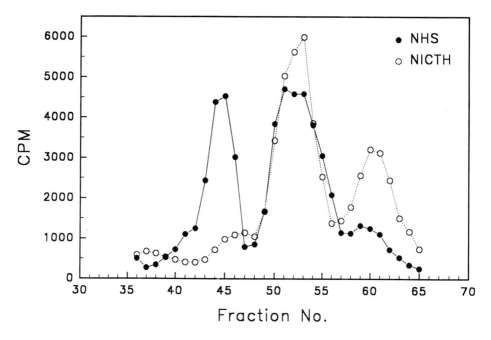

Fig. 3. Normal human serum (●) and NICTH serum (○) were incubated 18 h at 37°C with ^{125}I-proIGF-II E(1–21). Binding protein complexes were separated by FPLC Sepharose-12 column. Reprinted with permission from Daughday et al. [8].

normal enzymatic processing to the 7.5 kDa IGF-II peptide. Yang et al. [12] have performed transfection experiments with plasmids containing the cDNA for normal proIGF-II and with a mutant form in which the codon for Thr[75] (amino acid 8 of the E domain) was replaced with the codon for alanine. When transvected into NIH 3T3 cells the plasmid with the normal proIGF-II cDNA gave rise to a translation product which was normally processed to 7.5 kDa IGF-II, whereas the mutant plasmids when transvected into these fibroblasts gave rise to the mutant IGF-II which resisted processing to 7.5 kDa IGF-II. While there is no reason to believe that all the various tumors that can cause NICTH possess a mutation in Thr[75] which would result in defective protease processing, it is more likely that the enzymatic machinery required for normal O-linked glycosylation could be disorganized in these tumors.

IGF binding proteins in NICTH serum

The transport of "big" IGF-II in the serum of NICTH patients, differs greatly from the transport of IGF-II in normal serum. In normal serum 75–85% of the IGF-II immunoactivity circulates as a 150 kDa ternary complex with IGFBP-3 and acid labile subunit (ALS) [6]. In the serum of NICTH patients, however, the IGF-II immunoactivity is largely present as small MW binary complexes which are less than 50 kDa.

We first suspected that "big" IGF-II might be unable to activate the binding of ALS after it has bound to BP-3. In a collaborative study with Baxter [13] it was found that "big" IGF-II partially purified from the serum of NICTH patients, could form the 150 kDa complex when incubated with purified IGFBP-3 and ^{125}I-ALS. We subsequently obtained recombinant proIGF-II E(1—21) from Bjorn Hammerburg of Stockholm [14]. Recombinant ^{125}I-proIGF-II E(1—21) was incubated with 1 ml of normal or with 1 ml of NICTH serum for 17 h at 37°C in the presence of aprotinin and PMSF followed by FPLC through neutral Sepharose 12. This temperature and duration of incubation were selected because the incorporation of the labeled proIGF-II into the 150 kDa complex is extremely slow. We suspect that the amount of fully potent IGFBP-3 with available binding sites is very low. Despite the severe conditions of these experiments there was minimal degradation of the IGFs, IGFBP-3 or ALS. We found that both [125]IGF-II and ^{125}I-pro-IGF-II E(1—21) entered 150 kDa complexes of normal sera, but neither entered 150 kDa complexes of NICTH sera (Fig. 3).

We have concluded that the failure of NICTH sera to generate 150 kDa complexes is not attributable to proIGF-II E(1—21), but to deficiency of either IGFBP-3 or ALS.

NICTH serum contains a 2- to 3-fold increase in the concentration of IGFBP-2 [12]. A considerable portion of this IGFBP-2 may be secreted by the tumor itself. We have considered the possibility that IGFBP-2 might compete with IGFBP-3 for available IGF-II and thereby reduce the amount of IGF-II entering the 150 kDa complex. If this mechanism were responsible IGFBP-2 would lower the concentration of free IGF-II. To test this possibility, we have measured the concentration of free IGF-II immunoactivity in normal and NICTH sera by the method of Hizuka et al. [14]. In this method serum, diluted in water, is passed through a C-18 Sep-Pak. Protein bound IGFs pass through the column and free IGF is retained. The free IGFs are eluted in 70% ethanol, 0.1 M acetic acid. This method has been validated for free IGF-I and we have found it equally satisfactory for IGF-II. As we lack a "gold standard" method for comparison, there is no way to be sure that some of the measured IGF-II immunoactivity has been stripped from labile binding protein complexes. When this method was applied to 14 normal sera the free IGF-II immunoactivity, as measured by this method, was 761 ± 73 pmol/l. In contrast the free IGF-II of seven NICTH sera was 6458 ± 761 pmol/l. These results indicate that there is no lack of available IGF-II to bind to IGFBP-3.

Another possible defect in IGF binding with NICTH serum could be ALS deficiency. There is now conflicting evidence on this question. In our collaborative study with Baxter [13] it was found that the concentration of ALS in five NICTH sera varied from 3.0—17.4 mg/l with a mean of 10.9 mg/l. Although the mean is only 38% of normal, it should have been sufficient to form the 150 kDa complex in all but one of our cases.

More direct evidence that ALS may not be limiting in patients with NICTH was provided in a study with Baxter [10]. ^{125}I-IGF-II covalently linked to IGFBP-3 was

82

added to two NICTH sera. After incubation for 30 min at 22°C an aliquot was passed through Sepharose 12 FPLC. It was found that most of the labeled complex eluted as a 150 complex. This result must mean that there was sufficient ALS present in these sera to complex with IGF-II-BP3.

We have extended these studies by incubating ^{125}I-IGF-II with NICTH serum in the presence or absence of 10 µg of recombinant IGFBP-3. We found that there was no 150-kDa complex formed unless additional IGFBP-3 was added (Fig. 4), indicating that ALS was not limiting. With another NICTH serum we were unable to generate the 150 kDa complex. In a somewhat similar approach Zapf et al. [15] incubated [125]IGFBP-3 with four normal sera and three NICTH sera. The complexes formed were separated by Sephadex G-200 neutral columns. The normal sera generated labeled 150 kDa complexes while the NICTH sera did not. They concluded that the NICTH sera were deficient in ALS. We suggest that in some NICTH sera defective binding can result from ALS deficiency, whereas in other sera ALS is present in sufficient quantities to form the 150 kDa complexes and BP-3 appears to be limiting.

There is no lack of binding of IGF-II to IGFBP-3 in NICTH serum. We have shown this by acid stripping normal and NICTH serum. When equal aliquots of the stripped sera were incubated with ^{125}I-IGF-II and the binary complex immunoprecipitated with specific anti-IGFBP-3 serum. The immunoprecipitate from a NICTH serum contained 53% of the counts as did that from normal serum (Fig. 5).

As most of the IGFBP-3 in NICTH serum is not tied up in the 150 kDa complexes

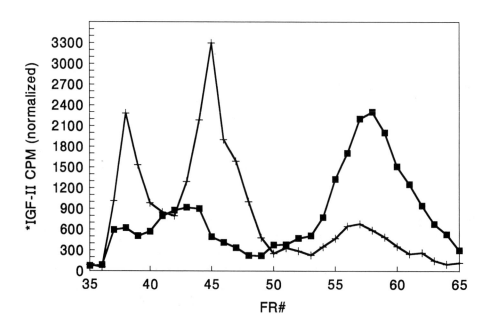

Fig. 4. One ml of NICTH serum was incubated with ^{125}I-IGF-II with (+) or without (■) the addition of 10 µg of recombinant nonglycosylated IGFBP-3 (Celtrix Pharmaceuticals Inc.) for 18 h at 37°C; 150-kDa binding-protein complexes were separated from smaller complexes by Sepharose-12 FPLC.

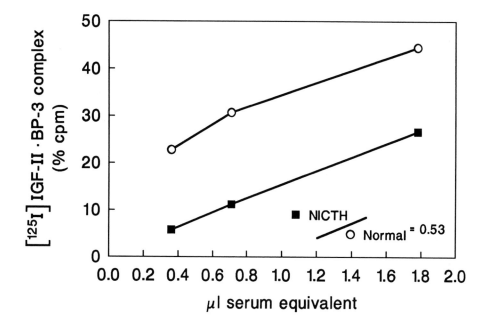

Fig. 5. Endogenous IGFs were stripped from 1 ml of normal serum (O) and NICTH serum (■) by passage through a Sephadex G-50 column in 0.1 M acetic acid. Binding protein fractions were pooled. Aliquots of each pool were incubated with rabbit anti-IGFBP-3 serum (Upstate Biotechnology Inc.) and immunoprecipitated anti-rabbit γ globulin serum (Pierce).

and after binding IGF's it should be able to bind ALS. The failure to do so suggests that NICTH IGFBP-3 is unable to undergo the allosteric change required for binding to ALS.

There is some support for this abnormal IGFBP-3 in NICTH sera in studies done with Baxter [13]. Three normal and five NICTH sera were first acid treated to remove ALS, but without removing IGFBP-3 binary complexes. The ability of these unlabeled complexes to compete with ^{125}IGF-I cross-linked with IGFBP-3 for binding to added purified ALS was measured. All the NICTH sera had much less activity than normal serum in blocking 150 kDa complex formation. A possible interpretation of these results is that the IGFBP-3 complex in NICTH sera can no longer bind to ALS normally. The abnormality could be the result of protease action on IGFBP-3.

The abnormalities of IGF binding proteins which have been discussed leads to an increase in free IGF-II related peptides and a predominance of low molecular binary complexes which more readily pass through the capillary membrane and reach target tissue receptors.

84

Acknowledgements

We thank Dr. Ellen Heath Monig for her suggestions and Ms. Nancy Ebsen for secretarial assistance. The work was supported by the National Institutes of Health, Grant PO1 HD 20815.

References

1. Phillips LS, Robertson DG. Metabolism 1993;42:1093–1101.
2. Zumstein PP, Luthi C, Humbel RE. Proc Natl Acad Sci USA 1985;82:3169–3172.
3. Gowan LK, Hampton B, Hill DJ, Schlueter RJ, Perdue JF. Endocrinology 1987;121:499–458.
4. Haselbacher GK, Irminger JC, Zapf J, Ziegler WH, Humbel RE. Proc Natl Acad Sci USA 1987;84: 1104–1106.
5. Daughaday WH, Emanuele MA, Brooks MH, Brooks H, Barbatto AL, Kapidia M, Rotwein P. N Engl J Med. 1988;319:1434–1440.
6. Daughaday WH, Kapidia M. Proc Natl Acad Sci USA 1989;86:6778–6782.
7. Hudgins RWK, Hampton B, Burgess WH, Perdue JF. J Biol Chem 1992;267:8153–8160.
8. Daughaday WH,Trivedi B, Baxter RC. Proc Natl Acad Sci USA 1993;90:5823–5827.
9. Perdue JF, Gowan LK, Hudgins WR, Scheuermann J, Foster B, Northcutt Brown A. In: Raizada MK LeRoith D (eds) Molecular Biology and Physiology of Insulin, IGFs and Their Receptors. New York: Plenum Publishing Corp 1991;45–46.
10. Daughaday WH, Trivedi B. J Clin Endocrinol Metab 1992;75:641–645.
11. Hortin GL, Trimpe BL. Anal Biochem 1990;188:271–277.
12. Yang C, Zhan X, Perdue JE. Program of the Annual Meeting of the Endocrine Society 1992;80 (abstract).
13. Baxter RC, Daughaday WH. J Clin Endocrinol Metab 1991;b73:696–702.
14. Hizuka N, Takano K, Asadawa K, Sukegawa I, Fukada I, Demura H, Iwashita M, Adachi T, Snizume K. Growth Reg 1991;1:51–55.
15. Zapf J, Futo E, Peter M, Froesch ER. J Clin Invest 1992;90:2574–2584.
16. Shapiro ET, Bell GI, Polonsky KS, Rubenstein AH, Kew MC, Tager HS. J Clin Invest 1990;85: 1672–1679.
17. Daughaday WH, Wu J-C, Lee S-D, Kapadia M. J Lab Clin Med 1990;115:552–562.
18. Fukada I, Hizuka N, Takano K, Asakawa-Yasumoto K, Shiizume K, Demura H. Endocrine J 1993; 40:111–119.

Receptors

Transmembrane signaling properties of the insulin and IGF-I tyrosine kinase receptors

Jeffrey E. Pessin

Department of Physiology and Biophysics, The University of Iowa, Iowa City, IA 52242, USA

Abstract. In addition to the classical homotypic insulin and IGF-I receptors that are composed of two identical $\alpha\beta$ half-receptors, recent data has suggested that several cell types contain receptors composed of two nonidentical $\alpha\beta$ half-receptors assembled into a mature $\alpha_2\beta_2$ insulin/IGF-I hybrid receptor complex. The unique immunogenic properties of these hybrid receptors has provided an important model to examine the molecular mechanism of ligand-stimulated transmembrane signaling. Biochemical and molecular biological studies of these insulin/IGF-I hybrid receptors have demonstrated that ligand-stimulated β subunit autophosphorylation occurs via an intramolecular trans-autophosphorylation mechanism. Further, this reaction occurs independent of which α subunit is ligand occupied. These data provide a molecular explanation for the negative-dominant phenotype observed in heterozygotic patients expressing kinase-defective insulin receptors from one allele. In addition, these observations provide important new insights into the mechanism of tyrosine kinase receptor transmembrane signaling.

Introduction

During the past 15 years substantial progress has been made in understanding the structural and functional properties of the insulin and IGF-I receptors. These cell surface glycoproteins are responsible for the specific binding of insulin and IGF-I, respectively, and transmitting this binding signal to intracellular actions [1–7]. Both these receptors are initially synthesized as Mr 155,000 $\alpha\beta$ polypeptide fusion precursor proteins, which undergo extensive co- and posttranslational modifications [8–12]. The precursor is processed from the endoplasmic reticulum through the trans-Golgi network resulting in the formation of intramolecular disulfide bonds linking the α and β subunits. Concomitant with this process, two $\alpha\beta$ fusion precursors dimerize followed by a proteolytic cleavage event which separates the α from the β subunit. Finally, the dimerized $\alpha\beta$ half-receptors become disulfide-linked through the α subunits coincident with the addition of terminal sialic acid residues and exposure of the native $\alpha_2\beta_2$ heterotetrameric receptor on the cell surface membrane.

Physiochemical studies have begun to dissect the modular functional domains of these receptors. Recent molecular studies have begun to define the domains responsible for insulin and IGF-I binding specificity. Although controversy exists in

---

Address for correspondence: Jeffrey E. Pessin, Department of Physiology and Biophysics, The University of Iowa, Iowa City, IA 52242, USA. Tel.: +1-319-335-7823. Fax: +1-319-335-7330.

the literature, most studies have localized the insulin binding domain to two discrete regions between amino acid residues 1–68 and 315–514 in the insulin receptor [13–22]. In contrast, the domain responsible for high affinity IGF-I binding to the IGF-I receptor is apparently localized to amino acid residues 191–290 [13–16,23,24].

The initial biochemical event associate with ligand binding is the specific autophosphorylation of the receptors on tyrosine residues. This autophosphorylation reaction, in turn, activates the tyrosine kinase activities of the receptors towards intracellular target substrates [25–30]. The major tyrosine autophosphorylation sites in the insulin receptor have been identified as Y960, Y1146, Y1150, Y1151, Y1316 and Y1322 [31–35]. The tyrosine phosphorylation sites in 1146-1151 region are necessary for the activation of substrate kinase activity, whereas the 1316 and 1322 tyrosine sites are thought to be involved in the regulation of mitogenesis [36–40]. Interestingly, mutations of the insulin receptor 960 tyrosine residue to phenylalanine does not alter insulin receptor expression, assembly, binding or autophosphorylation properties [41]. However, this mutation apparently inhibits interaction with downstream substrates and impairs insulin action. Although the precise locations and role of the individual IGF-I receptor autophosphorylation sites have not been experimental identified, the tyrosine residues in equivalent positions are likely candidates based upon the high degree of structural similarity with the insulin receptor [1–7]. In any case, β subunit autophosphorylation of both the insulin receptor and the IGF-I receptor results in activation of the exogenous substrate tyrosine kinase in vitro and in vivo [25–30].

Recently, the most proximal target for the insulin and IGF-I receptor tyrosine kinase activity has been identified [42–46]. This protein, termed insulin receptor substrate 1 (IRS1), is a ubiquitous cytoplasmic protein containing numerous potential tyrosine, serine and threonine phosphorylation acceptor sites. In analogy to the platelet-derived growth factor and EGF receptors, tyrosine phosphorylation of specific IRS1 tyrosine residues results in the generation of src homology 2 (SH2) domain binding site motifs [47]. Thus, intracellular signaling molecules containing specific SH2 domains will associate with the tyrosine phosphorylated IRS1 molecule generating a multi-subunited signaling or docking complex. It is thought that this signaling complex is responsible for the divergent downstream activation of numerous effector systems mediated by insulin and IGF-I binding to their receptors.

Insulin/IGF-I hybrid receptors

To probe the signaling properties of the insulin and IGF-I receptors, several years ago we initiated a series of studies examining the mechanism by which extracellular ligand binding can activate the intracellular tyrosine kinase domains. The approach taken was based upon previous immunological data demonstrating the presence of functional $\alpha_2\beta_2$ insulin/IGF-I hybrid receptors composed of an insulin $\alpha\beta$ half-receptor disulfide-linked with an IGF-I $\alpha\beta$ half-receptor in various cell types [48–53]. Based upon the established biosynthetic pathway for these receptors [1–3,8–12], and our ability to assembly receptor subunits in vitro [54,55], we hypothesized that the formation of insulin/IGF-I hybrid receptors would only occur following cotranslational processing. This speculation was confirmed in the vaccinia virus/bacteriophage T7 transient expression system used to coexpress various wild type and mutant insulin/IGF-I receptors [56,57]. In this system, the formation of various nonidentical αβ half-receptors into mature $\alpha_2\beta_2$ heterotetrameric receptors was shown to occur in a random manner dependent upon the relative levels of the two αβ precursors.

Utilizing both biochemical in vitro reconstitution and in vivo assembly of nonidentical αβ half-receptors, we were able to demonstrate that ligand binding primarily resulted in an intramolecular β subunit trans-autophosphorylation event [54–57]. The relationship between intramolecular cis- vs. trans-autophosphorylation is schematically represented in Fig. 1. As illustrated in this model, ligand occupancy of one α subunit can either activate the autophosphorylation of the β subunits by a cis- or trans-mechanism. In the former case, β subunit autophosphorylation results from one β subunit catalytic domain transferring phosphate from ATP to acceptor sites on the same β subunit. In the latter mechanism, one β subunit becomes kinase activated and transfers phosphate from ATP to tyrosine acceptor sites on the adjacent β subunit.

However, in these studies we were unable to examine the spatial relationship between ligand occupancy vs. β subunit autophosphorylation, since both αβ half-

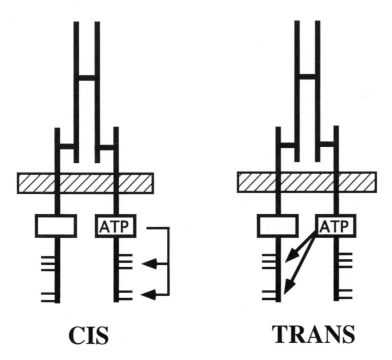

CIS   TRANS

Fig. 1. Schematic model for intramolecular cis- vs. intramolecular trans-autophosphorylation of the insulin receptor. Intramolecular cis-autophosphorylation (left) is represented by insulin activating the kinase activity and autophosphorylation of one β subunit. Intramolecular trans-autophosphorylation (right) is represented by insulin activating the kinase activity of one β subunit which in turn autophosphorylates the adjacent β subunit within a single $\alpha_2\beta_2$ heterotetrameric holoreceptor.

receptors were fully capable of binding ligand. To distinguish this relationship, we prepared several mutant insulin/IGF-I hybrid receptors each composed of one active and one kinase-defective $\alpha\beta$ half-receptor (Fig. 2). In these experiments, we initially utilized a hybrid receptor consisting of a truncated kinase-inactive insulin $\alpha\beta$ half-receptor ($\alpha\beta_{IR.A/K.\Delta43}$) assembled with a wild type IGF-I $\alpha\beta$ half-receptor (Fig. 2, lanes

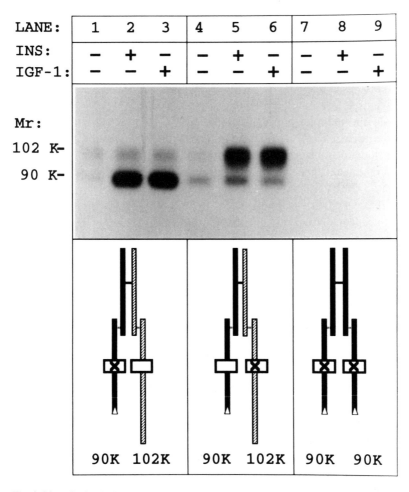

Fig. 2. Ligand stimulation of intramolecular trans-autophosphorylation in mutant/wild type insulin/IGF-1 hybrid receptors. 3T3442A fibroblasts were infected with the vTF3-7 recombinant vaccinia virus and transfected with 9 μg/150 mm dish pTM1-IR.A/K.Δ43 plus 3 μg/150 mm dish pTM1-IGFR.WT (lanes 1–3), 6 μg/150 mm dish of both pTM1-IR.Δ43 plus pTM1-IGFR.A/K (lanes 4–6) and 9 μg/150 mm dish pTM1-IR.A/K.Δ43 (lanes 7–9). The homotypic and insulin/IGF-1 hybrid receptors were partially purified as previously described [57]. Insulin/IGF-1 hybrid receptor, $\alpha\beta_{IR.A/K.\Delta43}$-$\alpha\beta_{IGFR.WT}$, (lanes 1–3), insulin/IGF-1 hybrid receptor, $\alpha\beta_{IR.\Delta43}$-$\alpha\beta_{IGFR.A/K}$, (lanes 4–6) and homotypic insulin receptor, $\alpha\beta_{IR.A/K.\Delta43}$-$\alpha\beta_{IR.A/K.\Delta43}$, were immunoprecipitated with the insulin receptor monoclonal antibody, 83–7, and subjected to autophosphorylation in the absence of ligand (lanes 1, 4 and 7), in the presence of 80 nM insulin (lanes 2, 5 and 8), or in the presence of 80 nM IGF-1 (lanes 3, 6 and 9). The receptor subunits were resolved by reducing SDS-polyacrylamide gel electrophoresis and autoradiography. Reprinted with permission from Frattali and Pessin [57].

1—3). In this hybrid receptor, labeling of the 90 kDa subunit was indicative of an intramolecular trans-autophosphorylation reaction pathway, whereas labeling of the 102 kDa β subunit represents intramolecular cis-autophosphorylation. Under basal conditions both the 90 kDa and 102 kDa β subunits were found to be autophosphorylated (Fig. 2, lane 1). In contrast, insulin primarily stimulated the labeling of the 90 kDa kinase-defective insulin receptor β subunit with little increase in labeling of the 102 kDa kinase-active IGF-I receptor β subunit (Fig. 2, lane 2). Surprisingly, IGF-I treatment also resulted in the predominant labeling of the 90 kDa kinase-defective insulin receptor β subunit (Fig. 2, lane 3).

To confirm these findings, we took a complementary approach to prepare hybrid receptor composed of a truncated kinase-active insulin αβ half-receptor ($\alpha\beta_{IR.\Delta43}$) assembled with a kinase-inactive IGF-I αβ half-receptor ($\alpha\beta_{IGFR.A/K}$). In this receptor species, labeling of the full length 102 kDa β subunit indicates intramolecular trans-autophosphorylation. In contrast, labeling of the 90 kDa kinase-active insulin receptor β subunit would be indicative of intramolecular cis-autophosphorylation. In this hybrid receptor, both insulin (Fig. 2, lane 5) and IGF-I (Fig. 2, lane 6) increased autophosphorylation of the kinase-inactive 102 kDa β subunit with little effect on the kinase-active 90 kDa β subunit. As expected, the homotypic, kinase-defective insulin receptor demonstrated no significant β subunit autophosphorylation in either the absence or presence of insulin or IGF-I (Fig. 2, lanes 7—9). Similarly, no significant β subunit autophosphorylation was observed within homotypic kinase-defective IGF-I receptors in either the basal state or in response to either ligand (data not shown). Taken together, these data strongly support a model in which insulin and IGF-I activate β subunit autophosphorylation by an intramolecular trans-autophosphorylation mechanism independent of which α subunit was ligand occupied.

These data are consistent with another study demonstrating that ligand occupancy of one insulin receptor α subunit activates the autophosphorylation of both β subunits roughly in a 60—40% ratio [58]. Thus, we proposed that a mechanism by which ligand occupancy of either α subunit results in the propagation of an intramolecular signal that can activate both β subunits to function as tyrosine-specific protein kinases. These activated β subunits initially function to transphosphorylate each other, resulting in the tyrosine phosphorylation of both β subunits as schematically illustrated in Fig. 3. Since hybrid receptors composed of one functional and one nonfunctional αβ half-receptors are substrate kinase inactive (55), we hypothesize that autophosphorylation of the 1146, 1150 and 1151 tyrosine residues of both β subunits are necessary for insulin-mediated signaling. This model also provides a molecular explanation for the negative dominant phenotype observed in patients expressing the insulin receptor from one normal allele and from one allele encoding a kinase-defective insulin receptor gene.

Conclusions

Recent molecular characterization of insulin and IGF-I receptors have provided a

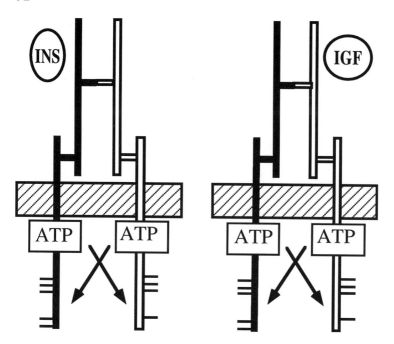

Fig. 3. Schematic representation of ligand-stimulated transmembrane autophosphorylation of insulin/IGF-1 hybrid receptors. In this model, ligand occupancy of either α subunit results in the activation of both β subunits such that a series of intramolecular autophosphorylation events occur. Under these conditions, both β subunits will become autophosphorylated followed by activation of receptor substrate kinase activity.

surprising complexity which may underlie many of the important physiological functions of these tyrosine kinase receptors. The presence of insulin/hybrid receptors in addition to classical homotypic insulin and IGF-I receptors suggests a unique function for this receptor species. Numerous studies have demonstrated that insulin is primarily a metabolic regulator whereas IGF-I primarily functions in the differentiation and mitogenic pathways [1—3]. Since the insulin/IGF-I hybrid receptors apparently bind IGF-I with a greater specificity than insulin suggests that these receptors may be more IGF-I-like than insulin-like [50,51,53,57]. However, as of yet there are no experimental data testing the biological signaling role of the insulin/IGF-I hybrid receptor. In addition, due to the unique immunogenic properties of these receptors, further molecular and biochemical analysis of subunit-subunit interactions should result in new and exciting information regarding the precise mechanisms of ligand-mediated transmembrane signaling.

Acknowledgements

This work was supported by research grant DK 33823 and DK 25295 from the National Institute of Health.

References

1. Rechler MM, Nissley SP. Annu Rev Physio 1985;47:425–442.
2. Goldfine ID. Endocrinol Rev 1987;8:235–255.
3. Jacobs S, Cuatrecasas P. Annu Rev Pharmacol Toxicol 1983;23:461–479.
4. Ebina Y, Ellis L, Jarnagin K, Edery M, Graf L, Clauser E, Ou JH, Masiarz R, Kan YW, Goldfine ID, Roth RA, Rutter WJ. Cell 1985;40:747–758.
5. Ulrich A, Bell JR, Chen EY, Herrera R, Petruzzelli LM, Dull TJ, Gray A, Coussens L, Liao YC, Tsubokawa M, Mason A, Seeburg PH, Grunfeld CL, Rosen OM, Ramachandran J. Nature 1985;313: 756–761.
6. Steele-Perkins G, Turner J, Edman JC, Hari J, Pierce SB, Stover C, Rutter WJ, Roth RA. J Biol Chem 1988;263:11486–11492.
7. Ullrich A, Gray A, Tam AW, Yang-Feng T, Tsubokawa M, Collins C, Henzel W, LeBon T, Kathuria S, Chen E, Jacobs S, Francke U, Ramachandran J, Fujita-Yamaguchi Y. EMBO J 1986;5:2503–2512.
8. Van Oberghen E, Kasuga M, LeCam M, Hedo JA, Itin A, Harrison LC. Proc Natl Acad Sci USA 1981;78:1052–1056.
9. Forsayeth JB, Maddux B, Goldfine ID. Diabetes 1986;35:837–846.
10. Hedo JA, Collier E, Watkinson A. J Biol Chem 1987;262:954–957.
11. Deutsch PJ, Wan CF, Rosen OM, Rubin CS. Proc Natl Acad Sci USA 1983;80:133–136.
12. Ronnett GV, Knutson P, Kohanski RA, Simpson TL, Lane MD. J Biol Chem 1984;259:4566–4575.
13. Andersen AS, Kjeldsen T, Wiberg FC, Christensen PM, Rasmussen JS, Norris K, Moller KB, Moller NPH. Biochemistry 1990;29:7363–7366.
14. Gustafson TA, Rutter WJ. J Biol Chem 1990;265:18663–18667.
15. Kjeldsen T, Andersen AS, Wiberg FC, Rasmussen JS, Schaffer L, Balschmidt P, Moller DB, Moller NPH. Proc Natl Acad Sci USA 1991;88:4404–4408.
16. Schumacher R, Mosthaf L, Schlessinger J, Brandenburg D, Ullrich A. J Biol Chem 1991;266:19288– 19295.
17. Zhang B, Roth RA. Proc Natl Acad Sci USA 1991;88:9858–9862.
18. Yip CC, Grunfeld C, Goldfine ID. Biochemistry 1991;30:695–701.
19. Yip CC, Hsu H, Patel RG, Hawley HM, Maddux BA, Goldfine ID. Biochem Biophys Res Commun 1988;157:321–329.
20. Rafaeloff R, Patel R, Yip CC, Goldfine ID, Hawley DM. J Biol Chem 1989;264:15900–15904.
21. Wedekind F, Baer-Pontzen K, Bala-Mohan S, Choli D, Zahn H, Brandenburg D. Biol Chem Hoppe-Seyler 1989;370:251–258.
22. Waugh SM, DiBella EE, Pilch PF. Biochemistry 1989;28:3448–3455.
23. Fabry M, Schaefer E, Ellis L, Kojro E, Fahrenholz F, Brandenburg D. J Biol Chem 1992;267:8950– 8956.
24. DeMeyts P, Gu JL, Shymko RM, Kaplan BE, Bell GI, Whittaker J. Mol Endocrinol 1990;4:409–416.
25. Rosen OM, Herrera R, Olowe Y, Petruzzelli LM, Cobb MH. Proc Natl Acad Sci USA 1983;80: 3237–3240.
26. Yu KT, Czech MP. J Biol Chem 1986;261:4715–4722.
27. Kohanski RA, Lane MD. Biochem Biophys Res Commun 1986;134:1312–1318.
28. Klein HH, Freidenberg GR, Kladde M, Olefsky JM. J Biol Chem 1986;261:4691–4697.
29. Flores-Riveros JR, Sibley E, Kastelic T, Lane MD. J Biol Chem 1989;264:21557–21572.
30. White MF, Shoelson SE, Keutmann H, Kahn CR. J Biol Chem 1988;263:2969–2980.
31. Tornqvist HE, Pierce MW, Frackelton AR, Nemenoff RA, Avruch J. J Biol Chem 1987;262:10212– 10219.
32. Tornqvist HE, Gunsalus JR, Nemenoff RA, Frackelton AR, Pierce MW, Avruch J. J Biol Chem 1987;263:350–359.
33. Tavare JM, Denton RM. Biochem J 1988;252:607–615.
34. Tavare JM, O'Brien RM, Siddle K, Denton RM. Biochem J 1988;253:783–788.

35. Feener EP, Backer JM, King GL, Wilden PA, Sun XJ, Kahn CR, White MF. J Biol Chem 1993;268: 11256—11264.
36. McClain DA, Maegawa H, Levy J, Huecksteadt T, Dull TJ, Ullrich A, Olefsky JM. J Biol Chem 1988;263:8904—8911.
37. Maegawa H, McCalin DA, Freidenberg G, Olefsky JM, Napier M, Lapari T, Dull TJ, Lee J, Ullrich A. J Biol Chem 1988;263:8912—8917.
38. Thies RS, Ullrich A, McClain DA. J Biol Chem 1989;264:12820—12825.
39. Ando A, Momomura K, Tobe K, Yamamoto-Honda R, Sakura H, Tamori Y, Kaburagi Y, Koshio O, Akanuma Y, Yazaki Y, Kasuga M, Kadowaki T. J Biol Chem 1992;267:12788—12796.
40. Myers MG Jr, Backer JM, Siddle K, White MF. J Biol Chem 1991;266:10616—10623.
41. White MF, Livingston JN, Backer JM, Lauris V, Dull TJ, Ullrich A, Kahn CR. Cell 1988;54:641—649.
42. Izumi T, White MF, Kadowaki T, Takaku T, Akanuma Y, Kasuga M. J Biol Chem 1987;262:1282—1287.
43. Rothenberg PL, Lane WS, Karasik A, Backer JM, White MF, Kahn CR. J Biol Chem 1991;266: 8302—8311.
44. Keller SR, Kitagawa K, Aebersold R, Lienhard GE, Garner CW. J Biol Chem 1991;266:12817—12820.
45. Sun XJ, Rothenberg P, Kahn CR, Backer JM, Araki E, Wilden PA, Cahill DA, Goldstein BJ, White MF. Nature 1991;352:73—77.
46. Myers MG Jr, Sun XJ, Cheatham B, Jachna BR, Glasheen EM, Backer JM, White MF. Endocrinology 1993;132:1421—1430.
47. Myers MG Jr, White MF. Diabetes 1993;42:643—650.
48. Soos MA, Siddle K. Biochem J 1989;263:553—563.
49. Soos MA, Whittaker J, Lammers R, Ullrich A, Siddle K. Biochem J 1990;270:383—390.
50. Soos MA, Field CE, Siddle K. Biochem J 1991;290:419—426.
51. Moxham CP, Duronio V, Jacobs S. J Biol Chem 1989;264:13238—13244.
52. Chin JE, Tavare JM, Ellis L, Roth RA. J Biol Chem 1991;266:15587—15590.
53. Garofalo RS, Barenton B. J Biol Chem 1992;267:11470—11475.
54. Treadway JL, Morrison BD, Goldfine ID, Pessin JE. J Biol Chem 1989;264:21450—21453.
55. Treadway JL, Morrison BD, Soos MA, Siddle K, Olefsky J, Ullrich A, McClain DA, Pessin JE. Proc Natl Acad Sci, USA 1991;88:214—218.
56. Frattali AL, Treadway JL, Pessin JE. J Biol Chem 1992;267:19521—19528.
57. Frattali AL, Pessin JE. J Biol Chem 1993;268:7393—7400.
58. Lee J, O'Hare T, Pilch PF, Shoelson SE. J Biol Chem 1993;268:4092—4098.

The insulin-like growth factors and their regulatory proteins
R.C. Baxter, P.D. Gluckman and R.G. Rosenfeld, editors

95

Hybrid and atypical insulin-like growth factor receptors

Maria A. Soos, Catherine E. Field, Barbara T. Navé and Kenneth Siddle
University of Cambridge, Department of Clinical Biochemistry, Addenbrooke's Hospital, Hills Road, Cambridge CB2 2QR, UK

Abstract. Insulin receptor/insulin-like growth factor (IGF) receptor hybrids are widely distributed in mammalian tissues. They bind IGF-I with high affinity (IC_{50}, 0.15 nM), but insulin with lower affinity (IC_{50}, 4 nM) and show co-operative interactions between receptor halves. Atypical IGFR are immunologically distinct from hybrid receptors, but closely related to classical IGFR. Unlike classical receptors they bind insulin with relatively high affinity (IC_{50}, 1.5 nM) as well as IGF-I (IC_{50}, 0.1 nM). They are not the product of a separate gene nor the result of alternative mRNA splicing, but rather result from post-translational or conformational modification of classical IGF receptors.

Introduction

The biological actions of insulin-like growth factors (IGFs) are mediated by the type I IGF receptor (IGFR) [1]. This is a member of a family of structurally and functionally related proteins which also includes the insulin receptor (IR) and insulin-receptor related receptor (IRR) [2–5]. These receptors show considerable similarity of amino acid sequence and share a common disulphide-linked $(\alpha\beta)_2$ subunit structure [2–7]. They have an intrinsic tyrosine kinase in the β subunit which is activated by ligand binding to the α subunit and is essential for their biological activity [2–8]. The IR binds insulin with high affinity and the IGFs with low affinity, whereas the type I IGFR binds IGFs with much higher affinity than insulin [1]. IGFs also bind with high affinity to the type II IGF/mannose-6-phosphate receptor. However, this is structurally unrelated to the IGFR/IR family, being composed of a single polypeptide chain without kinase activity and is not thought to mediate biological actions of IGFs [9,10]. The type I IGFR and IR are widely distributed in mammalian tissues, although they vary in concentration between different cell types. The IRR, on the other hand, is much more restricted in its tissue distribution and its ligand has yet to be identified [11–13].

Although each receptor is the product of a single gene, both IGF-I receptors and insulin receptors exhibit structural and functional heterogeneity. Structural diversity is known to arise by alternative splicing of mRNA [14–17] and, in cells expressing both type I IGF receptors and insulin receptors, by the formation of hybrid receptors [18–20]. It has also been suggested that receptor subtypes could be the product of as yet unidentified genes or the result of distinct posttranslational modifications of classical receptors [21–26]. Functional heterogeneity in terms of atypical ligand binding specificity has also been described in a variety of cell types. Both atypical insulin receptors, with relatively high affinity for the IGFs [27,28], and atypical IGF receptors, with relatively high affinity for insulin [29–31], have been reported, although the structural basis for this atypical binding behaviour is still unknown.

We describe here the results of some of our studies on hybrid and atypical IGF receptors. In this work we have made extensive use of large panels of receptor-specific monoclonal antibodies recognising known epitopes on the IR or IGFR [32–35]. We show that hybrid and atypical IGF receptors are distinct proteins which may be responsible for the "specificity spillover" of insulin and IGF-I.

IR/IGFR hybrids

Hybrid receptors are composed of disulphide-linked ($\alpha\beta$) halves of both the IGFR and IR in an asymmetric ($\alpha\beta$)($\alpha^*\beta^*$) structure. We first identified hybrids in human placental membranes and various cell lines as a subpopulation of high affinity IGF-I binding sites which reacted with all available IR monoclonal antibodies [18]. More recently we have shown that hybrids also react well with most IGFR monoclonal antibodies [36]. Indeed the characteristic feature of hybrids, which distinguishes them from classical receptors, is their reaction with both IR-specific and IGFR-specific antibodies. Although native receptors are similar in size to classical ($\alpha\beta$)$_2$ receptors, under reducing conditions, known to generate isolated ($\alpha\beta$) receptor halves, a smaller species is generated which still binds IGF-I, but which no longer reacts with IR-specific antibodies [18]. We have also shown the formation of hybrids between mouse IGFR and human IR in transfected NIH3T3 cells [19]. Most importantly, in these studies hybrid receptors could be detected in intact cells, ruling out any possibility that hybrids are generated as an artefact of solubilisation.

The existence of hybrids was independently proposed by Moxham et al. [20] from the immunological and structural heterogeneity of receptor β subunits after IGF-I stimulated autophosphorylation. Hybrid receptors have also been generated in vitro from isolated receptor halves [37]. Interestingly, analogous hybrids have been reported for other families of tyrosine kinase receptors, including the α and β forms of the platelet-derived growth factor receptor [38] and the epidermal growth factor receptor with the neu proto-oncogene [39]. However, in these cases hybrid formation is ligand dependent and noncovalent.

Although the existence of hybrid receptors is now well established, their physiological importance is not yet clear. To assess the potential significance of IR/IGFR hybrids, we have examined their distribution in normal tissues and analysed the ligand binding properties of purified receptors.

Tissue distribution of hybrid receptors

For our initial studies on the distribution of hybrid receptors, we used the rabbit as a model [40]. In these studies a surprisingly high percentage of IGF-I binding sites

Table 1. Tissue distribution of hybrid receptors in rabbit tissues

Tissue	Hybrids (% total IGFR)
Heart	90 ± 5
Skeletal muscle	86 ± 12
Fat	69 ± 9
Kidney	63 ± 8
Brain	55 ± 11
Lung	50 ± 8
Liver	40 ± 10
Speen	40 ± 10

behaved as hybrids in all tissues examined, varying from approximately 40% in liver and spleen to 90% in heart and muscle (Table 1). Preliminary experiments show a similar proportion of hybrids in the corresponding human tissues.

Rabbit tissues were homogenised in 50 mM Hepes/150 mM NaCl buffer pH 7.6. Microsomal membrane fractions were prepared and solubilised in 1% Triton X-100. Solubilised membranes were incubated with ^{125}I-IGF-I before addition of monoclonal antibody and precipitation with sheep anti-(mouse IgG) immunoadsorbent. ^{125}I-IGF-I bound to hybrids (determined with antibody IR 83–7) is expressed as a percentage of the total receptor-bound ^{125}I-IGF-I (determined with antibody IGFR 17–69). Results are the mean ± SD of three experiments.

Since there is little difference in the binding affinity of hybrids and type I IGF receptors for IGF-I (see below), these fractions probably approximate to the proportions of IGFR halves incorporated into hybrids. A direct comparison is not possible with insulin receptors because of differences in the ligand binding affinity of hybrids and insulin receptors (see below). However, in most of these tissues insulin receptors are probably in excess over type I IGF receptors, so hybrids must represent a smaller fraction of total insulin receptors than of type I receptors. There was no clear relationship between the fraction of IGF-I receptors attributable to hybrids and the ratio of IGF-I to insulin binding. This may reflect cellular heterogeneity of the tissues with an uneven distribution of type I IGF receptors and insulin receptors amongst the different cell types. More sophisticated studies on uniform populations of cells are necessary to establish whether hybrid formation is a spontaneous process which simply reflects the relative numbers of individual receptors or whether it is an active and perhaps regulated process. Ligand-induced hybrid formation in vitro, however, appears to involve a near random combination of receptor halves, with no clear preference for homologous rather than heterologous assembly [37].

Purification of hybrid receptors

A problem in assessing the properties of hybrids is that they always coexist with classical receptors. To study the properties of hybrids without interference from other receptors, we purified hybrids from detergent solubilised placental membranes using

98

Table 2. Ligand binding properties of purified receptors

Receptor	IC$_{50}$ (nM)			
	^{125}I-insulin		^{125}I-IGF-I	
	IGF-I	Insulin	IGF-I	Insulin
Hybrids	1.1 ± 0.6	4 ± 1	0.15 ± 0.05	65 ± 9
IR	43 ± 6	0.4 ± 0.1	—	—
IGFR	—	—	0.07 ± 0.04	250 ± 90

a two-step immunoaffinity protocol [36]. This made use of the observation that one group of IGFR monoclonal antibodies, recognising an epitope in the region 440–514 of the α subunit [33,35], reacted poorly with hybrids compared to classical type I IGF receptors. Presumably the epitope for these antibodies, exemplified by antibody 24–55, involves a conformation or juxtaposition of subunits which is present in type I IGF receptors, but not in hybrids. It was therefore possible to use immobilised antibody 24–55 to deplete solubilised placental membranes of classical type I IGF receptors, leaving the bulk of hybrids and all the insulin receptors in solution. Hybrid receptors were then separated from insulin receptors by binding to an IGFR-specific antipeptide antibody 1–2, followed by elution with free peptide. Classical type I IGF receptors and insulin receptors were also isolated using similar methods. The purified hybrid preparation was essentially free of classical receptors as judged by the ability of both IGFR-specific and IR-specific antibodies to deplete >85% of both IGF-I and insulin binding activity.

Ligand binding properties of purified receptors

The ligand binding properties of purified receptors were tested in competition studies [36]. The concentration of unlabelled insulin required to inhibit ^{125}I-insulin binding was 10-fold higher for hybrids than for insulin receptors, indicating that hybrids have a lower affinity for insulin than insulin receptors (Table 2). This is compatible with the recent proposal that high affinity insulin binding to the IR requires contact of insulin with both α subunits of the IR [41–43]. The displacement curve for ^{125}I-insulin with unlabelled IGF-I was rather shallow [36]. Some effect of IGF-I was observed at low ligand concentrations typical of binding to the type I IGFR, suggesting that IGF-I binding to the IGFR half has a "trans" effect on the affinity of the IR half. However, at the higher IGF-I concentrations inhibition may be due to direct competition for the insulin binding site.

Interestingly IGF-I binding to hybrids was not subject to the same constraints as insulin binding. The displacement curves for ^{125}I-IGF-I binding to hybrids and type I IGF receptors were similar [36]. In each case IGF-I was much more effective at competing for ^{125}I-IGF-I binding than insulin (Table 2). Thus the IGFR α subunits within hybrids and classical receptors display similar affinities for IGF-I and insulin. It is known that the determinants of high affinity ligand binding are located in different regions of type I IGF receptors and insulin receptors [35,41] and this may underlie the asymmetric binding properties of hybrids.

Binding of ^{125}I-insulin to purified insulin receptors and hybrids or ^{125}I-IGF-I to purified type I IGF receptors and hybrids, was measured in the presence of varying concentrations of unlabelled IGF-I or insulin. The concentration of unlabelled ligand necessary for half-maximal inhibition of ^{125}I-ligand binding (IC50) is shown here. Results are the means ± SD of three independent experiments.

Although we, and more recently others [44], found that hybrids purified from placenta bound insulin with lower affinity than IGF-I, it has been reported that hybrids reconstituted in vitro from isolated receptor halves bind similar amounts of insulin and IGF-I [37]. At present it is difficult to reconcile these discrepant findings, although they may partly reflect the use of different ligand concentrations, since the use of higher ligand concentrations would tend to reduce any effects of affinity differences. Another possibility is that purified hybrids and those formed in vitro differ in, for example, the formation of disulphide bonds or their conformation which then affects their ligand binding properties.

To further compare the properties of hybrid and classical receptors, and to investigate whether there are co-operative interactions between hybrid receptor halves, we tested the effect of receptor-specific antibodies on ligand binding and negative co-operativity of purified receptors. Receptor-specific monoclonal antibodies, known to modulate ligand binding to classical receptors [32,33], also modulated IGF-I binding to hybrids [40]. Thus an IGFR antibody 24—60, which inhibits IGF-I binding to type I receptors, inhibited 75% of IGF-I binding to hybrids while another antibody IGFR 26—3, which stimulates IGF-I binding to type I receptors, also gave a 1.5-fold stimulation of IGF-I binding to hybrids. These antibodies had no effect on ligand binding to insulin receptors. The IGFR half within hybrids, therefore, behaves similarly to classical receptors. IGF-I binding to hybrids was also modulated by IR antibodies. Two antibodies (47—9, 25—49), which inhibit insulin binding to insulin receptors, inhibited IGF-I binding to hybrids by 70—80%, while a third (18—146), which stimulates insulin binding to insulin receptors, gave a 1.5-fold stimulation of IGF-I binding to hybrids. These antibodies had no effect on ligand binding to classical type I IGF receptors. Modulation of IGF-I binding by IR antibodies must be due to a "trans" effect where antibody binding to the IR half of hybrids influences IGF-I binding to the IGFR half. This could reflect antibody induced conformational interactions between receptor halves. However, since antibodies are large molecules it is also possible that inhibitory antibodies binding to the IR half of hybrids act by sterically blocking IGF-I binding to the IGFR half.

It has been known for some time that dissociation of tracer amounts of labelled insulin from insulin receptors is accelerated in the presence of unlabelled insulin, arising from negative co-operativity [43]. More recently a similar effect of unlabelled IGF-I on the dissociation of ^{125}I-IGF-I from IGF-I receptors in cells has been reported [43]. To determine whether hybrids also exhibit negative co-operative interactions, the time course for dissociation of labelled ligand from purified receptors was measured (Fig. 1). As previously described by others for cell- or membrane-bound

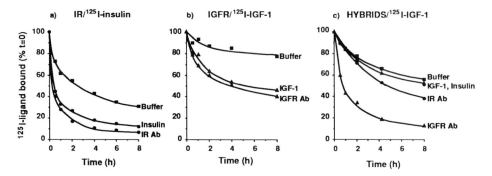

Fig. 1. Dissociation of ^{125}I-ligand from purified receptors. Receptors purified from human placenta were preincubated at 4°C with ^{125}I-insulin (IR) or ^{125}I-IGF-I (IGFR, hybrids) to form receptor/^{125}I-ligand complexes before a 100-fold dilution into buffer, unlabelled insulin, IGF-I or antibodies IGFR 24—60 or IR 25—49. Receptor-bound radioactivity was then determined at the indicated times and is expressed here as a percentage of that bound at zero time.

receptors [43,45], we found that dissociation of ^{125}I-insulin from purified insulin receptors was accelerated by unlabelled insulin and by inhibitory IR monoclonal antibodies (47—9, 25—49) relative to the buffer control (Fig. 1a). We also observed a similar acceleration of the dissociation of ^{125}I-IGF-I from purified type I IGF receptors by unlabelled IGF-I and by the IGFR antibody 24—60 (Fig. 1b). Interestingly, the dissociation of IGF-I from the IGFR was slower than that of insulin from the IR, consistent with the higher affinity of the IGFR for its ligand. Although IGF-I and insulin had little effect on the dissociation of IGF-I from purified hybrids, antibody IGFR 24—60 markedly accelerated the dissociation of IGF-I (Fig. 1c). Moreover IR-specific antibodies 47—9 and 25—49 also induced a small, but consistent, increase in dissociation of prebound IGF-I, implying that antibody binding to the IR half of hybrids is able to influence IGF-I already bound to the IGFR half, again suggesting co-operative interactions between receptor halves within hybrids.

The properties of hybrid receptors, therefore, do not appear to be simply the sum of their component parts. Although, as isolated from placenta, hybrids bind IGF-I with a comparable affinity to classical IGF receptors, they bind insulin with a much lower affinity than insulin receptors. There are co-operative interactions between receptor halves within hybrids as shown by the effect of low concentrations of IGF-I on insulin binding and the ability of IR-specific antibodies to modulate IGF-I binding and display negative co-operative properties. The IR half, however, appears more susceptible to transmodulation than the IGFR half. Unless their affinity for insulin is susceptible to modulation in vivo, hybrids are more likely to be responsive to IGF-I than insulin under physiological conditions. However, the sequestration of IR halves into less responsive hybrids could provide a mechanism for modulating insulin sensitivity.

Atypical IGF receptors

Atypical IGF receptors have been described in several cell types including L-6 myocytes, bovine neural retina cells and MCF-7 human breast cancer cells [29–31]. All these cell lines have few insulin receptors compared to IGF-I receptors. This is important for the detection of atypical IGF receptors, since the characteristic feature of these receptors is that they bind insulin as well as IGF-I with relatively high affinity and they are most easily identified by ^{125}I-insulin binding. Atypical IGF receptors can therefore only be detected in cells where the level of classical insulin receptors is sufficiently low that these do not contribute significantly to insulin binding. In all cases it is likely that atypical receptors represent only a subpopulation of total IGF-I receptors.

Immunological relationships of hybrids, atypical and classical IGF-I receptors

The structural basis for atypical receptors is still unknown. To determine whether atypical IGF receptors are distinct from hybrid receptors, immunodepletion studies were carried out using a large panel of IGFR-specific and IR-specific monoclonal antibodies recognising distinct regions on the receptors [32,33]. Atypical IGF receptors are clearly different from hybrid receptors by immunological criteria (Table 3).

Hybrid and classical receptors purified from human placenta and atypical IGFR from solubilised MCF-7 cells, were incubated with immobilised receptor-specific antibody. After centrifugation, to remove immunoreactive receptors, residual receptors were measured by ^{125}I-ligand binding. Results are the mean ± SD of five independent experiments for purified receptors and the mean of two experiments for atypical receptors.

Classical IGF receptors were depleted only by IGFR antibodies (e.g., 24–60) and classical insulin receptors only by IR antibodies (e.g., 83–14). In solubilised MCF-7 cells, a small percentage (10–15%) of the insulin binding was to classical insulin receptors and was removed by IR antibodies. The majority of the binding, however, was to atypical IGF receptors and was depleted only by IGFR antibodies. Very similar results were obtained with the other IGFR- and IR-specific antibodies. Atypical IGF receptors are thus structurally closely related to classical IGF receptors since they are immunologically indistinguishable. In contrast, purified hybrid

Table. 3. Immunodepletion of receptors

Immobilised antibody	Depletion (%)			
	Hybrids (^{125}I-IGF-I)	Classical IGFR (^{125}I-IGF-I)	Classical IR (^{125}I-insulin)	Atypical IGFR (^{125}I-insulin)
IGFR 24–60	94 ± 4	99 ± 2	1 ± 2	88
IR 83–14	97 ± 3	3 ± 3	99 ± 2	12

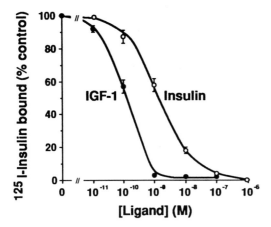

Fig. 2. Binding specificity of receptors solubilised from IGF-IR/3T3 cells. Binding of ^{125}I-insulin to WGA-purified receptors from IGF-IR/3T3 cells was measured at 4°C in the presence of the indicated concentrations of unlabelled IGF-I or insulin. Specific receptor-bound ^{125}I-insulin is expressed as a percentage of that in the absence of unlabelled ligand. Results are the means ± SD of five independent experiments.

receptors reacted with both IGFR-specific and IR-specific antibodies as shown by the ability of antibodies IR 83–14 and IGFR 24–60 to deplete most of the IGF-I binding (Table 3). Identical results were obtained with the other IR antibodies and with most IGFR antibodies. The exception was a group of IGFR antibodies, recognising the region 450–514 on the α subunit, which reacted well with classical and atypical IGFR but poorly with hybrids as discussed above.

Using a more limited panel of antibodies, others have also shown that atypical IGF receptors react with an IGFR-specific antibody, but not with IR-specific antibodies [31]. Atypical IGF receptors are thus clearly distinct from hybrid receptors, but are immunologically very closely related to classical IGF-I receptors.

Atypical IGF receptors in transfected cells

To determine whether atypical IGF receptors are derived from a different gene from classical receptors, human type I IGF receptors expressed in mouse fibroblasts (IGF-IR/3T3 cells) were examined for atypical behaviour. Although intact cells bound very little ^{125}I-insulin, significant insulin binding was found in soluble extracts. Specificity of ^{125}I-insulin binding to solubilised IGF-IR/3T3 cells was measured in competition studies using unlabelled IGF-I or insulin (Fig. 2).

Insulin binding was displaced by low concentrations of insulin (IC_{50} 2nM) as well as IGF-I (IC_{50} 0.2nM) and thus exhibited properties of atypical IGF receptors. In contrast, ^{125}I-insulin binding to insulin receptors is displaced by low concentrations of insulin and only by much higher concentrations of IGF-I, while the converse is true for IGF-I binding to classical IGF-I receptors [9]. Atypical IGF receptors could

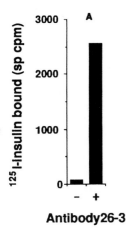
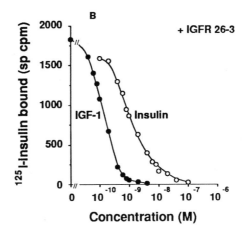

Fig. 3. Insulin binding to IGF-IR/3T3 cells in the presence of antibody IGFR 26–3. Binding of ^{125}I-insulin (20,000 cpm) to intact IGF-IR/3T3 cells was measured in the presence and absence of 10 nM antibody IGFR 26–3 (A). Specificity of ^{125}I-insulin binding in the presence of antibody was determined in competition experiments with unlabelled IGF-I and insulin (B). Specific receptor-bound radioactivity is shown after subtraction of nonspecific binding (120 cpm) measured in the presence of 1 μM insulin.

thus be detected in cells transfected with human IGFR cDNA, indicating that atypical IGF receptors are not derived from a different gene from classical receptors, nor as a result of alternative mRNA splicing.

Atypical binding behaviour could be induced in intact IGF-IR/3T3 cells by certain IGFR antibodies known to dramatically increase insulin binding to cells [33]. In the absence of antibody very little insulin binding was detected, but in the presence of antibody IGFR 26–3 it was dramatically stimulated up to 50-fold (Fig. 3). Insulin binding in the presence of antibody showed the same specificity as solubilised receptors, that is it was displaced by relatively low concentrations of unlabelled insulin and IGF-I. Scatchard analysis of the binding data showed that in the presence of antibody the affinity of insulin binding sites was similar to that reported for the IR itself and that the numbers of binding sites for IGF-I and insulin were comparable [33], indicating that the high affinity insulin binding was to the IGFR itself and not to the much smaller number of endogenous insulin receptors or hybrid receptors.

The binding properties of IGF-I receptors in the presence of these antibodies are strikingly similar to the atypical behaviour of the solubilised receptors. Interestingly, chimeras, in which the amino-terminal portion of the IR is substituted in the IGFR, also bind both insulin and IGF-I with high affinity [46]. It has been suggested that these binding properties may reflect the loss of IGFR sequences which are inhibitory to insulin binding rather than a positive contribution of the IR amino-terminus. An intriguing possibility, therefore, is that the high affinity insulin binding properties of atypical receptors may reflect the loss of inhibitory constraints on insulin binding due to posttranslational modification of classical receptors or their interaction with other proteins, resulting in subtle changes in conformation. Antibodies may stabilise a particular conformation, thus giving rise to a receptor with atypical behaviour.

Whatever the mechanism responsible for generating atypical receptors, the outcome should be to make the IGFR more responsive to insulin. To test this, we examined whether the IGFR antibody 26–3 could potentiate the mitogenic effect of insulin in transfected cells [33]. DNA synthesis was measured by the incorporation of radioactively labelled thymidine into TCA precipitable material, after incubating cells with varying concentrations of insulin or IGF-I. In the presence of antibody, IGF-I was 5–10-fold more potent in stimulating thymidine uptake than in its absence. Although in the absence of antibody insulin only stimulated DNA synthesis at very high concentrations, in the presence of antibody it was effective at about 50-fold lower concentrations. These results suggest that atypical IGF receptors are more responsive to insulin than classical type IGF receptors, and this could clearly be important in relation to the ability of insulin to act as a growth factor at physiological concentrations.

Conclusions

In conclusion, hybrid and atypical IGF receptors are distinct proteins which bind IGF-I with a similar affinity to classical type I IGF receptors, but insulin with a higher affinity than classical receptors. Although the structural basis for hybrid receptors is clear, further studies are necessary to understand the biochemical nature of atypical receptors. It also remains to be determined whether hybrid and atypical receptors have a physiological significance which is different from that of classical receptors. Indeed, it is still an open question whether classical type I IGF receptors and insulin receptors themselves show signalling differences [47–49]. Hybrids and/or atypical receptors may play a role in the "specificity spillover" of insulin (particularly in hyperinsulinaemic states) or IGF-I. Nevertheless, whatever their importance in vivo hybrid and atypical receptors are of interest in their own right because of the insights they provide into the structure and function of normal receptors.

Acknowledgements

We are grateful to Dr. A. Ullrich (Max-Planck Institut für Biochemie, Martinsreid, Germany) for the IGF-IR/3T3 cells. We also thank the Wellcome Trust and the British Diabetic Association for financial support.

References

1. Rechler MM, Nissley SP. Ann Rev Physiol 1985;47:425–442.
2. Ullrich A, Gray A, Tam AW, Yang-Feng T, Tsubokawa M, Collins C, Henzel W, Le Bon T, Kathuria S, Chen E, Jacobs S, Francke U, Ramachandran J, Fujita-Yamaguchi Y. EMBO J 1986;5:2503–2512.

3. Shier P, Watt VM. J Biol Chem 1989;264:14805−14608.
4. Yarden Y, Ullrich A. Ann Rev Biochem 1988;57:443−478.
5. Siddle K. Prog Growth Factor Res 1992;4:301−320.
6. Ebina Y, Ellis L, Jarnagin K, Edery M, Graf L, Clauser E, Ou J, Masiarz F, Kan YW, Goldfine ID, Roth RA, Rutter WJ. Cell 1985;40:747−758.
7. Ullrich A, Bell JR, Chen EY, Herrera R, Petruzzelli M, Dull TJ, Gray A, Coussens L, Liao Y-C, Tsubokawa M, Mason A, Seeburg PH, Grunfeld C, Rosen OM, Ramachandran J. Nature 1985;313:756−761.
8. Rosen OM. Science 1987;237:1452−1458.
9. Humbel RE. Eur J Biochem 1990;190:445−462.
10. Cohick WS, Clemmons DR. Ann Rev Physiol 1993;55:131−153.
11. Shier P, Watt VM. Mol Endocrinol 1992;6:723−729.
12. Zhang B, Roth RA. J Biol Chem 1992;267:18320−18328.
13. Reinhardt RR, Chin E, Zhang B, Roth RA, Bondy CA. Endocrinology 1993;133:3−10.
14. Yee D, Lebovic GS, Marcus RR, Rosen N. J Biol Chem 1989;264:21439−21441.
15. Mostaf L, Grako K, Dull TJ, Coussens L, Ullrich A, McClain DA. EMBO J 1990;9:2409−2413.
16. Yamaguchi Y, Flier JS, Yokota A, Benecke H, Backer JM, Moller DE. Endocrinology 1991;129:2058−2066.
17. Yamaguchi Y, Flier JS, Benecke H, Ransil BJ, Moller DE. Endocrinology 1993;132:1132−1138.
18. Soos MA, Siddle K. Biochem J 1989;263:553−563.
19. Soos MA, Whittaker J, Lammers R, Ullrich A, Siddle K. Biochem J 1990;270:383−390.
20. Moxham CP, Duronio V, Jacobs S. J Biol Chem 1989;264:13238−13244.
21. Ota A, Wilson GL, LeRoith D. Eur J Biochem 1988;174:521−530.
22. Garofalo RS, Rosen OM. Mol Cell Biol 1989;9:2806−2817.
23. Alexandrides TK, Smith RJ. J Biol Chem 1989;264:12922−12930.
24. Hainut P, Kowalski A, Giorgetti S, Baron V, Van Obberghen E. Biochem J 1991;273:673−678.
25. Garofalo RS, Barenton B. J Biol Chem 1992;267:11470−11475.
26. Moss AM, Livingston JN. Biochem J 1993;294:685−692.
27. Jonas HA, Cox AJ, Harrison LC. Biochem J 1989;257:101−107.
28. Jonas HA, Cox AJ. Biochem J 1990;266:737−742.
29. Burant CF, Treutelaar MK, Allen KD, Sens DA, Buse MG. Biochem Biophys Res Commun 1987;147:100−107.
30. Waldbillig RJ, Chader GJ. Biochem Biophys Res Commun 1988;151:1105−1112.
31. Milazzo G, Yip CC, Maddux BA, Vigneri R, Goldfine ID. J Clin Invest 1992;89:899−908.
32. Soos MA, Siddle K, Baron MD, Heward JM, Luzio JP, Bellatin J, Lennox ES. Biochem J 1986;235:199−208.
33. Soos MA, Field CE, Lammers R, Ullrich A, Zhang B, Roth RA, Andersen AS, Kjeldsen T, Siddle K. J Biol Chem 1992;267:12955−12963.
34. Zhang B, Roth RA. Proc Natl Acad Sci USA 1991;88:9858−9862.
35. Schumacher R, Soos MA, Schlessinger J, Brandenburg D, Siddle K, Ullrich A. J Biol Chem 1993;268:1087−1094.
36. Soos MA, Field CE, Siddle K. Biochem J 1993;290:419−426.
37. Treadway JL, Morrison BD, Goldfine ID, Pessin JE. J Biol Chem 1989;264:21450−21453.
38. Heidaran M, Pierce JH, Yu J-C, Lombardi D, Artrip JE, Fleming TP, Thomason A, Aaronson SA. J Biol Chem 1991;266:20232−20237.
39. Qian X, Decker SJ, Greene MI. Biochemistry 1992;89:1340−1344.
40. Soos MA, Navé BN, Field CE, Siddle K. Exp Clin Endocrinol 1993;101(suppl 2):10−11.
41. Yip CC. J Cell Biochem 1992;48:19−25.
42. Schäffer L. Exp Clin Endocrinol 1993;101(suppl 2):7−9.
43. De Meyts P. The structural basis of insulin and insulin-like growth factor-I (IGF-I) receptor binding and negative cooperativity, and its relevance to mitogenic versus metabolic signaling. Diabetologica (in press).

44. Kasuya J, Paz P, Maddux BA, Goldfine ID, Hefta SA, Fujita-Yamaguchi Y. Biochemistry 1993;32:13531—13536.
45. Forsayeth JA, Montemurro A, Maddux BA, DePirro R, Goldfine ID. J Biol Chem 1987;262:4134—4140.
46. Kjeldsen T, Andersen AS, Wiberg FC, Rasmussen JC, Schäffer L, Balschmidt P, Moller KB, Moller NPH. Proc Natl Acad Sci USA 1991;88:4404—4408.
47. Lammers R, Gray A, Schlessinger J, Ullrich A. EMBO J 1989;8:1369—1375.
48. Hofmann C, Goldfine ID, Whittaker J. J Biol Chem 1989;264:8606—8611.
49. Weiland M, Bahr F, Hohne M, Schürmann A, Ziehm D, Joost HG. J Cell Physiol 1991;149:428—435.

Transcriptional repression of the IGF-II and IGF-I receptor genes by tumor suppressor WT1: implications for normal kidney development and Wilms' tumor

Haim Werner, Charles T. Roberts Jr and Derek LeRoith

Diabetes Branch, NIDDK, National Institutes of Health, Bethesda, MD 20892, USA

Abstract. Transcription factor WT1 is a tumor suppressor gene product that is involved in the etiology and/or progression of a subset of Wilms' tumors. WT1 binds to specific *cis* elements in the promoter regions of the IGF-II and IGF-I receptor genes and suppresses the activity of both promoters. During kidney development, the expression patterns of the IGF-II and WT1 genes are complementary, i.e., stages and regions with high levels of WT1 mRNA exhibit low levels of IGF-II mRNA. Mutations of the WT1 gene are commonly seen in Wilms' tumors, which may result in derepression of the IGF-II and IGF-I receptor promoters; the high levels of locally produced IGF-II can interact with the overexpressed receptor, resulting in a mitogenic loop which may be important in the biology of Wilms' tumor.

Wilms' tumor as a paradigm of aberrant kidney differentiation

Wilms' tumor, or nephroblastoma, is a pediatric kidney cancer that affects 1 in 10,000 children, making it the most common abdominal malignancy in children. Wilms' tumors are often associated with other congenital malformations in syndromes such as Wilms' tumor, Aniridia, Genitourinary abnormalities and mental Retardation (WAGR), Denys-Drash and Beckwith-Wiedeman (BWS) [1].

Much of the interest in Wilms' tumor stems from the fact that it constitutes a paradigm for the relationship between malignancy and aberrant differentiation [2]. The tumor arises from embryonic metanephric blastema cells that would, under normal circumstances, differentiate into the various components of the kidney. Wilms' tumors may include stromal, epithelial and mesenchymal elements in a context of primitive glomerular and tubular structures, suggesting that the normal nephrogenic process has been interrupted [3].

WT1: a Wilms' tumor predisposition gene

Genetic analysis of WAGR patients revealed a gross constitutional deletion of chromosome band 11p13 in association with an alteration of the remaining allele, suggesting that this locus corresponds to a Wilms' tumor predisposition gene [4]. This hypothesis was further corroborated by the observation that approximately 20% of spontaneous Wilms' tumors show loss of heterozygosity for genetic markers at the

11p13 locus [5,6].

Cloning of the WT1 gene was achieved by several groups, employing different molecular strategies. Using a genomic DNA library prepared from a somatic cell hybrid, Call et al. [7] identified a clone that mapped to this region and that was subsequently used to isolate a number of cDNAs encoding WT1. An alternative approach was adopted by Gessler et al. [8] who used a chromosome jumping library to enrich for sequences containing CpG islands, some of which contained the WT1 locus.

WT1 mutations are present in ~10% of Wilms' tumors and in almost 100% of patients with Denys-Drash syndrome, a condition which includes nephroblastoma, streak gonads, ambiguous genitalia and nephropathy [9]. There is strong evidence that, in addition to the WT1 gene, other loci are involved in Wilms' tumors. Thus, 11p15 is the site of WT2, which may represent the gene locus involved in BWS. Another putative locus is on chromosome 16q and the existence of a further locus has been postulated to explain certain cases of familial Wilms' tumors [10].

WT1 gene structure and expression

The WT1 gene, located on chromosome 11p13, consists of ten exons spanning a region of 50 kb of genomic DNA [11]. The mRNA is generally 3.5 kb in length and is expressed in the kidney, gonadal ridge, spleen, brain and spinal cord during embryonic development and in the kidney, gonads and uterus in adults [12]. Full-length cDNAs have been isolated from various mammalian species and their sequences have been shown to be highly conserved [13,14]. The WT1 gene product is a nuclear protein of 52–54 kDa that contains four zinc fingers of the Kruppel C2-H2 class in its C-terminus; the four zinc fingers are encoded by exons 7–10, respectively [15] (Fig. 1).

The primary transcript of the WT1 gene is normally subject to alternative splicing of two different sequences: a 51-b sequence encoded by exon 5 and a 9-b sequence which results from the use of an alternative 5′ splice junction in exon 9. Inclusion of the exon 5 sequence adds 17 amino acids to the N-terminus, whereas the 9-b alternative splice adds three amino acids (KTS) between zinc fingers 3 and 4 [11]. The presence of the KTS sequence impairs binding to the consensus sequence, whereas the effect of the 17-amino acid insert is unknown [16,17]. Cells expressing WT1 can, therefore, contain four different mRNAs, the commonest being the transcript containing both extra sequences, and the least common being the mRNA transcript lacking both [18].

Recently, the presence of an abnormal WT1 transcript lacking exon 2 sequences was reported in Wilms' tumor, but not in normal WT1-expressing tissues [19]. This variant transcript encodes a functionally altered protein that lacks the transcriptional repressor effect of wild-type WT1 and, in fact, is thought to counteract the repression exerted by other WT1 variants.

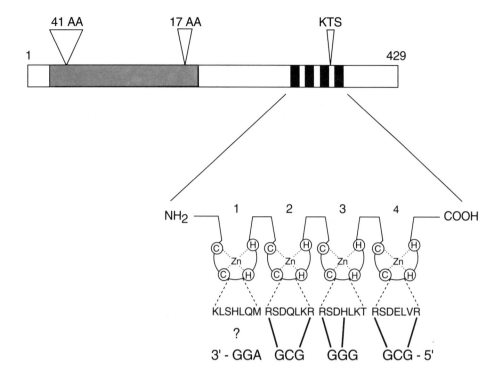

Fig. 1. Schematic representation of WT1. The WT1 protein has an N-terminus (dotted) rich in proline, glutamine, serine and glycine residues that is involved in transactivation (repression) of promoters with GCGGGGGCG elements. The C-terminus contains four zinc finger domains (closed rectangles), that are involved in DNA binding. Three alternatively spliced fragments have been described in WT1: the 123-bp exon 2, encoding a 41-amino acid segment that is deleted in cases of Wilms' tumor; the 51-bp exon 5, encoding a 17-amino acid segment and 3-amino acid (KTS) coding sequence between zinc fingers 3 and 4. The solid bars represent interactions between amino acids and nucleotide.

WT1 as a transcription factor

Characterization of the WT1 protein revealed some of the typical features of a transcription factor, i.e., a zinc finger domain located at the C-terminus that is involved in DNA binding and an N-terminus rich in proline, glutamine, serine and glycine residues [15]. These amino acids are generally found in the transactivation domains of many transcription factors such as Sp1 and CTF/NF1 [20].

WT1 belongs to the EGR family of transcription factors that are encoded by a family of immediate early genes whose transcription is rapidly induced by cell-surface stimuli such as growth factors and/or mitogens [21]. The major consensus binding sequence derived for this family of transcription factors is 5'-GCGG-GGGCG-3' [22]. This specific sequence has been found in the promoter region of various genes, including those encoding IGF-II, the IGF-I receptor, PDGF-A, CSF-1, TGF-β, EGR-1 and Pax-2 [23–25]. Zinc fingers 2, 3 and 4 bind a 3-bp sub-site, but it is still not clear whether the first zinc finger binds DNA.

The sequence-specific amino acid-nucleotide interactions are essentially all arginine-guanine except for the histidine-guanine interaction involving the third finger. The arginine exists in an arginine-serine-aspartic acid triplet at the knuckle of the finger (Fig. 1). As already mentioned, the transcriptionally active domain of the WT1 protein is the proline/glutamine-rich N-terminus that is responsible for transcriptional repression. This repression may depend on the expression of other proteins such as p53, since in Saos-2 osteosarcoma cells, which lack p53, WT1 activates transcription, whereas when p53 is coexpressed WT1 becomes a transcriptional repressor [26].

WT1 involvement in kidney development

Early stages of urogenital development include the pronephros (between the 3rd and 4th weeks of gestation) and mesonephros (between the 4th and 9th weeks); these stages are characterized by the induction of the mesenchyma into nephric tubules. At a later stage, the metanephros (blastema) wraps around the Wolffian duct-derived ureteric bud and the blastemal cells condense, epithelialize and form a renal vesicle. Further differentiation of these cells into tubular epithelium or glomerular epithelial cells (podocytes) occurs. As vascularization of Bowman's capsule occurs, these podocytes become involved in glomerular filtration.

The pattern of WT1 gene expression during normal human kidney development suggests that it may be a candidate gene involved in urogenital development. WT1 is expressed in the mesenchymal cells of the metanephros at the stage that they condense, epithelialize and differentiate into nephric tubules, whereas at later stages it is highly expressed by the podocytes. Thus, WT1 is not expressed during the proliferative phase of the blastemal mesenchyme, but is expressed primarily by developing epithelial cells [2,10,12,14].

The crucial role of WT1 in early urogenital development, has been recently demonstrated by experiments in which the murine WT1 gene was inactivated by targeting in embryonic stem cells [27]. WT1 deletion resulted in apoptosis of the metanephric blastema at day 11 of gestation, and failure of the ureteric bud to grow out from the Wolffian duct, suggesting that the events that induce the formation of the metanephric kidney require WT1.

Does WT1 suppress IGF-II gene expression during kidney development?

During development of the human kidney, the proliferating blastemal cells of the metanephros differentiate into the glomerulus and tubular epithelium, including proximal tubules, the loop of Henle and the collecting ducts. IGF-II is expressed at high levels by the undifferentiated blastema and the blastemal cells that are induced to condense around the ureteric bud [28]. IGF-II is not expressed by epithelial cells of the renal vesicles that differentiate from the early renal vesicle, but is expressed in stromal cells that are derived from the renal vesicle and in low amounts by the secretory and podocyte epithelia.

The expression of the IGF-I receptor gene in the developing kidney is highest around day 13 of gestation, which corresponds to the initial postinductive period of metanephric development. The levels of IGF-I receptor mRNA progressively decrease during subsequent stages of gestation. IGF-I receptor mRNA is distributed through the kidney parenchyma at day 13, with very high concentrations at the ureteric bud and its branches [29].

As mentioned in the previous section, WT1 transcripts are absent in undifferentiated blastemal cells, but begin to appear in the induced blastemal cells that form the early condensates and is easily detectable in epithelial cells of the renal vesicle and highly expressed by podocytes. Thus, the patterns of IGF-II and WT1 gene expression during human renal development appear to be complementary, suggesting an effect of WT1 on the regulation of IGF-II gene expression.

The regulatory regions of the IGF-II and IGF-I receptor genes

The complex IGF-II gene contains multiple promoters that are differentially utilized in a developmental and tissue-specific manner [30]. This multiple promoter usage results in IGF-II transcripts that range from 6.0–2.2 kb in length. The 6.0 kb IGF-II transcript in fetal kidney is the product of the P3 promoter. The P3 promoter (from nucleotide –295 to +135) is 81% GC and contains multiple potential WT1 consensus binding elements (5'-GCGGGGGCG-3'). Most of these lie 5' to the cap site, but some occur in the 5'-untranslated region (UTR). Sites both 5' and 3' to the transcription start site seem to be involved in the repression of IGF-II promoter activity by the WT1 gene product, as demonstrated using the purified WT1 zinc finger region protein in gel-shift and DNase I footprinting experiments [23].

The IGF-I receptor gene promoter is unusually GC-rich and lacks TATA and CAAT elements. The transcription start site is contained within an "initiator" motif, however, and there are multiple Sp1 consensus binding sites in the proximal promoter region and the 5'-UTR. These features have been previously described in other developmentally regulated genes, where it has been shown that accurate transcription occurs despite the absence of TATA and CAAT elements, due to the initiator sequence and the action of the Sp1 transcription factor [31].

In addition to Sp1 sites, the IGF-I receptor gene promoter contains multiple putative WT1 binding sites. Six of these sites lie in the proximal 500 nucleotide of the 5' flanking region and an equivalent number are present in the 5'-UTR. Coexpression in CHO cells of a luciferase reporter gene driven by the –476/+640 region of the IGF-I receptor gene promoter and a WT1 expression vector, resulted in almost total suppression of IGF-I receptor promoter activity [24]. Coexpression of other fragments of the IGF-I receptor gene promoter showed that this inhibition was proportional to the total number of WT1 binding sites in the construct. Gel-retardation

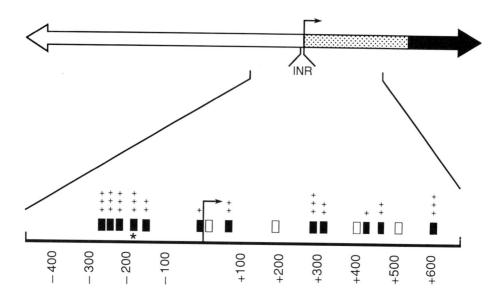

Fig. 2. Schematic representation of WT1 binding sites in the proximal promoter region of the IGF-I receptor gene. Mapping of WT1 sites was achieved by means of DNase I footprinting using labeled fragments of the promoter and the purified WT1 zinc finger domain protein. The translated sequence is black, the 5'-untranslated sequence is dotted and the 5'-flanking region is open. The arrow denotes the transcription start site within the initiator (INR) element. Footprinted sites are denoted by closed rectangles. Open rectangles represent putative WT1 sites which were not footprinted by WT1 protein under the conditions assayed. The asterisk is a perfectly conserved EGR/WT1 consensus sequence. The relative affinity of the different sites is shown by the + signs.

and DNase I footprinting experiments revealed that the purified zinc finger region of the WT1 protein specifically interacted with consensus binding sites both upstream and downstream of the initiator element, albeit with different affinities [32] (Fig. 2). Furthermore, the binding of the WT1 protein containing the KTS insert described above was markedly impaired, as compared with binding of the WT1 protein lacking the KTS sequence.

The involvement of IGF-II and the IGF-I receptor in Wilms' tumor

Several lines of evidence point to a significant role for the IGF-II/IGF-I receptor axis in the biology of Wilms' tumor. Early studies showed that Wilms' tumors contain high levels of IGF-II mRNA and protein, suggesting that this growth factor may be an important mitogenic agent in these tumors [33,34]. The IGF-II gene, which is expressed in human tissues from the maternal allele, has been shown to be frequently expressed from both alleles in Wilms' tumor and in BWS, suggesting that relaxation or loss of imprinting could represent a potential mechanism in carcinogenesis [35]. Additionally, BWS is characterized cytogenetically by paternal duplications of the

11p15.5 chromosomal region, a region which also contains the IGF-II gene [36].

Most of the biological actions of IGF-II are believed to be mediated by the IGF-I receptor. The role of the IGF-I receptor in Wilms' tumorigenesis is exemplified by experiments which showed that intraperitoneal administration of antibody αIR-3 − a monoclonal antibody against human IGF-I receptor − to nude mice bearing Wilms' tumor heterotransplants prevented tumor growth and resulted in partial tumor remission [37].

Further support for the notion that the IGF-I receptor plays an important role in the etiology of Wilms' tumor comes from recent studies which show that the IGF-I receptor gene, in addition to IGF-II, is overexpressed in Wilms' tumor [24]. Moreover, the levels of IGF-I receptor mRNA in individual tumors were inversely correlated with the levels of WT1 mRNA, thus corroborating the in vitro findings that the IGF-I receptor promoter, like the IGF-II promoter, is negatively regulated by WT1.

Since mutations of the WT1 gene commonly seen in Wilms' tumors often affect the zinc finger region, this may result in the derepression of IGF-II and IGF-I receptor promoters, leading to increased transcription and expression of both ligand and receptor proteins (Fig. 3). Paracrine activation of the IGF-I receptor by locally produced IGF-II may elicit a mitogenic event, which may be a key step in the etiology and/or progression of Wilms' tumor.

**REGULATION OF IGF-II AND IGF-I RECEPTOR GENE EXPRESSION
BY THE WT1 WILMS' TUMOR SUPPRESSOR GENE PRODUCT**

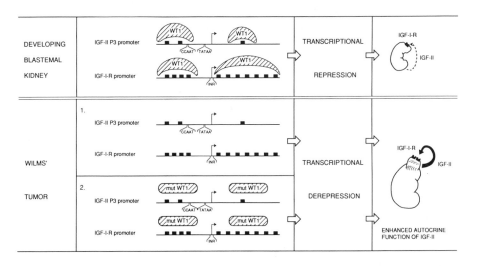

Fig. 3. Hypothetical model for the regulation of IGF-II and IGF-I receptor gene expression by WT1. During blastemal kidney development, WT1 protein binds specific *cis*-elements in the promoter regions of the IGF-II and IGF-I receptor genes. This results in repression of transcription from both genes, leading to a halt in cellular proliferation and, eventually, a program of cell differentiation is set in motion. In Wilms' tumor, the WT1 gene can be either deleted (such as in WAGR) or mutated, resulting in a defective protein unable to bind to the IGF-II and IGF-I receptor promoters. As a result, transcription from both genes is derepressed, leading to enhanced autocrine/paracrine action of IGF-II via the IGF-I receptor. This mitogenic loop may be a key step in the etiology of Wilms' tumor.

114

References

1. Haber DA, Housman DE. Adv Cancer Res 1992;59:41–68.
2. Rauscher FJ III. FASEB J 1993;7:896–903.
3. Beckwith JB, Kiviat NB, Bonadio JF. Pediatr Pathol 1990;10:1–36.
4. Riccardi VM, Sujanksy E, Smith AC, Francke U. Pediatrics 1978;61:604–610.
5. Orkin SH, Goldman DS, Sallan SE. Nature 1984;309:172–174.
6. Koufos A, Hansen MF, Lampkin BC, Workman ML, Copeland NG, Jenkins NA, Cavenee WK. Nature 1984;309:170–172.
7. Call KM, Glasser T, Ito CY, Buckler AJ, Pelletier J, Haber DA, Rose EA, Kral A, Yeger H, Lewis WH, Jones C, Housman DE. Cell 1990;60:509–520.
8. Gessler M, Poustka A, Cavenee W, Neve RL, Orkin SH, Bruns GAP. Nature 1990;343:774–778.
9. Coppes MJ, Campbell CE, Williams BRG. FASEB J 1993;7:886–895.
10. Van Heyningen V, Hastie ND. Trends Genet 1992;8:16–21.
11. Haber DA, Sohn RL, Buckler AJ, Pelletier J, Call KM, Housman DE. Proc Natl Acad Sci USA 1991; 88:9618–9622.
12. Pelletier J, Schalling M, Buckler AJ, Rogers A, Haber DA, Housman DE. Genes Devel 1991;5:1345–1356.
13. Sharma PM, Yang X, Bowman M, Roberts V, Sukumar S. Cancer Res 1992;52:6407–6412.
14. Buckler AJ, Pelletier J, Haber DA, Glaser T, Housman DE. Mol Cell Biol 1991;11:1707–1712.
15. Morris JF, Madden SL, Tournay OE, Cook DM, Sukhatme VP, Rauscher FJ III. Oncogene 1991;6: 2339–2348.
16. Madden SL, Cook DM, Morris JF, Gashler A, Sukhatme VP, Rauscher FJ III. Science 1991;253: 1550–1553.
17. Bickmore WA, Oghene K, Little MH, Seawright A, Van Heyningen V, Hastie ND. Science 1992;257:235–237.
18. Iluang A, Campbell CE, Bonetta L, McAndrews-Hill MS, Chilton-MacNeill S, Coppes MJ, Law DJ, Feinberg AP, Yeger H, Williams BRG. Science 1990;250:991–994.
19. Haber DA, Park S, Maheswaran S, Englert C, Re GG, Hazen-Martin DJ, Sens DA, Garvin AJ. Science 1993;262:2057–2059.
20. Pabo CO, Sauer RT. Annu Rev Biochem 1992;61:1053–1095.
21. Sukhatme VP. Am Soc Nephrol 1990;1:859–866.
22. Rauscher FJ III, Morris JF, Tournay OE, Cook DM, Curran T. Science 1990;250:1259–1262.
23. Drummond IA, Madden SL, Rowher-Nutter P, Bell GI, Sukhatme VP, Rauscher FJ III. Science 1992; 257:674–678.
24. Werner H, Re GG, Drummond IA, Sukhatme VP, Rauscher FJ III, Sens DA, Garvin AJ, LeRoith D, Roberts CT Jr. Proc Natl Acad Sci USA 1993;90:5828–5832.
25. Wang ZY, Madden SL, Deuel TF, Rauscher FJ III. J Biol Chem 1992;267:21999–22002.
26. Maheswaran S, Park S, Bernard A, Morris JF, Rauscher FJ III, Hill DE, Haber DA. Proc Natl Acad Sci USA 1993;90:5100–5104.
27. Kreidberg JA, Sariola H, Loring JM, Maeda M, Pelletier J, Housman D, Jaenisch R. Cell 1993;74: 679–691.
28. Yun K, Fidler AE, Eccles MR, Reeve AE. Cancer Res 1993;53:5166–5171.
29. Wada J, Liu ZZ, Alvares K, Kumar A, Wallner E, Makino H, Kanwar YS. Proc Natl Acad Sci USA 1993;90:10360–10364.
30. Soares MB, Turken A, Ishii D, Mills L, Episkopo UV, Cotter S, Zeitlin S. Efstratiadis A. J Mol Biol 1986;192:737–752.
31. Werner H, Bach MA, Stannard B, Roberts CT Jr, LeRoith D. Mol Endocrinol 1992;6:1545–1558.
32. Werner H, Rauscher FJ III, Sukhatme VP, Drummond IA, Roberts CT Jr, LeRoith D. J Biol Chem 1994;269:12577–12582.
33. Paik S, Rosen N, Jung W, You J-M, Lippman ME, Perdue JF, Yee D. Lab Invest 1989;61:522–526.
34. Reeve AE, Eccles MR, Wilkins RJ, Bell GI, Millow LJ. Nature (London) 1985;317:258–260.

35. Rainier S, Johnson LA, Dobry CJ, Ping AJ, Grundy PE, Feinberg AP. Nature 1993;362;747–749.
36. Koufos A, Grundy P, Morgan K, Aleck KA, Hadro T, Lampkin BC, Kalbakji A, Cavenee WK. Am J Hum Genet 1989;44:711–719.
37. Gansler T, Furlanetto R, Gramling TS, Robinson KA, Blocker N, Buse MG, Sens DA, Garvin AJ. Am J Pathol 1989;135:961.

Signal structures on the mannose 6-phosphate/IGF-II receptor

Thomas Braulke[1], Christian Körner[1], Olaf Rosorius[1] and Bernd Nürnberg[2]

[1]*Institut für Biochemie II, Universität Göttingen, 37073 Göttingen; and* [2]*Institut für Pharmakologie, Universitätsklinikum Rudolf Virchow, Freie Universität Berlin, 14195 Berlin, Germany*

Abstract. We investigated the role of two distinct structural determinants of the mannose 6-phosphate (M6P) /IGF-II receptor cytoplasmic tail, namely the phosphorylation and the G-protein activator regions, in receptor tail-protein interactions and signal transduction, respectively. The specific phosphorylation of serine residues 82 and 157 by a casein kinase II is required for the tail interaction with a cytosolic protein of 35 kDa (referred to as TIP 35). The interaction of two other 35 kDa and 91 kDa proteins salt-washed from membranes were independent of receptor tail phosphorylation. The assembly of both cytosolic and membrane associated TIP 35 in a 130–150 kDa complex is necessary for interaction with the receptor tail and is inhibited upon ATP hydrolysis. Zn^{2+} chelate chromatography revealed that either TIP 35 or another component of the 130–150 kDa complex belong to the class of Zn^{2+}-binding proteins.

Wild-type or truncated human M6P/IGF-II receptor mutants lacking the proposed G_{i2} activator region were purified from overexpressing mouse L-cells and reconstituted with purified trimeric G_{o1} or G_{i2} proteins or with the respective $G\alpha$ monomers and $\beta\gamma$ complexes in phospholipid vesicles. The addition of IGF-II failed to stimulate the GTPγS binding to G proteins in vesicles containing the wild-type or mutant receptor. The possible structural requirements in the M6P/IGF-II receptor tail necessary to achieve responsiveness to IGF-II are discussed.

Introduction

Mannose 6-phosphate (M6P)-containing lysosomal enzymes and IGF-II bind at different sites to a common receptor. About 90% of the M6P/IGF-II receptors are localized in intracellular membranes and mediate the transport of newly synthesized lysosomal enzymes between the trans Golgi network (TGN) and endosomes where the low pH induces the dissociation of the receptor ligand complexes. The lysosomal enzymes move to lysosomes whereas the M6P/IGF-II receptors return to the Golgi for another transport cycle. The M6P/IGF-II receptors in intracellular membranes are in a continuous rapid exchange with receptors at the cell surface which are involved in binding, internalization and transport of extracellular M6P-containing ligands and IGF-II to the lysosome [1,2]. Both transport routes from the TGN and from the plasma membrane to endosomes are mediated by clathrin-coated vesicles containing HA I and HA II adaptins, respectively [3], and require additional cytosolic and membrane-associated proteins [4]. It has been shown that signal structures localized

Address for correspondence: Thomas Braulke, Institute of Biochemistry II, Gosslerstraße 12d, D-37073, Göttingen, Germany. Fax: +49-551-395979.

in the cytoplasmic tail are necessary for M6P/IGF-II receptor routing (for review see [5]). Thus, a tyrosine-containing internalization signal representing residues 24–29 of the receptor-tail, has been identified which is recognized by HA II adaptins [6,7]. A second signal required for efficient sorting of lysosomal enzymes in the TGN includes a dileucine motif at the carboxyl terminus [8]. Furthermore, a sequence of 14 amino acids corresponding to residues 123–136 of the human M6P/IGF-II receptor tail has been reported to be responsible for the IGF-II induced coupling to and activation of G_{i2}-proteins (for review see [9]). The 14 amino acid region is interchangeable with a β_2 adrenergic receptor sequence resulting in an activation of adenylate cyclase stimulating G_s-protein [10]. However, despite a number of reports indicating that cellular responses to IGF-II, like the stimulation of amino acid uptake in human myoblasts [11] or the Na^+/H^+ exchange and inositol triphosphate production in canine kidney proximal tubular cells [12,13] are mediated by the M6P/IGF-II receptor, other studies give differing results. The use of (1) various antibodies against IGF-I and M6P/IGF-II receptors [14–16]; (2) mutants of IGF-II which bind specifically to one or the other receptors [17,18]; and (3) targeted mutagenesis in mice [19], indicate that biologic responses to IGF-II are mediated via interaction with the IGF-I or with an additional receptor.

In addition, it has been suggested that posttranslational modifications such as phosphorylation/dephosphorylation are involved in M6P/IGF-II receptor trafficking. Thus the insulin-induced redistribution of M6P/IGF-II receptors from internal membranes to the cell surface, is associated with a decrease in the phosphorylation state of M6P/IGF-II receptors in the plasma membrane [20]. Two serine residues within the receptor tail, which are transiently phosphorylated by a casein kinase II (CK II), have been shown to promote the recruitment of HA I adaptins to Golgi membranes and to be required for complex formation with a 35 kDa cytosolic protein [21,22]. In contrast, two other membrane-associated proteins appear to interact with the M6P/IGF-II receptor tail independently of phosphorylation.

In order to elucidate the biological significance of these interactions we further characterized the proteins. Additionally, we have used purified M6P/IGF-II receptor and a receptor mutant truncated in the cytoplasmic tail for reconstitution experiments with isolated G-proteins to investigate the role of the M6P/IGF-II receptor in signal transduction.

Materials and Methods

Materials

Recombinant IGF-II was a gift from W. Märki (Ciba Geigy, Basel). Oligonucleotides were synthesized on an Applied Biosystem model 381 A solid phase synthesizer. The cDNA of human M6P/IGF-II receptor and mouse L-cells deficient in M6P/IGF-II receptor were kindly provided by William S. Sly (St. Louis University, St. Louis) and Stuart Kornfeld (Washington University, St. Louis).

Antibodies

The monoclonal antibody 2C2 directed against the human M6P/IGF-II receptor [23] was iodinated with IODO-GEN. Antisera against the human liver M6P/IGF-II receptor and the recombinant M6P/IGF-II receptor-tail were raised in goat and rabbits, respectively. Antiserum against the synthetic peptide corresponding to the last 15 C-terminal amino acids (peptide 15C) of the human M6P/IGF-II receptor-tail, was obtained by immunizing rabbits with the peptide coupled to keyhole limpet hemocyanin.

DNA constructs and transfection

The M6P/IGF-II receptor tail (amino acids 2329–2492) was expressed in *Escherichia coli* and purified as described [24]. Oligonucleotide-directed mutagenesis was carried out [25] to introduce a stop codon into the cDNA sequence at position 2403 (amino acid 75 of the cytoplasmic tail; StL75). The mutation and the receptor-tail construct were verified by dideoxynucleotide sequencing. The wild-type and mutant M6P/IGF-II receptor cDNA were cloned in the expression vector pBHE. Mouse L-cells deficient in M6P/IGF-II receptors were transfected with the pBHE plasmids and pSV2 neo (neomycin resistance) plasmid (10:1) using the calcium phosphate technique. Selection was performed with 0.8 mg/ml neomycin. Stable colonies were isolated and screened for M6P/IGF-II receptor expression by measuring the binding of iodinated 2C2 antibodies in saponin-permeabilized cells and immunoprecipitation of receptors [26].

M6P/IGF-II receptor and G proteins

The wild-type and mutant M6P/IGF-II receptor were purified to a single protein from overexpressing mouse L-cells using phosphomannan affinity columns [27] in the absence of divalent cations. The receptors were eluted with 10 mM M6P, concentrated and dialyzed in ultrafiltration thimbles (Schleicher & Schüll, exclusion size 25,000), pretreated with 1 M glycine solution, pH 7.4. The purity of M6P/IGF-II receptors and the intactness of the cytoplasmic receptor tails were assessed after SDS-PAGE by silver staining or Western blotting with different receptor antibodies. $G\alpha_{o1}$, $G\alpha_{i2}$ and $\beta\gamma$ complexes as well as heterotrimeric G_{o1} and G_{i2} proteins were purified from bovine brain [28].

Assays

Cross-linkage analysis using the purified M6P/IGF-II receptor-tail [^{32}P]labeled by casein-kinase II and cytosolic or salt-washed membrane proteins, were carried out as described previously [22]. Reconstitution of purified wild-type and mutant M6P/IGF-II receptor and G proteins into phospholipid vesicles and GTPγS binding, were carried out according to Nishimoto et al. [29].

120

Results

M6P/IGF-II receptor tail interacting proteins

Interactions between the M6P/IGF-II receptor tail and cytosolic or membrane-associated proteins were monitored in a rapid in vitro assay. The receptor domain was first phosphorylated by casein kinase II and $[\gamma^{32}P]ATP$ to label the tail at physiologically used serine residues 82 and 157 [21]. The $[^{32}P]M6P/IGF$-II receptor tail was then incubated at 30°C with cytosolic fractions or proteins salt-washed from brain membranes, cross-linked by means of bis(sulfosuccinimidyl) suberate (BS3) and analyzed by SDS-PAGE and autoradiography. When cytosolic fractions were used the major cross-link product had an apparent molecular mass of 58 kDa. After subtraction of the 23 kDa corresponding to the phosphorylated M6P/IGF-II receptor tail the apparent molecular mass of this tail interacting protein was 35 kDa (TIP 35). By cross-linkage of $[^{32}P]$ M6P/IGF-II receptor tail with salt-washed membrane proteins

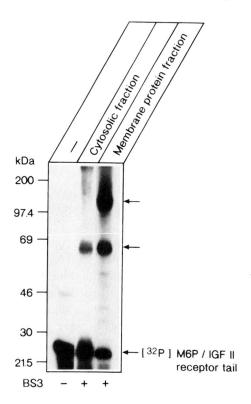

Fig. 1. The $[^{32}P]$labeled M6P/IGF II receptor tail was incubated either with rat brain cytosolic proteins fractionated on a DEAE-Sephacel column or with salt-washed membrane proteins cross-linked by BS3 and analyzed by SDS-PAGE and autoradiography. In controls the $[^{32}P]$labeled M6P/IGF II receptor-tail was incubated without BS3 in the absence of additional proteins. The positions of the $[^{32}P]$ M6P/IGF II receptor tail and of the major 58 kDa and 114 kDa cross-link products are indicated by arrows. The positions of the molecular mass markers (kDa) are indicated.

two interacting proteins with molecular masses of 35 and 91 kDa (TIP 35-M and TIP 91-M) were detected (Fig. 1) [22]. The interaction of the cytosolic TIP 35 with the M6P/IGF-II receptor tail had been shown to depend on tail phosphorylation only by casein kinase II, whereas the receptor tail phosphorylated at two different serine residues by a protein kinase A failed to cross-link to TIP 35 [22]. Inhibition studies with nonphosphorylated M6P/IGF-II receptor tails, however, had shown that TIP 35-M and TIP 91-M interact with different structural determinants than the cytosolic TIP 35. Both cytosolic and membrane associated TIP 35 are parts of higher molecular mass complexes of approximately 130–150 kDa [22].

The presence of a low concentration (0.1 μM) of ATP during the incubation of cytosolic proteins with the [32P] M6P/IGF-II receptor tail, completely prevented the formation of the cross-link product with TIP 35 (Fig. 2). Neither GTP, GTPγS nor ADP (not shown) at this concentration altered the cross-linking formation, whereas the nonhydrolyzable ATP analog AMPPNP inhibited the cross-linkage only at 1000-fold higher concentrations. The interactions of TIP 35-M and TIP 91-M with the receptor tail were also ATP-sensitive (not shown).

The presence of divalent cations during the incubation of the [32P] M6P/IGF-II receptor tail with cytosolic proteins increased the formation of the 58 kDa cross-link

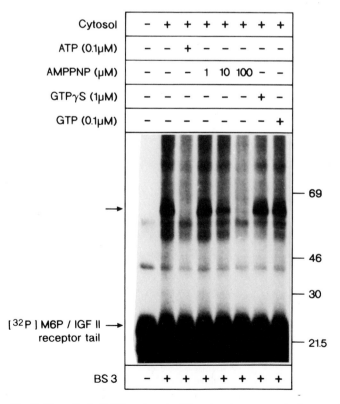

Fig. 2. The effect of different nucleotides at various concentrations on the formation of the cross-link product between the [32P] M6P/IGF II receptor tail and TIP 35 was examined as described in Fig. 1.

product whereby Zn^{2+} (1.5 mM) stimulated the cross-linkage 14- to 18-fold. The interaction with TIP 35-M and TIP 91-M was stimulated similarly by Zn^{2+} (not shown).

To examine whether TIP 35 is a Zn^{2+}-binding protein, a cytosolic fraction from rat brain was applied to Zn^{2+}-chelate agarose, and following washing, bound proteins were either eluted with: (1) increasing concentrations of imidazole in equilibrium buffer; (2) a pH-gradient; or (3) EDTA. The eluted fractions were dialyzed and tested for cross-linking. Cytosolic TIP 35 bound to the Zn^{2+}-chelate matrix and was specifically eluted with imidazole (20 mM) at low pH (pH 6.0) or with 25 mM EDTA (Fig. 3). The results indicate that either the cytosolic TIP 35 or another component of the 130–150 kDa complex belong to the class of Zn^{2+}-binding proteins.

Does IGF-II induce coupling of G-proteins to M6P/IGF-II receptor?

Previous studies by Nishimoto and his colleagues [30,31] have shown that a stretch of 14 amino acids (residues 123–136) (Fig. 4A) of the human M6P/IGF-II receptor tail is responsible for the IGF-II-induced coupling to G-proteins. To examine the G-protein coupling properties of M6P/IGF-II receptors, mutant receptor was reconstituted in phospholipid vesicles with trimeric G_{o1}- and G_{i2}-proteins or with purified $G\alpha_{o1}$- and $G\alpha_{i2}$-monomers together with $\beta\gamma$ complexes. A mutant was produced that possessed only the first 74 amino acids (StL75) of the cytoplasmic tail by introducing

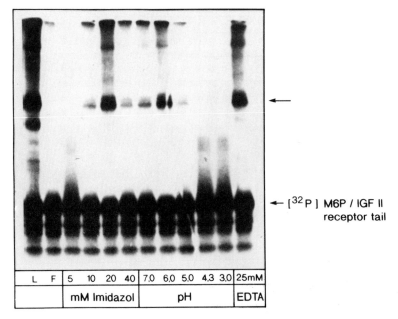

$\leftarrow$ [^{32}P] M6P / IGF II
receptor tail

L	F	5	10	20	40	7,0	6,0	5,0	4,3	3,0	25mM
			mM Imidazol					pH			EDTA

Fig. 3. Cytosolic fractions of rat brain were applied to three Zn-chelate-Sepharose 6B columns and following washing either eluted with increasing concentrations of imidazole; with phosphate/citrate buffer (pH 7-3) or with 25 mM EDTA. The eluted fractions were dialyzed and tested for cross-linking as described in Fig. 1. L = an aliquot of the loaded cytosolic fraction; F = flow through fraction.

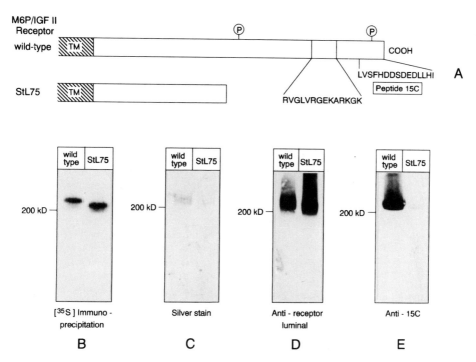

Fig. 4. (A) Schematic presentation of human wild-type M6P/IGF II receptor tail and mutant form StL75 showing the putative G protein binding region (residues 123–136) and the casein kinase II phosphorylated serine residues 82 and 157. Peptide 15C is a 15 amino acid peptide located at the carboxy terminus of the tail. The StL75 mutant form was generated by replacing the leucine (residue 75) codon with a stop codon. (B) Fluorograph of immunoprecipitated human wild-type and StL75 M6P/IGF II receptors from overexpressing radioactive-labeled mouse L-cells deficient for the M6P/IGF II receptor. (C, D, E) Wild type and StL75 M6P/IGF II receptors after purification visualized by silver staining (C), or antibody-ECL staining after electrotransfer to nitrocellulose by means of a receptor antibody directed against the luminal domain (D) or against peptide 15C (E).

a stop codon in leucine 75 (Fig. 4A). The human wild-type and mutant M6P/IGF-II receptor was stably expressed in mouse L-cells deficient in M6P/IGF-II receptors. By immunoprecipitation of M6P/IGF-II receptors from metabolically labeled over-expressing L-cells the truncation in the StL75 mutant was confirmed resulting in a faster electrophoretic mobility (Fig. 4B).

The wild-type and mutant M6P/IGF-II receptor were purified from overexpressing L-cells by phosphomannan chromatography. It should be noted that under the commonly used conditions of purification, the receptor can loose parts of its cytoplasmic tail indicated by failing reactivity with an antibody directed against the last 15 amino acids of the human M6P/IGF-II receptor (peptide 15C) (Fig. 4A). The same observation was reported previously [32]. For purification of an intact M6P/IGF-II receptor, divalent cations had to be omitted from all buffers and substituted by EDTA and a variety of protease and phosphatase inhibitors. Under

124

these conditions a wild-type M6P/IGF-II receptor with a complete cytoplasmic tail was purified as shown by its reactivity with the 15C antibody (Fig. 4E). The purified truncated StL75 receptor showed the characteristic gel shift compared with the wild-type receptor by silver staining (Fig. 4C) or in a Western blot using an antibody

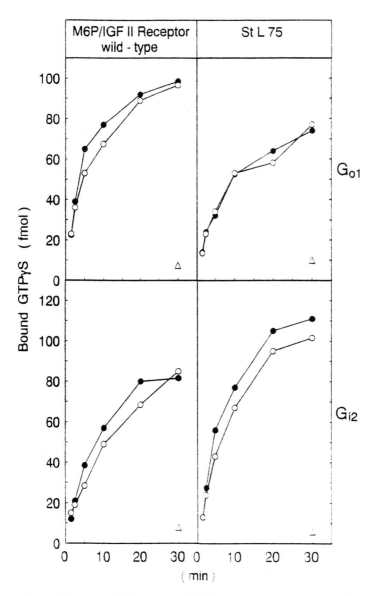

Fig. 5. Wild-type or StL75 mutant M6P/IGF II receptors reconstituted with trimeric G_{o1} or G_{i2} proteins, were incubated for the indicated period with 120 nM [^{35}S] GTPγS in the absence (O) or presence (●) of 100 nM IGF II. Each point is the mean of duplicates. The GTPγS binding to G proteins of a representative experiment out of 2–3 is shown. Δ, GTPγS binding in the presence of 100 μM unlabeled GTPγS.

directed against the luminal domain of the M6P/IGF-II receptor (Fig. 4D), whereas the anti-C 15 antibody did not react with the StL75 receptor (Fig. 4E).

At first the wild-type or mutant M6P/IGF-II receptor (33 pmol) were reconstituted with the trimer forms of either G_{o1} or G_{i2} (12 pmol) into phospholipid vesicles. The presence of M6P/IGF-II receptors in reconstituted vesicles was shown by antibody reactivity in Western blot, $[^{125}I]IGF$-II cross-linking and binding of $[^{125}I]$ pentamannose 6-phosphate coupled bovine serum albumin (not shown). The amount of functionally active G-protein was confirmed by quantitative GTPγS binding. In these experiments each two different wild-type M6P/IGF-II receptor and StL75 receptor preparations, one preparation of G_{o1} and two preparations of G_{i2} were tested. The binding of GTPγS was followed in the absence or presence of 100 nM IGF-II for up to 30 min (Fig. 5). In the presence of IGF-II the rate of GTPγS binding to wild-type receptor/G_{o1} vesicles was slightly increased (up to 1.2-fold). With wild-type receptor/G_{i2} a maximum 1.3-fold stimulation of binding by IGF-II was observed. However, in StL75/G_{i2} vesicles an up to 1.3-fold increase in GTPγS binding in response of IGF-II was also observed during the time course. In StL75/G_{o1} vesicles IGF-II did not affect the GTPγS binding rate compared with controls. The rate and the highest amount of GTPγS binding to the vesicles, attained after 20–30 min of incubation, were not altered by the reconstitution of receptors (not shown). In vesicles in which wild-type M6P/IGF-II receptor was reconstituted with purified monomer $G\alpha_{o1}$ or $G\alpha_{i2}$ and βγ-dimers, the GTPγS binding in the presence of IGF-II in either case was not different to trimeric G-protein experiments (not shown). Thus, taken together the results indicate that the binding of IGF-II to both the wild-type M6P/IGF-II receptor and a receptor mutant lacking the proposed G-protein binding region failed to significantly stimulate the GTPγS binding to G_{o1} or G_{i2} proteins.

Discussion

The M6P/IGF-II receptor-dependent transport of newly synthesized lysosomal enzymes from the Golgi to the lysosome and of lysosomal enzymes and IGF-II from the cell surface to endosomes is mediated by clathrin-coated vesicles. The vesicle formation involves the sequential binding of the heterotetramer HA I or HA II adaptor proteins to Golgi or plasma membranes, respectively, and of clathrin triskeletons [33]. The cytoplasmic domain of the M6P/IGF-II receptor phosphorylated by a casein kinase II like-kinase, functions as an efficient binding site for HA I adaptors to Golgi membranes and may contribute together with the carboxyterminal dileucine motif to the sorting of lysosomal enzymes along the clathrin-dependent pathway [21,34,35]. Phosphorylation of the cytoplasmic tail of the M6P/IGF-II receptor catalyzed by a casein kinase II serves also as a signal structure for the specific interaction with a 35 kDa cytosolic protein (TIP 35), which does not bind GTP and is a noncovalently linked component of a higher molecular mass complex [22]. The M6P/IGF-II receptor tail interacts only with TIP 35 if it is part of the complex. In the present report we could show that TIP 35 or an associated protein of the complex is a Zn^{2+}-binding protein and that the amount of TIP 35 cross-linked to the receptor tail was increased in the presence of Zn^{2+}. It is still not known whether Zn^{2+} ions directly affect the receptor tail-TIP 35 interaction or stabilize the 130–150 kDa complex resulting in an increased efficiency of cross-linking. Furthermore, the cross-linking of the M6P/IGF-II receptor tail to TIP 35 was completely abolished by low concentrations of ATP, but not by the nonhydrolyzable nucleotide AMPPNP. This suggests that either phosphorylation processes or simple ATP hydrolysis lead to a dissociation of the 130–150 kDa complex. The biological significance of phosphorylation-dependent interaction of the M6P/IGF-II receptor tail with TIP 35 for transport functions has not been determined.

The involvement of an ATP-sensitive higher molecular complex in vesicle targeting is not without precedent. The N-ethylmaleimide-sensitive fusion protein (NSF), a soluble tetramer of 76 kDa, participates in both constitutive and regulated intracellular fusion processes. Three monomeric soluble NSF attachment proteins (SNAPs) with molar masses of 35, 36 and 39 kDa are necessary for NSF binding to membranes to assemble with SNAP receptors (SNARE) to a 20S particle. NSF is an ATPase, and binding and hydrolysis of ATP are critical in determining the stability of the 20S particle [36]. Whether the phosphorylated M6P/IGF-II receptor tail can function as a vesicular SNARE remains to be elucidated. The phosphorylated M6P/IGF-II receptor may not only direct clathrin-coated vesicles from the TGN to endosomes, but could serve as a sorting signal within the endosomal compartment as reported for the polymeric immunoglobulin receptor [37].

The M6P/IGF-II receptor is phosphorylated in vivo at 4–5 different serine residues in its cytoplasmic tail [24]. Apart from the two casein kinase II-phosphorylated serine residues 82 and 157, the locations of the three other phosphorylation sites and the respective kinase(s) are unknown. It is therefore tempting to speculate whether these phosphorylation sites are involved in additional receptor-protein interactions. The interaction of TIP 35-M and TIP 91-M with the M6P/IGF-II receptor is phosphorylation independent [22]. Preliminary competition studies using synthetic peptides corresponding to different regions of the human M6P/IGF-II receptor tail revealed that only peptide 18–37 inhibited the formation of cross-link products with both TIP 35-M and TIP 91-M. The amino acid region 18–37 contains the signal for rapid internalization (residues 24–29) suggesting that TIP 35-M and/or TIP 91-M may be involved in receptor endocytosis. Finally, the interaction of the M6P/IGF-II receptor tail with cytosolic TIP 35 or TIP 35-M/TIP 91-M was not affected by the phosphorylated or nonphosphorylated 46 kDa M6P receptor tail, respectively (unpublished results), a second transport receptor for lysosomal enzymes. These results indicate that the M6P/IGF-II receptor can specifically interact with cytosolic and/or membrane-associated proteins which may be important for M6P/IGF-II receptor functions different to those of the 46 kDa M6P receptor, e.g., endocytosis of lysosomal enzymes [5] or distinct endosomal distribution [39].

In our investigations into the M6P/IGF-II receptor — G protein interaction in phospholipid vesicles we obtained no evidences that IGF-II induces the coupling to G_{i2}-proteins. There were no differences in GTPγS binding to G_{i2} reconstituted in vesicles with the purified wild-type M6P/IGF-II receptor or a truncated mutant receptor lacking the putative G protein-coupling sequence. Additionally, in no case did the presence of M6P/IGF-II receptors in phospholipid vesicles affect the kinetics of GTPγS binding to reconstituted G_{i2} or G_{01} proteins. One may consider that different G protein preparations explain the contrasting data of Nishimoto and colleagues [29–31]. The identical purification procedure despite the species and organ source of G proteins [29–31], the regulatory capabilities of the used G proteins examined by reconstitution in living cells [39,40] and the failing effects of IGF-II on lipid vesicles reconstituted with receptors and purified $G\alpha_{o1}$, $G\alpha_{i2}$ and $\beta\gamma$ complexes, respectively argue against the possibility. In addition, different $\beta\gamma$ complex composition in the G protein preparations used in the two laboratories which might activate, inhibit or antagonize the α subunit [41] can be excluded, because the purified $\beta\gamma$ complexes used here for reconstitution with $G\alpha$ monomers contain total $\beta\gamma$ dimers. Secondly, the used M6P/IGF-II receptor preparations in the two laboratories might be different. We purified the wild-type and mutant receptor from overexpressing mouse L-cells under optimized conditions, preventing the proteolytic cleavage of parts or the total cytoplasmic receptor tail which was monitored using antibodies directed against the last 15 carboxyterminal amino acids. Both the wild-type and mutant M6P/IGF-II receptors were competent in binding M6P-containing ligands and IGF-II with similar affinities (C. Körner, unpublished results).

It is likely that differences in the entirety of purified M6P/IGF-II receptor are responsible for the divergent observations which might also be consistent with the data obtained recently with chimeric M6P/IGF-II receptors. Takahashi et al. [10] have observed that in COS-7 cells expressing a M6P/IGF-II receptor construct containing a G_s binding region in its cytoplasmic tail the basal adenylate cyclase activity was elevated which was further stimulated in response to IGF-II. The authors proposed that in wild-type M6P/IGF-II receptors the binding of IGF-II interrupts the interaction between a suppressor and the G-protein coupling region resulting in G-protein activation. On the other hand Okamoto et al. [42] have found that the failure of IGF-II to trigger the coupling of the receptor to G_{i2} in quiescent BALB/c3T3 cells could be restored by priming the cells with PDGF and EGF or by transfection with viral *ras* p21. It is possible that under these conditions the cytoplasmic M6P/IGF-II receptor tail is modulated, e.g., dephosphorylated and achieves structural responsiveness to IGF-II. It has been shown, that hyperphosphorylated M6P/IGF-II receptors at the cell surface of fibroblasts, due to an inhibition of phosphatase 2A, is accompanied by an inhibition of IGF-II-stimulated receptor redistribution [26]. Thus, the simple loss of distinct posttranslational modifications during the purification procedure could result in IGF-II-responsive M6P/IGF-II receptors, whereas e.g., completely phosphorylated receptors cannot be changed to an activated conformation. Further studies are necessary to elucidate whether the structural, reversible modifications may contribute to IGF-II-induced coupling of M6P/IGF-II receptors to G proteins.

128

Acknowledgements

The authors thank Dr. W.S. Sly for providing the cDNA of the human M6P/IGF-II receptor. We are grateful to Dr. O.G. Issinger for recombinant casein kinase II. We thank M. Uhde for excellent technical assistance and Dr. V. Armstrong and A. Thiel for their help with the manuscript. The study was supported by the Deutsche Forschungsgemeinschaft (Sonderforschungsbereich 236/B 11 and SFB 366/A 7), the Fonds der Chemischen Industrie and the Graduiertenkolleg "Signal mediated transport of proteins and vesicles" Göttingen.

References

1. Kornfeld S, Mellman I. Annual Rev Cell Biol 1989;5:483–525.
2. Czech MP. Cell 1989;59:235–238.
3. Robinson MS. Trends Cell Biol 1992;61:307–330.
4. Zerial M, Stenmark H. Curr Opin Cell Biol 1993;5:613–620.
5. Kornfeld S. Annu Rev Biochem 1992;2:293–297.
6. Canfield W, Johnson KF, Ye RD, Gregory W, Kornfeld S. J Biol Chem 1991;266:5682–5688.
7. Glickman JN, Conibear E, Pearse BMF, EMBO J 1989;8:1041–1047.
8. Johnson KF, Kornfeld S. J Cell Biol 1992;119:249–257.
9. Nishimoto I. Mol Reprod Devel 1993;35:398–407.
10. Takahashi K, Murayama Y, Okamoto T, Yokota T, Ikezu T, Takahashi S, Giambarella U, Ogata E, Nishimoto I. Proc Natl Acad Sci USA 1993;90:11772–11776.
11. Shimizu M, Webster C, Morgan DD, Blau HM, Roth R. Am J Physiol 1986;215:E611–E615.
12. Mellas J, Gavin IJR, Hammerman MR. J Biol Chem 1986;261:14437–14442.
13. Rogers SA, Hammerman MR. J Biol Chem 1989;264:4273–4276.
14. Kiess W, Haskell JF, Lee L, Greenstein LA, Miller BE, Aarons AL, Reckler MM, Nissley SP. J Biol Chem 1987;262:12745–12751.
15. Hartmann H, Meyer-Albert A, Braulke T. Diabetologica 1992;35:216–223.
16. Conover CA, Misra P, Hintz RL, Rosenfeld RG. Biochem Biophys Res Commun 1986;139:501–508.
17. Sakano K, Enjoh T, Numata F, Fujiwara H, Marumoto Y, Higashihashi N, Sato Y, Perdue JF, Yamaguchi YF. J Biol Chem 1991;266:20626–20635.
18. Buergisser DM, Roth BV, Giger R, Lüthi C, Weigl S, Zarn J, Humbel RE. J Biol Chem 1991;266:1029–1033.
19. Liu JP, Baker J, Perkins AS, Robertson EJ, Efstratiadis A. Cell 1993;75:59–72.
20. Corvera S, Folander K, Clairmont KB, Czech MP. Proc Natl Acad Sci USA 1988;85:7567–7571.
21. Le Borgue R, Schmidt A, Mauxion F, Griffith G, Hoflack B. J Biol Chem 1993;268:22552–22556.
22. Rosorius O, Issinger OG, Braulke T. J Biol Chem 1993;268:21470–21473.
23. Braulke T, Gartung C, Hasilik A, von Figura K. J Cell Biol 1987;104:1735–1742.
24. Rosorius O, Mieskes G, Issinger OG, Körner C, Schmidt B, von Figura K, Braulke T. Biochem J 1993;292:833–838.
25. Sayers J, Eckstein F. In: Creighton TE (ed) Protein Function: A Practical Approach. Oxford: IRL Press, 1989;275–295.
26. Braulke T, Mieskes G. J Biol Chem 1992;267:17347–17353.
27. Stein M, Meyer HE, Hasilik A, von Figura K. Biol Chem Hoppe-Seyler 1987;368:927–936.
28. Nürnberg B, Spicher K, Harhammer R, Bosserhoff A, Frank R, Hilz H, Schultz G. Purification of a novel G protein α_o-subtype from mammalian brain. Biochem J (in press).
29. Nishimoto I, Murayama Y, Katada T, Ui M, Ogata E. J Biol Chem 1989;264:14029–14038.
30. Okamoto T, Katada T, Murayama Y, Ui M, Ogata E, Nishimoto I. Cell 1990;62:709–717.

129

31. Nishimoto I, Ogata E, Okamoto T. J Biol Chem 1991;266:12747–12751.
32. Meresse S, Ludwig T, Frank R, Hoflack B. J Biol Chem 1990;265:18833–18842.
33. Schmid SL. Curr Opin Cell Biol 1993;5:621–627.
34. Meresse S, Hoflack B. J Cell Biol 1993;120:67–75.
35. Chen HJ, Remmler J, Delaney JC, Messner DJ, Lobel P. J Biol Chem 1993;268:22338–22346.
36. Söllner T, Whiteheart SW, Brunner M, Erdjument-Bromage H, Geromanos S, Tempst P, Rothman JE. Nature 1993;362:318–324.
37. Casanova JE, Breitfeld PP, Ross SA, Mostov KE. Science 1990;248:742–745.
38. Klumperman J, Hille A, Veenendaal T, Oorschot V, Stoorvogel W, von Figura K, Geuze HJ. J Cell Biol 1993;121:997–1010.
39. Hescheler J, Rosenthal W, Trautwein W, Schultz G. Nature 1987;325:445–447.
40. Friedrichs P, Nürnberg B, Schultz G, Hescheler J. FEBS Lett 1993;334:322–326.
41. Clapham DE, Neer EJ. Nature 1993;365:403–406.
42. Okamoto T, Asano T, Harada S, Ogata E. Nishimoto J. J Biol Chem 1991;266:1085–1091.

Does IGF-I ever act through the insulin receptor?

F.J. Ballard[1], Paul E. Walton[1], Frank R. Dunshea[2], Geoffrey L. Francis[1] and Frank M. Tomas[1]

[1]*Cooperative Research Centre for Tissue Growth and Repair, Adelaide, SA 5000; and [2]Victorian Institute of Animal Science, Werribee, VIC 3030 Australia*

Abstract. Research with cultured cells has shown that both the short-term "metabolic" effects of IGF-I as well as the longer-term "growth" effects are generally mediated via the IGF-I receptor. This evidence has been derived from the use of antibodies to the IGF-I receptor which block the "metabolic" effects of IGF-I, by measurements with specific cell lines that contain the IGF-I, but not the insulin receptor, by cells that have genetic defects in insulin binding, but exhibit unaltered IGF-I "metabolic" responses, by IGF-I receptor transfectants which show enhanced IGF-I short-term effects, as well as through a series of indirect methods such as experiments in which IGF-I potency is retained following down-regulation of the insulin receptor. This conclusion is also supported by experiments in vivo, including the demonstration of the "metabolic" hypoglycemic response to IGF-I in insulin-resistant states in rodents and humans, as well as by a series of studies using streptozotocin-diabetic rats in which insulin and IGF-I exert qualitatively different effects, even though both factors restore overall growth to a similar extent. Finally, the recent gene knockout experiments are best interpreted as IGF-I exhibiting all its actions via the IGF-I receptor. While all of these results suggest that the answer to the question posed in the title is "NO", it is likely that IGF-I can act through the insulin receptor in certain insulin hypersensitive cell types which contain very low numbers of IGF-I receptors. Under these conditions, however, very high IGF-I concentrations are required that are unlikely to occur in vivo.

Introduction

Intravenous injections of IGF-I lead to hypoglycemic responses with potencies that are 5—7% of those observed with insulin. This finding in several mammalian species, together with other insulin-like short-term effects of IGF-I and the observation that IGF-I binds to the insulin receptor, albeit weakly, has led to the view that IGF-I exerts its "metabolic" effects via the insulin receptor. Further support for this hypothesis has been based on measurements showing that much higher concentrations of IGF-I are required to stimulate metabolic effects in adipocytes than found with insulin, while the reverse applies to growth effects in fibroblasts [1]. A corollary of these findings has been a search for analogues of IGF-I that bind less well than IGF-I to the insulin receptor, on the assumption that such analogues will produce a lesser degree of hypoglycemia than IGF-I and, hence, will have greater therapeutic potential.

Address for correspondence: F.J. Ballard MD, CRC for Tissue Growth and Repair, P.O. Box 10065, Gouger Street, Adelaide, SA 5000, Australia.

In this overview, we have examined the evidence on whether IGF-I ever acts through the insulin receptor, including results obtained both with cultured cells and in vivo. Since insulin binds to the type 1 IGF receptor (henceforth termed the IGF-I receptor) with approximately the same relative affinity as IGF-I to the insulin receptor, we also comment on the related question: "Does insulin ever act through the IGF-I receptor?"

The insulin receptor family

The insulin and IGF-I receptors are tetrameric proteins consisting of two ligand-binding α subunits which are linked by disulphide bonds to two transmembrane β subunits that possess intrinsic tyrosine kinase activity. The two receptors share 50% sequence homology and exhibit a remarkably similar range of metabolic and growth actions when stimulated by their respective ligands [2]. The two receptors show limited cross specificities in that insulin or IGF-I bind with 0.1 to 1% affinities to the heterologous receptor [2]. Atypical insulin receptors have also been described that demonstrate relatively greater IGF-I binding [3]. Although the molecular nature of the atypical insulin receptor has not been established, a hybrid receptor has been described that is comprised of αβ halves of the insulin receptor assembled into a tetramer with αβ halves of the IGF-I receptor. Recently the binding characteristics of the insulin, IGF-I and hybrid receptors, have been compared after each had been affinity purified. Interestingly, the hybrid receptor behaved very similarly to IGF-I receptors with respect to IGF-I binding and competition by IGF-I or insulin, while insulin binding was approximately 10-fold lower than to the insulin receptor. These results suggest that the hybrids are more responsive to IGF-I than to insulin under physiological conditions [4].

The responses produced following insulin or IGF-I binding differ between cell types, but include "metabolic" effects such as stimulation of glucose uptake, amino acid uptake, glycogen deposition and lipogenesis as well as the inhibition of gluconeogenesis and lipolysis. Longer term "growth" responses are stimulations of protein and DNA synthesis, an inhibition of protein breakdown and differentiation functions such as the induction of specific enzymes. Although the "metabolic" effects have traditionally been recognised as more typical of insulin and the "growth" effects more typical of IGF-I, the receptor specificities do not themselves provide information as to whether IGF-I ever exerts its metabolic effects via the insulin receptor or perhaps via a hybrid receptor. Another receptor, the insulin receptor-related receptor, can probably be eliminated from consideration, because although it has considerable sequence homology to the IGF-I and insulin receptors [5], it does not appear to bind with either insulin or IGF-I [6].

IGF-I and insulin actions on isolated cells

A number of approaches have been explored using isolated cells to resolve the

Table 1. Summary of cell culture evidence that the "metabolic" effects of IGF-I are generally mediated via the IGF-I receptor rather than the insulin receptor

Experiment	Reference
Antibodies against the IGF-I receptor block both "growth" and "metabolic" effects of IGF-I in some cells and mimic both classes of effects in others.	J.S. Flier et al. [7] R.L. Chaiken et al. [8] H. Kato et al. [11]
Cells transfected with IGF-I receptors exhibit enhanced "metabolic" effects.	G. Steele-Perkins et al. [12] H. Kato et al. [11]
Cells that show poor insulin sensitivity exhibit potent IGF-I "metabolic" effects.	P.J. Bilan et al. [14]
IGF-I "metabolic" effects are normal in cells with insulin receptor defects.	T. Sasaoka et al. [16] J.A. Maassen et al. [17]
Down-regulation of the insulin receptor desensitises insulin, but not IGF-I effects.	M. Cascieri et al. [15]
Antibodies against the insulin receptor block insulin, but not IGF-I effects.	T. Kadowaki et al. [10]

question as to whether IGF-I exerts its "metabolic" effects via the insulin or IGF-I receptor. One method involves measurements of "metabolic" and "growth" effects of IGF-I made in the presence of the antibody αIR-3 that blocks IGF-I binding to the IGF-I receptor, but not binding to the insulin receptor. In several cell types this antibody has been shown to inhibit both IGF-I "metabolic" and "growth" responses, but to have minimal effects on insulin action except when the hormone was added at very high concentrations [7–10]. In cells with stably transfected IGF-I receptors, both "metabolic" and "growth" effects of IGF-I were inhibited by αIR-3 [11]. We note that this study and an earlier one [12] demonstrate enhanced "metabolic" effects of IGF-I in cells with additional transfected IGF-I receptors (Table 1). On the other hand, αIR-3 did not inhibit IGF-I or insulin mediated glucose transport in adipocytes [11]. These results can be reconciled because adipocytes require about 1000-fold higher concentrations of IGF-I than insulin to produce comparable responses, consistent with IGF-I acting through the insulin receptor in this insulin hypersensitive cell type. Likewise the blocking of insulin effects by αIR-3 at extremely high insulin concentrations in fibroblasts [8] is consistent with insulin acting through the IGF-I receptor under these conditions.

Experiments that examined insulin and IGF-I mediated responses after blocking the insulin receptor gave analogous results. Thus insulin, but not IGF-I, induced short-term effects that were blocked as expected in carcinoma cells [10], while the actions of both factors were inhibited in adipocytes [11], presumably because the effects are via the insulin receptor.

Cells that show poor insulin sensitivity exhibit potent IGF-I "metabolic" effects, as shown in L6 myoblasts [14] and in BC3H1 myocytes in which the insulin receptor had been down regulated [15]. In the latter experiment the insulin stimulation of glucose uptake was substantially blunted. Together these results are not consistent with IGF-I acting via the insulin receptor. A further approach which leads to the same conclusion involves the use of cells derived from patients with insulin receptor defects. Specifically, in two studies in which insulin and IGF-I effects on glucose and amino acid transport were compared in fibroblasts isolated from severely insulin-resistant Leprechaunism patients, insulin, but not IGF-I-mediated effects, were blunted [16,17].

Hypersensitive insulin responses have been established for a range of metabolic and growth effects in the rat H35 hepatoma. Half maximum insulin effects are observed at pM concentrations, while 1000-fold higher concentrations of IGF-I are required to elicit equivalent effects [18]. The IGF-I responses in these cells are clearly exerted through the insulin receptor because the IGF-I receptor is not present [19]. We note that in this cell line the "growth" effects of insulin occur following binding to the insulin receptor [19].

We have recently compared the relative potencies of insulin, IGF-I and IGF-I analogues to compete for insulin binding to the H35 hepatoma receptor and to inhibit intracellular protein breakdown. The results (Table 2) not only confirm the earlier experiments showing extreme poor IGF-I binding and potency, but establish that analogues of IGF-I, which do not associate with IGF binding proteins, retain the very low potency of IGF-I. Thus the insensitivity to IGF-I cannot be the result of the cells producing large amounts of binding proteins which would sequester the growth factor.

Table 2 also includes a series of experiments in which the area under the plasma glucose curve was measured after the administration of insulin, IGF-I, LR^3IGF-I, R^3IGF-I and des(1−3)IGF-I to conscious pigs. The hypoglycemic response produced by the three analogues which associate poorly with IGF binding proteins is far greater than the relative potencies of the analogues when acting via the insulin receptor. This difference argues that the "metabolic" effects of IGF-I are not mediated via that receptor.

Table 2. The relative hypoglycemic potencies of IGF-I, IGF-I analogs and insulin related to their binding and actions mediated through the insulin receptor

Peptide	Relative hypoglycemic effect[a]	Insulin receptor IC_{50} (nM)	Insulin receptor mediated action[b] ED_{50} (pM)
Insulin	100	0.24	5.1
IGF-I	5.5	130	3000
LR^3IGF-I	19	105	550
R^3IGF-I	21	120	530
Des(1-3)IGF-I	23	120	760

[a]Measured after intravenous injection of a bolus to pigs. [b]Inhibition of protein breakdown in H35 hepatoma cells.

Table 3. In streptozotocin diabetic rats both IGF-I and insulin restore growth and N-balance to normal, while only insulin ameliorates aspects of carbohydrate, lipid and protein metabolism

Measurement	Untreated	Insulin (1.2 mg/kg/d)	IGF-I (4.6 mg/kg/d)
N-retention (g/7 day)	0.73 ± 0.18	1.73 ± 0.17[a]	1.55 ± 0.07[a]
Glucose excretion (mmol, day 7)	106.1 ± 10.8	1.3 ± 0.8[b]	109.5 ± 4.2
Plasma glucose (mM, day 7)	22.9 ± 0.5	9.6 ± 3.3[a]	21.6 ± 0.6
3-MH excretion (μmol/kg/d, days 6 and 7)	9.1 ± 0.5	7.1 ± 0.4[a]	10.2 ± 0.5
Carcass fat (g/kg)	37.6 ± 2.8	92.5 ± 4.8[b]	30.0 ± 2.5

[a] $p < 0.01$; [b] $p < 0.001$ vs. untreated group.

IGF-I and insulin effects in diabetic rats

IGF-I has been shown to restore the weight gain of streptozotocin diabetic rats to the same extent as observed with insulin [20,21]. In both studies plasma glucose was approximately normalised by insulin, but not affected by IGF-I. In addition to this difference, glucosuria was almost completely prevented by insulin, while the rate of muscle protein breakdown as assessed by 3-methylhistidine (3-MH) excretion was reduced by insulin. Carcass fat was substantially increased by insulin. IGF-I was ineffective in every one of these measurements, even though it produced the same degree of overall anabolic response (Table 3).

We have carried out another experiment which was designed to test whether IGF-I and insulin exerted additive or synergistic effects in diabetic rats. This study was similar to that reported by Tomas et al. [21] except that insulin was administered subcutaneously via osmotic pumps, i.e., in the same way as IGF-I. The experiment confirmed the differences shown in Table 3 and in addition identified several other effects (Fig. 1) that are incompatible with insulin and IGF-I acting through a common receptor.

The body weight change produced by a very high dose of IGF-I, 500 μg/d, was not quite as good as that obtained with 85 μg insulin/d (Fig. 1), while partly additive effects were seen at suboptimal insulin doses. The weights of epididymal fat pads in these male rats were markedly increased following insulin administration, but only negligible effects were observed with IGF-I alone and none when IGF-I was infused at the same time as insulin.

Perhaps the most interesting changes in tissue weights were noted with liver and kidney (Fig. 1). Thus, fractional liver weights were increased by insulin, whereas IGF-I either produced no effect or led to slight decreases. The opposite applied to the kidney, an organ whose weight was decreased by insulin, but increased by IGF-I (Fig. 1).

Spleen and thymus weights have been shown to increase markedly when IGF-I was administered to rats under a number of physiological conditions [22,23]. Here we see that both IGF-I and insulin increased the fractional weights of these tissues (Fig. 1), but that the response produced by insulin was generally less than by

136

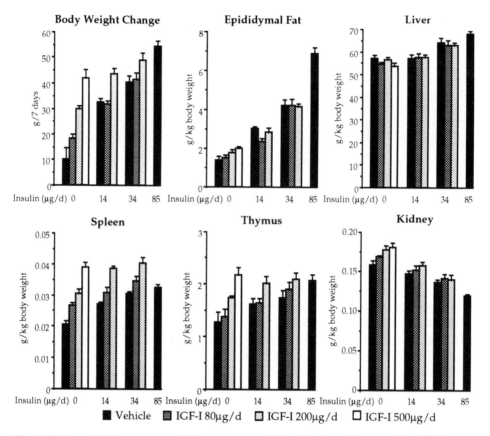

Fig. 1. Body weight changes over a 7-day treatment period and fractional tissue weights following the administration of IGF-I, insulin or combinations of the two factors to streptozotocin diabetic rats. The experiment was carried out as described previously [21] except that both insulin and IGF-I were infused by osmotic pumps.

IGF-I. Although not shown in Fig. 1, the plasma concentration of IGF-I was increased following insulin administration, so that the effects on thymus and spleen could have been secondary to increases in plasma IGF-I.

The mechanisms responsible for the divergent responses produced by insulin and IGF-I on diabetic rats remain unknown. However, it seems likely that the lack of IGF-I effect on fat deposition or on blood glucose may be a consequence of low IGF-I receptor numbers in adipose tissue and liver. While IGF-I must surely be increasing tissue glucose uptake in order to achieve a substantial increase in body growth, hepatic glucose output may not be altered. If IGF-I did bind significantly to insulin receptors that are abundant in these tissues, we would have expected insulin-like responses. The inability of IGF-I to inhibit muscle protein breakdown in diabetic rats is more puzzling, because IGF-I can markedly reduce 3-MH excretion under other conditions [24].

IGF-I and insulin effects during insulin-resistant states

Studies of insulin-resistant states in both rats and humans provide strong evidence that IGF-I can elicit "metabolic" effects other than through the insulin receptor. Thus Jacob et al. [25] and Rossetti et al. [26] showed that IGF-I administration to insulin-resistant rats was able to stimulate glucose uptake from the blood to the same extent as in normal animals. The insulin response was severely impaired.

Likewise the administration of IGF-I to patients with the insulin-resistant conditions of Mendenhall's syndrome [27], type A insulin resistance [28,29], diabetic ketoacidosis [30] and Leprechaunism [29] produced at least partial amelioration of their hyperglycemia, although the rates of glucose utilization may have been lower than in normal subjects [28].

Conclusions

Most of the experiments in cultured cells and in vivo argue that the receptor responsible for mediating the "metabolic" effects of IGF-I is the IGF-I receptor. The exceptions are cells such as adipocytes and the rat H35 hepatoma, which are both hypersensitive to insulin and have sparse or absent IGF-I receptors. In these cells IGF-I acts via the insulin receptor, but only at extremely high concentrations. Recent genetic evidence from IGF-I and IGF-I receptor gene knockout mice confirms our conclusion, because animals with IGF-I and IGF-I receptor double mutants have phenotypes that are indistinguishable [31]. If IGF-I had been acting through a second receptor, the authors reason that the phenotype of the double mutant should have been more severe.

References

1. King GL, Kahn CR. Nature 1981;292:644–646.
2. Czech MP, Annu Rev Physiol 1985;47:357–381.
3. Jonas HA, Cox AJ, Harrison LC. Biochem J 1989;257:101–107.
4. Soos MA, Field CE, Siddle K. Biochem J 1992;290:419–426.
5. Shier P, Watt VM. J Biol Chem 1989;264:14605–14608.
6. Zhang B, Roth RA. J Biol Chem 1992;267:18320–18328.
7. Flier JS, Usher P, Moses AC. Proc Natl Acad Sci USA 1986;83:664–668.
8. Chaiken RL, Moses AC, Usher P, Flier JS. J Clin Endocrinol Metab 1986;63:1181–1185.
9. Furlanetto RW, DiCarlo JN, Wisehart C. J Clin Endocrinol Metab 1987;64:1142–1149.
10. Kadowaki T, Koyasu S, Nishida E, Sakai H, Takaku F, Yahara I, Kasuga M. J Biol Chem 1986;261: 16141–16147.
11. Kato H. Faria TN, Stannard B, Roberts CT Jr, Le Roith D. J Biol Chem 1993;268:2655–2661.
12. Steele-Perkins G, Turner J, Edman JC, Hari J, Pierce SB, Stover C, Rutter WJ, Roth RA. J Biol Chem 1988;263:11486–11492.
13. Sinha MK, Buchanan C, Leggett N, Martin L, Khazanie PG, DiMarchi R, Pories WJ, Caro JF. Diabetes 1989;38:1217–1225.
14. Bilan PJ, Mitsumoto Y, Ramlal T, Klip A. FEBS Lett 1992;298:285–290.

138

15. Cascieri MA, Chicchi GC, Hayes NS, Strader CD. Biochim Biophys Acta 1986;886:491—499.
16. Sasaoka T, Kobayashi M, Takata Y, Ishibashi O, Iwasaki M, Shigeta Y, Goji K, Hisatomi A. Diabetes 1988;37:1515—1523.
17. Maassen JA, van der Zon GCM. Eur J Biochem 1990;190:553—557.
18. Gunn JM, Clark MG, Knowles SE, Hopgood MF, Ballard FJ. Nature 1977;266:58—60.
19. Mottola C, Czech MP. J Biol Chem 1984;259:12705—12713.
20. Scheiwiller E, Guler H-P, Merryweather J, Scandella C, Maerki W, Zapf J, Froesch ER. Nature 1986; 323:169—171.
21. Tomas FM, Knowles SE, Owens PC, Chandler CS, Francis GL, Ballard FJ. Biochem J 1993;291: 781—786.
22. Guler H-P, Zapf J, Scheiwiller E, Froesch ER. Proc Natl Acad Sci USA 1988;85:4889—4893.
23. Ballard FJ, Tomas FM, Read LC, Knowles SE, Owens PC, Lemmey AB, Martin AA, Wells JRE, Wallace JC, Francis GL. In: Spencer EM (ed) Modern Concepts of Insulin-like Growth Factors. New York: Elsevier, 1991;617—627.
24. Tomas FM, Knowles SE, Owens PC, Chandler CS, Francis GL, Read LC, Ballard FJ. Biochem J 1992;282:91—97.
25. Jacob RJ, Sherwin RS, Bowen L, Fryburg D, Fagin KD, Tamborlane WV, Shulman GI. Am J Physiol 1991;260:E262—E268.
26. Rossetti L, Frontini S, DiMarchi R, DeFronzo RA, Giaccara A. Diabetes 1991;40:444—448.
27. Quin JD, Fisher BM, Paterson KR, Inoue A, Beastall GH, MacCuish AC. N Engl J Med 1990; 323:1425—1426.
28. Schoenle EJ, Zenobi PD, Torresani T, Werder EA, Zachmann M, Froesch ER. Diabetologia 1991; 34:675—679.
29. Kuzuya H, Matsura N, Sakamoto M, Makino H, Sakamoto Y, Kadowaki T, Suzuki Y, Kobayashi M, Akazawa Y, Nomura M, Yoshimasa Y, Kasuga M, Goji K, Nagataki S, Oyasu H, Imura H. Diabetes 1993;42:696—705.
30. Usala A-L, Madigan T, Burguera B, Sinha MK, Caro JF, Cunningham P, Powell JG, Butler PC. N Engl J Med 1992;327:853—857.
31. Liu J-P, Baker J, Perkins AS, Robertson EJ, Efstratiadis A. Cell 1993;75:59—72.

Binding proteins

Similarities in the regulation of hIGFBP-1 and PEPCK gene expression

David R. Powell, Phillip D.K. Lee and Adisak Suwanichkul

Department of Pediatrics, Baylor College of Medicine, Houston, TX 77030, USA

Abstract. Regulation of human insulin-like growth factor binding protein-1 (hIGFBP-1) expression is similar to that of phosphoenolpyruvate carboxykinase (PEPCK), a key enzyme in gluconeogenesis. Both genes are expressed primarily in liver and kidney. As with PEPCK, hepatic expression of hIGFBP-1 is regulated by multiple hormones primarily at the level of transcription and many *cis* elements important to this regulation are located in the first 460 basepairs (bp) 5' to the transcription start site. Comparison of their organization and function suggests that the PEPCK and hIGFBP-1 promoters use similar *cis* elements and *trans*-acting factors in a different spatial organization to achieve similar effects.

Introduction

Insulin-like growth factor binding protein-1 (IGFBP-1) is a soluble 25 kDa protein which binds IGFs with high affinity [1]. Hepatocytes are the primary source of circulating hIGFBP-1. Levels of hIGFBP-1 fluctuate during the day, rising during a fast and falling with meals [1]. This regulation is probably the result of hormonal influences [1], since cortisol raises [2], while insulin inhibits [3,4] serum hIGFBP-1 levels. In rats, glucocorticoids increase hepatic IGFBP-1 expression, while in diabetic animals insulin lowers this expression [5,6]. In cultured hepatocytes, IGFBP-1 expression is inhibited by insulin [7—12], but is stimulated by dexamethasone [7,8,13] and by agents which mimic glucagon by raising intracellular cAMP levels [7,9,10,14]. This pattern is similar to the multihormonal regulation of hepatic PEPCK, a key enzyme in gluconeogenesis [15—17] and suggests that IGFBP-1 participates in glucose counterregulation. The recent demonstration that IGFBP-1 infusion into rats results in a transient rise in serum glucose levels, [18] supports this hypothesis and implies that an important function of IGFBP-1 is to bind serum IGFs and thereby block IGF-mediated glucose uptake during fasting.

The multihormonal regulation of IGFBP-1 expression is at the level of transcription [8,10,11—14], similar to that shown for PEPCK [19]. This suggests that the effects of these hormones on hIGFBP-1 transcription may be conferred by *cis* elements located in the first few hundred bp 5' to the transcription start site, as

Address for correspondence: David R. Powell, Texas Children's Hospital, Clinical Care Center, MC# 3-2482, 6621 Fannin St., Houston, TX 77030, USA.

occurs with PEPCK transcription [20–23]. This manuscript compares and contrasts what is known about the organization and function of the PEPCK and hIGFBP-1 promoters and concludes that these two promoters use similar *cis* elements and *trans*-acting factors in a different spatial organization to achieve similar effects.

Experimental procedures

Plasmid constructs

A 1.3 kilobase (kb) fragment of human genomic DNA which contains sequence spanning from −1205 to +68 bp relative to the hIGFBP-1 mRNA capsite was inserted into the promoterless pCAT(An) vector to create p1205CAT as described previously [24]. Plasmid pRShGRα [25], which expresses human glucocorticoid receptor (hGR) under the control of the Rous Sarcoma Virus long terminal repeat (RSV LTR), was kindly provided by Dr. Ronald M. Evans, The Salk Institute for Biological Studies, La Jolla, CA, USA. Plasmid pPKA [14,26], which expresses the catalytic subunit of cAMP-dependent protein kinase A (PKA), was kindly provided by Dr. Masa-aki Muramatsu, University of Tokyo, Tokyo, Japan. Plasmid pPEPCKCAT, constructed as described previously [26], was a generous gift of Dr. Richard W. Hanson, Case Western Reserve University, Cleveland, OH. The CCAAT/Enhancer Binding Protein (C/EBP)α expression vector was constructed as described [27].

Cell culture and DNA transfection

Maintenance and transfection of HEP G2 human hepatoma cells has been described [24,28]. Cells were transfected with 5 μg of chloramphenicol acetyltransferase (CAT) plasmid containing hIGFBP-1 promoter fragments and with 1 μg of the hGR expression vector pRShGRα. One μg of pRSVL plasmid, which contains the RSV LTR upstream to the luciferase reporter gene [29], was cotransfected to control for transfection efficiency. Some cells were also transfected with 4 μg of either pPKA or a control vector, as described previously [14], or with 2 μg of either C/EBPα expression vector or a control vector. Transfected cells were washed in phosphate-buffered saline (PBS) and then incubated with serum-free medium (Dulbecco's modified Eagle's medium supplemented with 5 mM L-glutamine, 50 units/ml penicillin, and 50 μg/ml streptomycin) ± dexamethasone (Sigma) and insulin (kindly provided by Eli Lilly Co.).

CAT and luciferase assays

CAT assays were performed by the method of Gorman et al. [30], and luciferase assays were performed by the method of de Wet et al. [29], as described previously [24].

Preparation of nuclear extracts

Nuclear extracts were prepared from $1-3 \times 10^8$ HEP G2 cells harvested after a 2 h incubation in serum-free medium, as described previously [28]. The extract was divided into 100 μl aliquots and then stored in liquid N_2.

Gel mobility shift assay

The 33-bp DNA fragment AB, which encodes the native IGFBP-1 promoter sequence from −124 to −97 bp and contains the putative insulin responsive element (IRE), was released from plasmid pTKCAT with *Bam*HI [28]. This fragment was labeled with [α-^{32}P]dATP using Klenow polymerase. The probe was purified in a 6% non-denaturing polyacrylamide gel, cut out and then eluted at room temperature for 2 h in 10 mM Tris HCl, pH 8.0, 1 mM EDTA, 50 mM NaCl.

One fmol of AB probe was incubated at room temperature with 2 μl nuclear extract, 3 μg poly(dG-dC) and with either a 200-fold excess of single-stranded (ss) oligonucleotide AB, ss oligonucleotide ABas, or concatamerized double-stranded (ds) DNA fragment AB, in 4 mM Tris-HCl, 12.5 mM HEPES, pH 7.9, 1 mM EDTA, 1 mM dithiothreitol, 12.5% glycerol and 198 mM KCl; the total volume was 15 μl. After a 30 min incubation, the mixture was separated on a 6% nondenaturing polyacrylamide gel using a high ionic strength Tris-glycine [31] gel buffer. Electrophoresis was carried out for 1 h at 225V, after which the gels were dried and autoradiographed.

Results and Discussion

The role of HNF-1

Cis elements and *trans*-acting factors which may participate in hIGFBP-1 and PEPCK gene transcription are shown schematically in Fig. 1. Some are involved in basal or

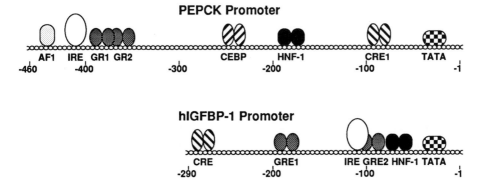

Fig. 1. Schematic representation of *cis* elements and *trans*-acting factors which may participate in hIGFBP-1 and PEPCK gene transcription. See text for details.

tissue-specific expression of these genes, while others confer the regulatory effects of cAMP, glucocorticoids and/or insulin to hIGFBP-1 and PEPCK gene transcription.

HNF-1 is a transcription factor, expressed primarily in liver and kidney, which transactivates the promoters of many genes expressed in these two tissues; indeed, this finding suggests that HNF-1 is one of a few master regulatory proteins required to produce the hepatic phenotype [32]. An HNF-1 binding site located from −79 to −53 bp 5′ to the hIGFBP-1 transcription start site, is absolutely required for activity of hIGFBP-1 promoter constructs transfected into HEP G2 cells [24]. Further studies have found that HNF-1 activates transcription of the hIGFBP-1 promoter through this *cis* element [33]. In addition, an HNF-1 binding site is located ~200 bp 5′ to the PEPCK transcription start site, well within the PEPCK promoter region which is sufficient to confer tissue-specific expression to a reporter gene in transgenic mice [34]. These observations suggest that HNF-1 may play a significant role in the liver- and kidney-specific expression of IGFBP-1 and PEPCK genes.

The effect of cAMP (glucagon)

Incubating cultured hepatocytes with cAMP and/or cAMP analogues increases IGFBP-1 protein levels, mRNA levels and activity of a construct containing the first 1205 bp of the hIGFBP-1 promoter [7,10,14]. The same effects were observed in HEP G2 cells, overexpressing the catalytic subunit of cAMP-dependent PKA, the protein which mediates the intracellular effects of cAMP [14,35]. It is likely that cAMP is a second messenger for glucagon; in support of this hypothesis, glucagon raises IGFBP-1 protein levels in medium conditioned by human fetal liver explants [9].

A series of deletion and site-directed mutations of the hIGFBP-1 promoter have identified a cAMP response element (CRE) which confers a modest 2- to 3-fold increase in hIGFBP-1 promoter activity brought about by PKA or cAMP + theophylline [14]. This element, located from −273 to −249 bp 5′ to the transcription start site, binds CRE binding protein or CREB (Fig. 1), and mutations which block CREB binding also diminish cAMP- or PKA-mediated increases in hIGFBP-1 promoter activity. CREB has also been implicated in conferring the effect of cAMP to the PEPCK promoter. CRE1, located ~90 bp 5′ to the PEPCK transcription start site (Fig. 1), binds CREB and by itself confers a modest 2- to 3-fold increase in promoter activity brought about by cAMP or PKA in HEP G2 cells [26], similar to the effect observed with the hIGFBP-1 CRE.

Unlike the hIGFBP-1 promoter, the PEPCK promoter contains elements in addition to the CREB binding site which contribute to the ~30-fold rise in promoter activity mediated by cAMP. The most important of these elements is located ~240 bp 5′ to the transcription start site and binds C/EBPα [26]. C/EBPα can be shown to confer the cAMP effect to the PEPCK promoter, which it binds at −240 bp and also at CRE1, which has a 7/8 bp match with the consensus C/EBP sequence [26]. Despite this role in cAMP-mediated activation of the PEPCK promoter, C/EBPα does not appear to activate the hIGFBP-1 promoter. HEP G2 cells transfected with the hIGFBP-1 promoter construct p1205CAT and cotransfected with the C/EBPα expression vector had only 80 ± 27% of the promoter activity of control cells not expressing C/EBPα, while additional cells transfected with the PEPCK promoter showed a 4-fold rise in activity in the presence of C/EBPα (N = 3 independent experiments). This failure of C/EBPα to stimulate hIGFBP-1 results partly from the fact that the hIGFBP-1 CRE has only a 5/8 bp match with the consensus C/EBP sequence [14].

The effect of glucocorticoids

Glucocorticoids raise serum IGFBP-1 protein levels and, in rats, raise hepatic IGFBP-1 mRNA levels [2,5]. In rat H4IIE hepatoma cells, the synthetic glucocorticoid dexamethasone raises IGFBP-1 protein and mRNA levels [7,8,11] by stimulating a 4.6- to 7.5-fold rise in IGFBP-1 gene transcription [8,11]. These increases are comparable to the dexamethasone-mediated rise in activity of IGFBP-1 promoter construct p1205CAT when this construct is cotransfected into HEP G2 cells with plasmid pRShGRα, which overexpresses the glucocorticoid receptor (GR), suggesting that DNA elements conferring glucocorticoid stimulation to the hIGFBP-1 promoter reside in the first 1205 bp 5′ to the transcription start site (Suwanichkul A, Morris SL, Allander SV, Powell DR; manuscript submitted).

Glucocorticoids regulate gene transcription by forming hormone-GR complexes which bind, apparently as dimers, to glucocorticoid response elements (GREs) with consensus sequence (T/G)GTACAnnnTGTTCT [36,37]. This binding then stimulates transcription, apparently by permitting the transactivation domain(s) of the GR to contact components of the initiation complex involved in basal transcription and perhaps also by permitting the GR to alter chromatin structure [37–39].

Recent studies identified two GREs which bind GR and are necessary to confer the effect of dexamethasone to the hIGFBP-1 promoter (Fig. 1); interestingly, loss of either GRE1 or GRE2 results in complete loss of promoter response to dexamethasone (Suwanichkul A, Morris SL, Allander SV, Powell DR; manuscript submitted). Many genes including PEPCK require multiple GREs to confer the effect of glucocorticoids, particularly if the GREs reside far from the transcription start site, and the likely cooperative interaction between GRE1 and GRE2 is also well described for multiple GREs in other genes [22,36,40,41]. The striking loss of dexamethasone effect after elimination of either GRE1 or GRE2 is unusual, but reminiscent of the significant loss of dexamethasone effect observed when either GR1 or GR2 of the PEPCK promoter (Fig. 1) was deleted [22]. This dramatic loss of activity may be explained by the fact that these four GRE sequences differ markedly from consensus, which may lead to binding affinities which are too low to allow transactivation from a single GRE.

An IRE which confers insulin inhibition of basal IGFBP-1 promoter activity [27], may also be necessary for maximal glucocorticoid stimulation (Suwanichkul A, Morris SL, Allander SV, Powell DR; manuscript submitted). This is similar to other genes where glucocorticoid/GR/GRE complexes must interact with other *trans*-acting

146

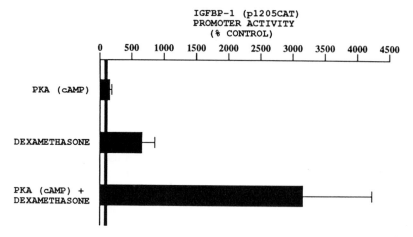

Fig. 2. Synergistic activation of hIGFBP-1 promoter construct p1205CAT by cAMP and glucocorticoids. HEP G2 cells were cotransfected with p1205CAT and with the GR expression vector pRShGRα. Some plates were also cotransfected with a vector expressing PKA, which reproduces the effects of cAMP. Plates were incubated ± 0.1 µM dexamethasone for 18 h, after which hIGFBP-1 promoter activity was estimated by assaying cellular protein for CAT activity. The effect of dexamethasone and/or PKA (cAMP) is presented as % control value, with control values emphasized as a solid black line at 100%. Estimates of hIGFBP-1 promoter activity represent the mean ± SD of three independent experiments.

factors bound to specific *cis* elements to achieve a maximal glucocorticoid-mediated increase in gene transcription [22,42–44]. In the case of the PEPCK gene, maximal glucocorticoid effect requires not only GR1 and GR2, but also accessory factor 1 (AF1) and AF2 elements and the proteins which they bind [22]; of interest, AF2 has been identified as an IRE [21,45], further increasing the similarity between the hIGFBP-1 and PEPCK promoters. The ability of other factors to act synergistically with the glucocorticoid/GR/GRE complex may depend on the sequence of the GRE [44]. Thus, GREs, such as GRE1 and GRE2 which have sequence quite different from consensus, may require that additional transcription factors help to stabilize glucocorticoid/GR/GRE binding before glucocorticoids can stimulate a significant increase in gene transcription.

The effect of cAMP/glucocorticoid combination

As shown in Fig. 2, the combination of dexamethasone and PKA (cAMP) results in a 3-fold greater stimulation of hIGFBP-1 promoter activity than the sum of individual dexamethasone and PKA stimulatory effects. This synergism was also noted when HEP G2 cells were incubated with dexamethasone ± cAMP and theophylline, and affected not only promoter activity, but also levels of hIGFBP-1 protein in conditioned medium [46]. These results differ from those observed with PEPCK, where the effects of dexamethasone and cAMP on gene transcription [19] and promoter activity [20] appeared to be additive rather than synergistic. However, the results are of interest in light of recent studies showing that maximal glucocorticoid stimulation of PEPCK promoter activity cannot be achieved in the absence of the CREB binding site at ~–90 bp, an affect which may require a protein-protein interaction between CREB and GR [47].

The effect of insulin

Serum levels of hIGFBP-1 inversely correlate with insulin levels and this insulin effect appears to dominate over the stimulatory effects of glucocorticoids and glucagon [1,3,4]. In diabetic rats, insulin lowers IGFBP-1 expression by rapidly decreasing the rate of hepatic gene transcription [6,48]. These observations are supported by in vitro studies using cultured hepatocytes, which show that the effects of insulin dominate over those of cAMP and dexamethasone and that insulin acts by inhibiting IGFBP-1 gene transcription [7–12,46].

Transfection studies in HEP G2 cells originally showed that elements conferring the inhibitory effect of insulin are present in the first 1205 bp of the hIGFBP-1 promoter [10]. Recent studies found that the ability of insulin to inhibit basal hIGFBP-1 promoter activity is conferred through a 25 bp region, which is 100% conserved in rat and mouse promoters and which has two A–T rich, 8 bp elements exhibiting dyad symmetry [27]. These two 8 bp sequences were designated the A element (–118 CAAAACAA –111) and the B element (–108 TTATTTTG –101). Site-directed mutagenesis of both the A and B elements of this IRE in the same 1205 bp hIGFBP-1 promoter construct abolished the inhibitory effect of insulin on promoter activity; in addition the native IRE, but not the AB mutant, conferred the inhibitory effect of insulin on the heterologous thymidine kinase (TK) promoter [27]. Gel mobility shift assay identified an IRE binding protein (IREBP) in HEP G2 nuclear extract which specifically binds the native, but not the mutant IRE. In Fig. 3, a gel mobility shift assay shows this IREBP binding to a 33 bp DNA probe containing the 25 bp hIGFBP-1 IRE, and demonstrates that the IREBP can be competed off by a 200-fold excess of ds, concatamerized IRE, but not by a similar excess of ss sense or antisense IRE oligonucleotides. A second protein, tentatively designated nonspecific binding protein (NSBP)2, will require further study since it, too, may be specifically competed by the IRE.

Recent studies indicate that the hIGFBP-1 IRE can confer the entire inhibitory effect of insulin on glucocorticoid-mediated increases in hIGFBP-1 promoter activity (Suwanichkul A, Morris SL, Allander SV, Powell DR; manuscript submitted). These studies used constructs containing deletion and site-directed mutations of the IRE to show that both the A and B elements of the IRE are required to confer maximal inhibition by insulin and that most of this inhibition is conferred by the A element alone; a similar trend was noted in studies looking at inhibition of basal promoter activity by insulin [27]. As mentioned above, these studies also suggested that the IRE is necessary for maximal stimulation of the hIGFBP-1 promoter by gluco-corticoids. The importance of the IRE in glucocorticoid action is consistent with the central location of the IRE between GRE1 and GRE2 (Fig. 1).

148

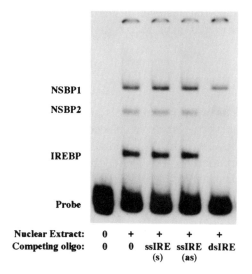

Nuclear Extract:	0	+	+	+	+
Competing oligo:	0	0	ssIRE	ssIRE	dsIRE
			(s)	(as)	

Fig. 3. IREBP binds to ds but not ss DNA encoding the hIGFBP-1 IRE: Gel mobility shift assay. The 33 bp DNA fragment AB, which encodes native IGFBP-1 promoter sequence from −124 to −97 bp and contains the IRE, was labeled with [α-^{32}P]dATP and used as probe. One fmol of AB probe was incubated at room temperature without (0) or with (+) HEP G2 nuclear extract, and without (0) or with a 200-fold excess of either ss sense oligonucleotide AB (ssIRE (s)), ss antisense oligonucleotide ABas (ssIRE (as)), or ds and concatamerized DNA fragment AB (dsIRE). Samples were separated, and the gel treated, as was described in Experimental procedures. NSBP1 and NSBP2, nonspecific binding proteins 1 and 2.

An IRE has been identified in the PEPCK promoter (Fig. 1) which allows insulin to partially inhibit glucocorticoid- and cAMP-mediated stimulation of PEPCK promoter activity in H4IIE cells [21,45]. The PEPCK and hIGFBP-1 IREs shares several characteristics:
— the sequence of the 10 bp PEPCK IRE (−416 TGGTGTTTTG −407) shares 7 and 6 bp, respectively, with the A and B elements of the hIGFBP-1 IRE. Thus, not only is the hIGFBP-1 A element more responsive to insulin than the B element, it is also more closely related to the PEPCK IRE. It seems likely that the PEPCK IRE and IGFBP-1 A element share important determinants allowing them to bind specific proteins needed to confer the inhibitory effect of insulin;
— as with the hIGFBP-1 IRE, the PEPCK IRE can confer the inhibitory effect of insulin to the TK promoter [21];
— as with the hIGFBP-1 IRE, the PEPCK IRE is required for maximal promoter stimulation by glucocorticoids [22]; and
— the protein which confers the insulin effect to either promoter is unknown.
Multiple proteins bind the PEPCK IRE [21], but none have been identified as a likely candidate to confer insulin inhibition, and the IREBP is not yet characterized. It is possible that the responsible protein has not yet been visualized due to characteristics (weak or heterodimeric binding; low abundance; lability) which have made detection difficult with the techniques employed to date.

Current understanding of the mechanisms behind the tissue-specific and hormonal regulation of hIGFBP-1 and PEPCK gene transcription is limited. However, comparison of hIGFBP-1 and PEPCK promoter structure and function suggests that these promoters have converged during evolution, retaining similar *cis* elements and *trans*-acting factors which, despite a somewhat different spatial organization, interact to achieve a similar overall regulation in liver and kidney by glucocorticoids, cAMP and insulin. In fact, the *cis* elements may share unusual characteristics which allow unique function. For example, weak GREs may be essential in such promoters to allow insulin inhibition; otherwise, a strong GRE might preferentially confer glucocorticoid stimulation which cannot be overcome by insulin. At present, it appears that the IREs are central to the hormonal regulation of each promoter. Thus, further insight into the regulation of hIGFBP-1 and PEPCK gene transcription will be best achieved by characterizing the IRE binding proteins and by investigating how these proteins are influenced by insulin, glucocorticoids and cAMP to regulate transcription.

Acknowledgements

This project was supported by National Institutes of Health RO1 DK-38773 (to DRP).

References

1. Lee PDK, Conover CA, Powell DR. Proc Soc Exp Biol Med 1993;204:4—29.
2. Conover CA, Divertie GD, Lee PDK. Acta Endocrinol 1993;128:140—143.
3. Conover CA, Butler PC, Wang M, Rizza RA, Lee PDK. Diabetes 1990;39:1251—1256.
4. Lee PDK, Jensen MD, Divertie GD, Heiling VJ, Katz HH, Conover CA. Metabolism 1993;42:409—414.
5. Luo J, Reid RE, Murphy LJ. Endocrinology 1990;127:1456—1462.
6. Ooi GT, Orlowski CC, Brown AL, Becker RE, Unterman TG, Rechler MM. Mol Endocrinol 1990;4:321—328.
7. Unterman TG, Oehler DT, Murphy LJ, Lacson RG. Endocrinology 1991;128:2693—2701.
8. Straus DS, Burke EJ, Marten NW. Endocrinology 1993;132:1090—1100.
9. Lewitt MS, Baxter RC. J Clin Endocrinol Metab 1989;69:246—252.
10. Powell DR, Suwanichkul A, Cubbage ML, DePaolis LA, Snuggs MB, Lee PDK. J Biol Chem 1991;266:18868—18876.
11. Orlowski CC, Ooi GT, Brown DR, Yang YW-H, Rechler MM. Mol Endocrinol 1991;5:1180—1187.
12. Mohn KL, Melby AE, Tewari DS, Laz TM, Taub R. Mol Cell Biol 1991;11:1393—1401.
13. Orlowski CC, Ooi GT, Rechler MM. Mol Endocrinol 1990;4:1592—1599.
14. Suwanichkul A, DePaolis LA, Lee PDK, Powell DR. J Biol Chem 1993;268:9730—9736.
15. Beale EG, Hartley JL, Granner DK. J Biol Chem 1982;257:2022—2028.
16. Yoo-Warren H, Cimbala MA, Felz K, Monahan JE, Leis JP, Hanson RW. J Biol Chem 1981;256:10224—10227.
17. Andreone TL, Beale EG, Bar RS, Granner DK. J Biol Chem 1982;257:35—38.
18. Lewitt MS, Denyer GS, Cooney GJ, Baxter RC. Endocrinology 1991;129:2254—2256.
19. Sasaki K, Cripe TP, Koch SR, Andreone TL, Petersen DD, Beale EG, Granner DK. J Biol Chem 1984;259:15242—15251.

150

20. Magnuson MA, Quinn PG, Granner DK. J Biol Chem 1987;262:14917—14920.
21. O'Brien RM, Lucas PC, Forest CD, Magnuson MA, Granner DK. Science 1990;249:533—537.
22. Imai E, Stromstedt P-E, Quinn PG, Carlstedt-Duke J, Gustafsson J-A, Granner DK. Mol Cell Biol 1990;10:4712—4719.
23. Friedman JE, Yun JS, Patel YM, McGrane MM, Hanson RW. J Biol Chem 1993;268:12952—12957.
24. Suwanichkul A, Cubbage ML, Powell DR. J Biol Chem 1990;265:21185—21193.
25. Giguere V, Hollenberg SM, Rosenfeld MG, Evans RM. Cell 1986;46:645—652.
26. Liu J, Park EA, Gurney AL, Roesler WJ, Hanson RW. J Biol Chem 1991;266:19095—19102.
27. Pei D, Shih C. Mol Cell Biol 1991;11:1480—1487.
28. Suwanichkul A, Morris SL, Powell DR. J Biol Chem 1993;268:17063—17068.
29. deWet JR, Wood KV, de Luca M, Helinski DR, Subramani S. Mol Cell Biol 1987;7:725—737.
30. Gorman CM, Moffat LF, Howard BH. Mol Cell Biol 1982;2:1044—1051.
31. Lee T-C, Chow K-L, Fang P, Schwartz RJ. Mol Cell Biol 1991;11:5090—5100.
32. Mendel D, Crabtree G. J Biol Chem 1991;266:677—680.
33. Powell DR, Suwanichkul A. DNA Cell Biol 1993;12:283—289.
34. Roesler WJ, Vandenbark GR, Hanson RW. J Biol Chem 1989;264:9657—9664.
35. Taylor SS. J Biol Chem 1989;264:8443—8446.
36. Jantzen H-M, Strahle U, Gloss B, Stewart F, Schmid W, Boshart M, Miksicek R, Schutz G. Cell 1987;49:29—38.
37. Beato M. Cell 1989;56:335—344.
38. Yoshinaga SK, Peterson CL, Herskowitz I, Yamamoto KR. Science 1992;258:1598—1604.
39. Yamamoto KR. Ann Rev Genet 1985;19:209—252.
40. Grange T, Roux J, Rigaud G, Pictet R. Nucl Acid Res 1989;17:8695—8709.
41. Schmid W, Strahle U, Schutz G, Schmitt J, Stunnenberg H. EMBO J 1989;8:2257—2263.
42. Schule R, Muller M, Otsuka-Murakami H, Renkawitz R. Nature 1988;332:87—90.
43. Nitsch D, Boshart M, Schutz G. Proc Natl Acad Sci USA 1993;90:5479—5483.
44. Schule R, Muller M, Kaltschmidt C, Renkawitz R. Science 1988;242:1418—1420.
45. O'Brien RM, Bonovich MT, Forest CD, Granner DK. Proc Natl Acad Sci USA 1991;88:6580—6584.
46. Powell D, Lee PDK, DePaolis LA, Morris SL, Suwanichkul A. Growth Reg 1993;3:11—13.
47. Imai E, Miner JN, Mitchell JA, Yamamoto KR, Granner DK. J Biol Chem 1993;268:5353—5356.
48. Ooi GT, Tseng LY-H, Tran MQ, Rechler MM. Mol Endocrinol 1992;6:2219—2228.

©1994 Elsevier Science B.V. All rights reserved
The insulin-like growth factors and their regulatory proteins
R.C. Baxter, P.D. Gluckman and R.G. Rosenfeld, editors

The gene regulation of insulin-like growth factor binding protein-2 (IGFBP-2)

Jürg Schwander, Eiji Kutoh, Jean-Luc Mary and Lukas Ritz

Molecular Endocrinology Lab 405, Zentrum für Lehre und Forschung, Kantonsspital, 4031 Basel, Switzerland

Abstract. The resonance of insulin-like growth factor binding protein-2 (IGFBP-2) in the concert of the IGF-system is starting to be defined. IGFBP-2 expression is tissue and species specific. In humans not many forms of regulation of the serum concentration are known. People treated with IGF-I and individuals carrying malignancies, have been shown to have elevated IGFBP-2 serum levels and in cerebral involvement with neoplasias elevated CSF concentrations. Different compartments with independent IGFBP-2 concentration and regulation can be defined (fetal/mother, milk, CSF). The IGFBP-2 genes in three species have a high degree of homology. In the rat the gene is regulated by Sp1 and Rb (Retinoblastoma gene product).

Introduction

Insulin-like growth factor binding protein-2 (IIGFBP-2) has been primarily defined in the rat, where most of the regulatory studies have been accomplished. It belongs to the smaller size binding-proteins that are thought to be able to permeate with or without bound IGF's from the intravascular to the interstitial space and vice versa. Ontogenetically it is present in serum before the ternary complex of IGFBP-3 appears. It has been shown to be expressed early in embryogenesis in mouse embryonic stem cells. For IGF-I it has a lower affinity, by an order of magnitude, than what was established for IGFBP-3. Its affinity for IGF-II is about 5—10 times higher. So far no specific or unique function in the concert of the IGF-system has been attributed to this binding protein. The goal of this presentation is to review what is known on the regulation of the expression of this binding protein and especially about its gene regulation. In addition it should focus the attention towards preliminary and new, but unpublished work of different groups.

Today two different approaches are possible to analyze the regulation of the production of a protein. What could be described as a deductive way starts with the observation of the localization of formation and the concentration of a protein or its message in different tissues or bodily fluids ex vivo or in cell cultures. The inductive approach will primarily study the gene structure and try to locate areas of interest e.g., known sequences for binding of regulatory proteins and test their function by proving the association of proteins to those DNA elements (Gelshift and DNase-protection assay) and by transfection experiments of gene fragments linked to reporter genes. These results will be limited, of course, to the small stretch of the gene studied and as well to the cell-type used in the transfection experiments or for the extraction of nuclear extracts. The biological value of these observations thereafter needs to be established in other systems to be generalizable. In addition the link will have to be made to physiological or pathophysiological regulation mechanisms found in earlier studies.

Both approaches have been performed for the IGFBP-2 gene by various groups including the authors' laboratory. However, so far the deductive way has not produced results that could be satisfactorily explained by the unveiling of molecular mechanisms, nor could the results obtained by the inductive way be conclusively connected to known regulation mechanisms for IGFBP-2.

Function of IGFBP-2

A broad array of publications have predominantly shown negative effects of IGFBP-2 on IGF's cellular action with a few exceptions [1,2].

Three new pieces of important information on the IGFBP-2 function where either published recently or are only available in preliminary or unpublished form.

Reeve et al. showed that IGFBP-2 could be crosslinked to the cell membranes of cells from certain human small cell lung cancer cell lines (SCLC) and not to the membranes of cells derived from nonsmall cell lung cancers (NSCLC). It was suggested, although not proven, that this membrane associated binding protein might modify IGF action in these cells in analogy to what was earlier found for IGFBP-3 or IGFBP-5 [3,4]. The possibility that IGFBP-2 might have an effect of its own on these cells has not been excluded. The structure of the cell surface, therefore, is decisive whether IGFBP-2 can bind to the cell or not. From earlier experiments it is known that in these lung tumour cell lines the expression of IGFBP-2 is induced and that therefore the binding protein might have an even more pronounced effect on the cells in conjunction with the appropriate change of the cell surface [5]. Cellular changes might regulate the binding protein effect.

Preliminary results of infusion experiments of hIGFBP-2 in goats performed by Prosser et al. indicated that a slight elevation of the concentration of this binding protein increases, as has been expected, the IGF-I shift from serum to interstitium. The dynamics seem to be similar for IGFBP-2 and IGF-I, suggesting the transport of IGF-I with IGFBP-2 (C. Prosser, personal communication). This illustrates that the change of concentration of IGFBPs is followed by a redistribution of the IGFs and thereby most probably by a change in metabolic rate of these growth factors that might or might not be overcome by the regulation of the production (feed back). This is the first in vivo proof of an effect of IGFBP-2 on the redistribution of the IGFs. This effect will be important predominantly in the adult organism where there exists an extensive intravascular pool of IGFs, bound to the ternary IGFBP-3 complex, that can be redistributed.

We have shown earlier, that the message of IGFBP-2 is found early in embryogenesis in mouse stem cells [6]. Later its expression pattern has been followed throughout embryogenesis in the rat and has been shown to be complementary to IGF-II [7,8]. However, other IGFBPs also appear early in embryogenesis. A gene-deletion of IGFBP-2 in mice has not produced any apparent deficiencies in the heterozygous or homozygous animals [9] (J. Pintar personal communication). First obvious anatomical changes were located in the brain: absence of the corpus callosum and an enlarged ventricular system. At the time it was unclear whether these changes were related to the gene knockout or to the specific strain of mice used, that frequently have cerebral malformations. A further more detailed histological analysis will be performed on these knockout animals to look for less obvious morphological changes. Therefore the absence of IGFBP-2 does not lead to the serious developmental consequences expected by the observed expression pattern in embryonic and fetal development.

Several hypotheses can be brought forward to try to explain these findings. First, IGFBP-2 has no important function at all. This statement can be easily dismissed when the observed defects in cerebral anatomy are verified.

One additional argument for its biological importance might be that states of total absence of IGFBP-2 in serum had not been found in more than 1000 serum-determinations of IGFBP-2. We encountered two females with very low serum levels. They both had no obvious health problems. So far we have not been able to check their family members for the occurrence of a genetically induced reduction of the serum levels of this binding protein.

A second argument might be that other IGFBPs could substitute for the lack of IGFBP-2 and that its absence therefore did not result in major deleterious consequences. A support for this hypothesis could come from the observed biological redundancy reflected in the number of the binding proteins and from a slight compensatory increase of mRNA for IGFBP-4 and IGFBP-5 in homozygous mice after gene-deletion of IGFBP-2 (J. Pintar, personal communication). This argument also does not get too much backup by our current knowledge of the IGF-binding proteins. We know, as will be discussed later in more detail for IGFBP-2, that the expression pattern of these binding proteins is ontogenetically different and tissue specific and that therefore a compensatory local replacement would seem improbable [9]. There are also marked differences in gene structure, especially in the regulatory areas and different properties of the proteins that make a substitution hypothesis improbable.

A final solution of this discussion will only be possible when the functions of these binding proteins will be better defined.

Regulation of IGFBP-2

Most studies on the regulation of the IGFBP-2 gene have been performed in the rat and quantity of message and protein were usually determined. Transcriptional regulation could therefore not be distinguished from change in message stability and translational or posttranslational events have often not been studied carefully. These limitations, however, do not reduce the value of the work that was already done. A few statements can summarize these published effects.

There are only a small number of ways to regulate IGFBP-2 expression. Two generalizable rules can be extracted from these results. First, the mode of expression is tissue-specific with the exception of the ontogenetic regulation. Second, caution is demanded to extrapolate findings from one species to another, since there is more and more evidence that most of the effects are species specific.

To better characterize these effects a selection of publications are reviewed.

Ontogenetic or developmental regulation

The fetal adult switch. IGFBP-2 is expressed in most fetal tissues and then develops the specific adult pattern of expression [6,10]. This pattern had been observed already in the beginning of the binding protein research area when individual binding proteins had not been defined [11,12]. The molecular mechanism of this effect that is observed in different species, like pig [13], has not been elucidated up to now. In humans a similar switch was found by measuring the serum concentration [14,15].

These finding can be interpreted as an indication that the expression of IGFBP-2 changes around birth in several species and that this could be regarded to be a general effect of yet unknown importance.

The experimental "metabolic regulation"

Hepatic. The liver is the best studied site of IGFBP-2 expression. Insulin negatively regulates or suppresses the extracted mRNA for IGFBP-2 and the secreted protein in hepatocytes [16]. An increase of IGFBP-2 message is seen in livers, in a pathophysiological state of insulin depletion, in rats, with streptozotocin induced diabetes. This effect is reversible by insulin substitution [17]. A similar effect is seen in fasting animals [18].

In humans there is no indication that a correspondent regulation exists. No suppression of the IGFBP-2 concentration has been seen in an individual with hypoglycemia due to hypersecretion of insulin (insulinoma) [14]. No systematic change of the IGFBP-2 concentration was found in untreated or intensely treated type II diabetics. And there was no negative correlation between C-peptide and IGFBP-2 serum levels. In 32 samples of well and insufficiently treated type I diabetics, there was, in analogy to the first findings, no correlation between IGFBP-2, C-peptide and blood glucose (J. Schwander et al., unpublished results).

Retinoic acid stimulates IGFBP-2 message in the rat liver, this effect is suppressible by insulin and reaches its maximum within 6 h [19]. We have localized a retinoic acid response element on the rat gene that will need further characterization (E. Kutoh et al., work in progression).

cAMP has a small neglectible effect and T3 has no influence on the expression of IGFBP-2 in the liver (C. Schmid, personal communication).

Bone. The second example that has been well studied comes from another tissue of cell culture system: the fetal rat calvarial osteoblasts. To illustrate the tissue specific effects, the effect of selected metabolic stimulators will be compared to the effects in the liver. In the rat osteoblast culture system IGFBP-2 is very well expressed and is one of the quantitvely major IGFBP's. This again seems to be in contrast with human osteoblasts that produce only minor amounts of IGFBP-2, if any. There, and in mouse osteoblasts, IGFBP-5, and its truncated form, seem to play a major role in IGF regulation [4,20].

In the rat bone several stimulators for the IGFBP-2 production have been identified. Strong stimulation is seen with cAMP and T3 (C. Schmid, personal communication and [21]) insulin, if anything, increases the concentration of IGFBP-2 message slightly and retinoic acid decreases the signal on Northern blots [19].

All four effects that were cited (cAMP, retinoic acid, T3 and insulin) diverge in their effects between rat liver and rat fetal osteoblasts.

This example strongly argues for a tissue specific regulation of the concentration of message and protein of IGFBP-2. This observation of specific regulation can be generalized to other tissues and to other binding proteins. In bone cells IGFBP-2 inhibits the IGF-I induced DNA-synthesis [22].

Cell densities

Early on in our experiments Jean Margot observed that when he was working with BRL3A cells, IGFBP-2 message levels were quite variable from one experiment to another. This happened with cells of the same passage and identical culture conditions. We then counted the cells and found that the amount of message/cell would decrease with decreasing cell numbers in culture (more than 20 times difference between 10^4 and 10^5cells/cm^2). Since we planned to continue to work with this cell line we tried to analyze those facts more closely and found that the transcriptional as well as the posttranscriptional regulation was changed in this setting (J. Margot et al., submitted for publication). Whether this effect can be reproduced in other cell types has not been established yet. However, these results should render researchers working on IGFBP-2 in cell cultures cautious and force them to closely monitor the cell numbers in their experiments, since a significant effect could be mimicked by a relatively small change in the amount of cells.

IGFBP-2 in man

Different compartments. The indication that the IGFBP-2 production in man might also be regulated in a tissue specific way, comes from the studies of different fluids or different compartments. IGFBP-2 here was measured by radioimmunoassay as described in [14]. There was no correlation found between the IGFBP-2 concentration of the umbilical cord serum and serum from the mother, between serum from the mother and her milk and recently between serum and CSF (Fig. 1) [14,23–25].

156

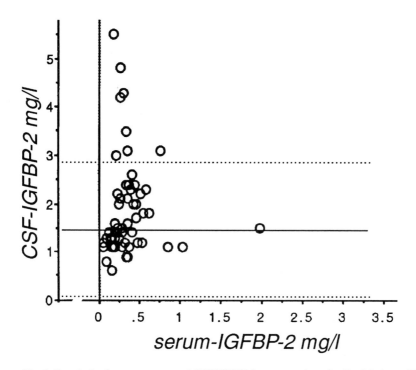

Fig. 1. Correlation between serum and CSF IGFBP-2 concentrations. In 61 adult (age >18 and >75 years) patients, samples of serum and CSF were obtained within 1 h. They were assayed for IGFBP-2 in a RIA [14]. "Normal" CSF concentrations (CSF's with normal cell count and protein concentration) are indicated mean: (solid line) ± 2 SD (dashed lines). There was no correlation found between serum and CSF concentration [25].

IGF-I treatment. IGFBP-2 in serum, increases during the in vivo treatment with IGF-I dose dependently [26] (P.D. Zenobi, personal communication). A similar effect has been established in vitro in a mammary cancer cell-line (MCF-7) [27]. What physiological significance is attributable to these findings remains, for the moment, unclear.

IGFBP-2 and neoplasia. Early on, when we started to measure IGFBP-2 in serum of patients coming into hospital, we found elevated levels in patients carrying solid and nonsolid malignant tumours [14], these findings were corroborated by the results of another group [15]. In addition it was shown that treatment of leukemias with at least temporary recovery, resulted in normalization of the IGFBP-2 levels (W.F. Blum, personal communication). Preliminary results also tell us that IGFBP-2 is elevated in CSF in presence of solid malignancies and probably also during brain involvement in lymphomas or in leukemia [25].

The question whether IGFBP-2 is taking part in the regulation of the malignant transformation and the maintenance of tumour growth or whether it is an accompanying marker of the development and the extension of some malignancies remains still unsettled.

Table 1. Comparison of the three IGFBP-2 genes characterized. Results were taken out of [29–31]

Gene structure	Human	Rat	Mouse
4 Exons	568	476	470 n
	220	224	227 n
	141	141	141 n
	496	472	516 n
3 Introns	27	32	24 kb
		686	n
		1793	n
No TAT or CAAT element			

IGFBP-2 genes

Gene structure

IGFBP-2 genes of the three species rat, mouse and man have been defined [28-31]. These genes are characterized by 4 exons and a large first intron (Table 1). All these genes contain no TATA or CAAT element, but contain GC rich regions. In this respect the gene shows some similarity to the gene of another binding protein, IGFBP-6, that has a similar promotor structure [32].

The homology between the three IGFBP-2 genes is very high for specific areas 5' of ATG. In particular all these three genes contain three GC boxes that have been shown to be regulatory elements. Two additional GC boxes are found in the mouse gene. There are no specific sequences for known glycosylation sites in the protein.

Large introns (over 23 kb), like the first intron in the IGFBP-2 gene, are uncommon and very often result from the insertion of repetitive elements. The event of insertion of these elements provides a tool to analyze the ontogeny in a gene family that most probably arose from gene duplication like the IGFBP or IGF-genes. IGFBP-5 is the only gene at present with a large first intron of about 10 kb [33]. The data from the 3 IGFBP-2 genes suggest that their divergence happened before the mammalian radiation. Further analysis of the IGFBP-5 gene will be needed to suggest a common regulation.

The chromosomal localization of the human IGFBP-2 gene is on chromosome 2 region 2q33-q34 [31,34]. In the mouse it is located on chromosome 1 [30].

In the human and the mouse it has been shown that the IGFBP-5 gene is located tail to tail close to the IGFBP-2 gene (D.R. Powell and P. Rotwein, personal communication).

Analysis of the promotor area

Since there were no TATA or CAAT elements in the promotor area, the importance of the fully conserved GC-rich element in all three genes for transcriptional activation was very suggestive. When we then analyzed the gene by transfecting constructs of the 5′ flanking region linked to reporter genes into BRL-3A cells, we found evidence for several regulatory elements (Fig. 2). Activating elements between –579

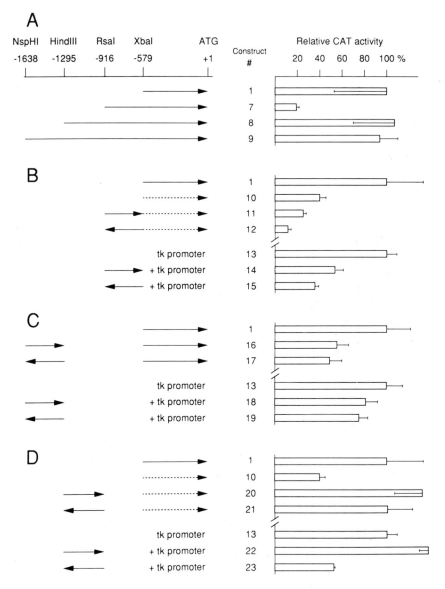

Fig. 2. Multiple elements regulate the rat IGFBP-2 gene. The gene fragments indicated by arrows were linked to a CAT reporter gene and transfected into BRL-3A cells as described earlier [29]: A) represents results of gene fragments of different length; B) Experiments with the inhibitory element (–579 to –916) including its influence on a thymidine kinase promotor; C) Shows results with a second potential silencer area (–1295 to –1638); D) Enhanced activity is found in this fragment (–916 to –1295) (J.B. Margot unpublished results).

and +1 as well as between −1295 and −916 and inhibitory elements between −579 and −916 and less certain between −1296 and −1638 of the rat genomic sequence. Similar elements could be defined on the human gene (J. Margot, unpublished data).

The analysis of the most 3′ element demonstrated the importance of the three GC elements closest to ATG. Without their presence transcription could not be activated. Sp1 an ubiquitous transfection factor interacted with these areas in the gel shift assay. This association was specific since it could be inhibited by anti-Sp1 antiserum and excess of the respective DNA fragments. In Drosophila cells, that are devoid of the transcription factor Sp1 coexpression of Sp1 and the GC-boxes further proved that they were necessary for transcriptional activation [29]. These results were on the whole confirmed and extended by DNase protection in footprinting experiments by another group [35].

Sp1 is known to be an ubiquitous transcription factor in mammalian cells, with a substantial flexibility of DNA binding and therefore does not seem to be an ideal candidate for a specific regulation of a gene. We therefore turned our attention to several other elements on the gene to see whether they could explain some of the regulation pattern found in in vivo or in cell culture experiments.

A silencer area

In the course of the analysis of the gene, we found that the transcriptional activation of the CAT or luciferase gene of the construct containing IGFBP-2 gene fragment (−916 to +1) was only 20% of the shorter (−579 to +1) and the longer (−1260 to +1) elements. We therefore concluded that the sequence (−916 to −580) was responsible for the inhibition. A deletion of this fragment in the −1260 to +1 construct led to a doubling of the transcriptional activation confirming the inhibitory effect of that gene segment. In addition this negative element inhibited transcriptional activation when it was linked to a thymidine kinase promotor in both orientations. Further PCR deletion led to a definition of two areas between −733 and −688 that were involved in that effect. Factors out of the nuclear extracts form BRL-3A cells, were found in gel shift assays to interfere with these sequences. The sequence examination of these two repressor elements showed that they both contained a target sequence for the retinoblastoma gene (pRb) product complex, a well characterized tumour suppressor. Overexpression of Rb in BRL-3A cells resulted in a dose dependent IGFBP-2 repression (E. Kutoh, submitted for publication).

Rb is a ubiquitous factor that in concert with other factors forms a DNA binding complex. It binds in its unphosphorylated from to the DNA and inhibits the cell to go through the cell cycle and therefore has a suppressor effect on cell proliferation. Phosphorylation inhibits its interaction and enhances the proliferation potentials of cells.

Earlier observations demonstrating that IGFBP-2 is often expressed in fetal development in areas of rapid proliferation [7,36] and that its message or protein formation is often found to be increased in neoplastic tissues [37] could be explained by such gene regulation. It remains to be seen in cell cultures whether Rb is

160

expressed in these cells and in what state of phosphorylation it occurs. Transformed cells would have to be screened as well for Rb-mutations.

From our earlier transfection experiments we know that the IGFBP-2 gene has many more regulatory elements that will have to be analyzed for their physiological importance. However, the discovery of this silencer element could form the first link between the analysis of the gene for regulatory elements and observations of gene regulation made in vivo and in cell culture system for the IGFBP-2 gene.

Acknowledgements

This work was made possible by grant No. 3200-037314.93 of the Swiss National Science Foundation and by a grant from the Cancer League Basel.

References

1. Rechler MM. Vitam Horm 1993;47:1−114.
2. Bourner MJ, Busby WH, Siegel NR. J Cell Biochem 1992;48:215−226.
3. Reeve JG, Morgan J, Schwander J, Bleehen NM. Cancer Res 1993;53:4680−4685.
4. Mohan S. Growth Reg 1993;3:67−70.
5. Reeve JG, Brinkman A, Hughes S, Mitchell J, Schwander J, Bleehen NM. J Natl Cancer Inst 1992;84:628−634.
6. Schwander J, Mary J-L, Landwehr J, Böni M, Margot J, Binkert C. In: Drop SLS, Hintz RL (eds) Insulin-like Growth Factor Binding Proteins. Amsterdam, New York, Oxford: Excerpta Medica, 1989;125−131.
7. Wood TL, Streck RD, Pintar JE. Development 1992;114:59−66.
8. Streck RD, Wood TL, Hsu MS, Pintar JE. Dev Biol 1992;151:586−596.
9. Wood TL, Rogler L, Streck RD, Cerro J, Green B, Grewal A, Pintar J. Growth Reg 1993;3:5−8.
10. Rechler MM, Brown AL, Ooi GT, Orlowski CC, Tseng LY, Yang YW. Adv Exp Med Biol 1991; 293:137−148.
11. White RM, Nissley SP, Moses AC, Rechler MM, Johnsonbaugh RE. J Clin Endocrinol Metab 1981; 53:49−57.
12. White RM, Nissley SP, Short PA, Rechler MM, Fennoy I. J Clin Invest 1982;69:1239−1252.
13. Kampman KA, Ramsay TG, White ME. Comp Biochem Physiol 1993;104:415−421.
14. Schwander J, Mary JL. Growth Reg 1993;3:104−108.
15. Blum WF, Horn N, Kratzsch J, Jorgensen JO, Juul A, Teale D, Mohnike K, Ranke MB. Growth Reg 1993;3:100−104.
16. Böni-Schnetzler M, Schmid C, Mary J-L, Zimmerli B, Meier PJ, Zapf J, Schwander J, Froesch ER. Mol Endocrinol 1990;4:1320−326.
17. Böni-Schnetzler M, Binz K, Mary J-L, Schmid C, Schwander J, Froesch ER. FEBS Lett 1989;251: 253−256.
18. Brown AL, Chiarotti L, Orlowski CC, Mehlman T, Burgess WH, Ackerman EJ, Bruni CB, Rechler MM. J Biol Chem 1989;264:5148−5154.
19. Schmid C, Schlaepfer I, Waldvogel M, Meier PJ, Schwander J, Boeni-Schnetzler M, Zapf J, Froesch ER. FEBS Lett 1992;303:205−209.
20. Andress DL, Birnbaum RS. J Biol Chem 1992;267:22467−22472.
21. Schmid C, Schlapfer I, Futo E, Waldvogel M, Schwander J, Zapf J, Froesch ER. Acta Endocrinol (Copenh) 1992;126:467−473.

22. Feyen JH, Evans DB, Binkert C, Heinrich GF, Geisse S, Kocher HP. J Biol Chem 1991;266:19469–19474.
23. Eriksson U, Duc G, Froesch ER, Zapf J. Biochem Biophys Res Commun 1993;196:267–273.
24. Breier BH, Milsom SR, Blum WF, Schwander J, Gallaher BW, Gluckman PD. Acta Endocrinol 1993; 129:427–435.
25. Schwander J, Mary J-L, Ritz L. (in prep).
26. Zapf J, Schmid C, Guler HP, Waldvogel M, Hauri C, Futo E, Hossenlopp P, Binoux M, Froesch ER. J Clin Invest 1990;86:952–961.
27. Adamo ML, Shao ZM, Lanau F, Chen JC, Clemmons DR, Roberts CT Jr, Leroith D, Fontana JA. Endocrinology 1992;131:1858–1866.
28. Brown AL, Rechler MM. Mol Endocrinol 1990;4:2039–2051.
29. Kutoh E, Margot JB, Schwander J. Mol Endocrinol 1993;7:1205–1216.
30. Landwehr J, Kaupmann K, Heinrich G, Schwander J. Gene 1993;124:281–286.
31. Binkert C, Margot JB, Landwehr J, Heinrich G, Schwander J. Mol Endocrinol 1992;6:826–836.
32. Zhu X, Ling N, Shimasaki S. Biochem Biophys Res Commun 1993;191:1237–1243.
33. Zhu X, Ling N, Shimasaki S. Biochem Biophys Res Commun 1993;190:1045–1052.
34. Ehrenborg S, Vilhelmsdotter S, Bajalica S, Larson C, Stern I, Koch J, Bondum-Nielsen K, Luthman H. Biochem Biophys Res Commun 1991;176:1250–1255.
35. Boisclair YR, Brown AL, Casola S, Rechler MM. J Biol Chem 1993;268:24892–24901.
36. Wood TL, Brown AL, Rechler MM, Pintar JE. Mol Endocrinol 1990;4:1257–1263.
37. Reeve JG, Schwander J, Bleehen NM. Growth Reg 1993;3:82–84.

Transcriptional regulation of the rat IGFBP-1 and IGFBP-2 genes

Matthew M. Rechler, Dae-Shik Suh, Yves R. Boisclair, Alexandra L. Brown and Guck T. Ooi

National Institute of Diabetes and Digestive and Kidney Diseases, National Institutes of Health, Bethesda, MD 20892, USA

Introduction

The biological activity of insulin-like growth factors (IGFs), like that of most cytokines, differs from that of most polypeptide hormones in that it is modulated by interactions with nonreceptor binding proteins in addition to binding to receptors (reviewed in [1]). For example, transforming growth factor-β occurs as an inactive latent complex with its NH_2-terminal propeptide and fibroblast growth factor is potentiated by binding to heparan sulfate proteoglycans. The six IGF-binding proteins (IGFBPs) for the insulin-like growth factors are bifunctional adaptor molecules that provide a versatile regulatory system, binding to the IGFs on the one hand and interacting with cellular and extracellular components on the other.

In in vitro assays, all of the IGFBPs inhibit IGF action. In particular situations all IGFBPs, except IGFBP-4 and -6, have been reported to potentiate IGF action and some may have IGF-independent actions [1,2]. In vivo, the IGFBPs appear to have unique functions. IGFBP-3 uniquely binds to an acid-labile subunit that forms the major IGF-carrying 150 kDa complex in plasma. IGFBP-1 exhibits dynamic metabolic regulation and may participate in glucose counterregulation. IGFBP-2 mRNA is expressed near sites of rapid proliferation in the embryo and is increased at sites of brain injury. Tissue-specific expression of the IGFBPs may target IGFs to specific tissues.

IGFBP activity is regulated at many levels: synthesis (including transcription, mRNA abundance and translation), posttranslational modifications (such as phosphorylation, glycosylation and proteolysis) and interactions with the extracellular matrix or cell surface. This article will describe recent studies in our laboratory on the transcriptional regulation of rat IGFBP-1 and IGFBP-2 gene expression.

Rat IGFBP-1 promoter regulation

Insulin is the predominant regulator of plasma IGFBP-1 in diverse conditions such as diabetes and fasting [3]. IGFBP-1 levels vary inversely with the insulin concentration. Glucagon and corticosteroids increase plasma IGFBP-1 [3,4].

Similar changes occur at the level of transcription and mRNA abundance in rat liver. IGFBP-1 transcription is increased in streptozotocin-diabetic rat liver and normalized within 1 h of insulin treatment [5—7]. Parallel changes occur in IGFBP-1 mRNA abundance, reflecting its short half-life. The changes in transcription are sufficient in magnitude to account for the changes in mRNA levels.

The H4-II-E rat hepatoma cell line provides a model system with which to investigate the mechanism for this transcriptional regulation. IGFBP-1 transcription and IGFBP-1 mRNA are increased by the synthetic glucocorticoid, dexamethasone and decreased by insulin [5]. Cyclic AMP [8] and phorbol esters [9] also increase IGFBP-1 mRNA in H4-II-E cells. Although stimulation of rat IGFBP-1 transcription by cyclic AMP and phorbol esters has not been studied in H4-II-E cells, both agents stimulate transcription of the human IGFBP-1 promoter [10,11].

We recently reported that fusing a 1004 bp fragment of the rat IGFBP-1 5'-flanking region (nt –925 to +79 with respect to the cap-site, +1) to a promoterless firefly luciferase reporter gene, enables it to be regulated by dexamethasone, insulin, cyclic AMP and phorbol esters [12]. The plasmid was transfected into H4-II-E cells using the cationic liposome method, the cells incubated 8—12 h in serum-containing medium followed by 16 h in serum-free medium, after which test agents were added for 24 h. Dexamethasone increased luciferase activity 25-fold; cyclic AMP and phorbol 12-myristate 13-acetate (PMA) gave a 3—4-fold increase. Insulin inhibited luciferase activity in the presence of each stimulatory agent by >90%. Dominant inhibition by insulin also has been observed in intact cells [8,13].

To determine the regions of the proximal promoter responsible for the regulation of promoter activity, transient transfection experiments were performed using a series of 5'-deletion mutants. The results are summarized in Fig. 1. Deletion of the region from nt –925 to nt –327 was without effect (not shown). Stimulation by cyclic AMP and phorbol esters was lost when the region between nt –327 and –235 was deleted.

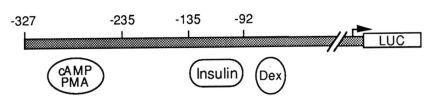

Fig. 1. Regions of the rat IGFBP-1 promoter that are required for stimulation of promoter activity by cyclic AMP, phorbol esters (PMA) and dexamethasone (Dex) and the inhibition of promoter activity by insulin. Rat IGFBP-1 promoter fragments having 5' ends at nt –327, –235, –135 or –92 and the same 3' end at +79, were prepared by PCR amplification using Vent DNA polymerase. They were coupled to a promoterless firefly luciferase gene (LUC) and transfected into the H4-II-E cell line using lipofectin [12]. Prior to assay, the serum-containing medium was replaced with serum-free medium containing 0.1% bovine serum albumin and incubated overnight. The agents to be tested were then added for 24 h, following which cells were lysed for determination of luciferase activity. A human growth hormone expression plasmid was cotransfected to correct for differences in transfection efficiency.

The results are summarized in the schematic diagram. The ellipses below indicate the regions whose deletion abolished the stimulation by cyclic AMP and PMA or the inhibition by insulin. Dexamethasone stimulation persisted in the nt –92 deletion. The cap-site, +1, is indicated by an arrow.

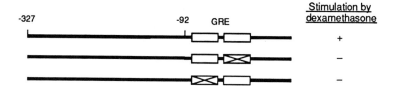

Fig. 2. Effect of site-mutagenesis of the right and left half-sites of the glucocorticoid response element (GRE) of the rat IGFBP-1 promoter (nt –91 to –77) on dexamethasone stimulation of promoter activity. Mutants were constructed in a nt –327 to nt +79 promoter fragment. The hexanucleotide half-sites of the wild-type GRE are shown by open boxes and mutated sites are indicated by an "X". Mutation of either half-site abolished dexamethasone stimulation of rat IGFBP-1 promoter activity.

The responsible sites have not yet been delineated. Unlike the human IGFBP-1 promoter [10], the rat IGFBP-1 promoter does not have a cyclic AMP response element. It does have a potential AP-2 site that might mediate the stimulation by both cyclic AMP and phorbol esters. This site is located between nt –292 and –285 in the complementary strand and is identical to the AP-2 consensus sequence [14] at seven of eight nucleotides. An AP-1 site, that might mediate the phorbol ester response, is also present between nt –308 and –302 (five of seven nt homology). Inhibition by insulin was not abolished until the region between nt –135 and –92 was deleted. Stimulation by dexamethasone persisted even in the nt –92 construct.

A sequence resembling the consensus glucocorticoid response element (GRE), (T/G)GTACANNNTGT(C/T)C(C/T), [15]) was present between nt –91 and nt –77 in the rat IGFBP-1 promoter [12]. The left hexanucleotide half-site (TGAACA, nt –91 to –86) and the right half-site (GGATCC, nt –82 to –77), retain Gs in the second position and Cs in the fifth position. These residues are highly conserved in other GREs and G2 and G5 (complementary strand) are involved in binding the glucocorticoid receptor (GR) [15]. To establish that this potential GRE was involved in dexamethasone stimulation, the right and left half-sites were separately altered by site-mutagenesis (Fig. 2) [12]. Mutation of either half-site abolished the stimulation of rat IGFBP-1 promoter activity by dexamethasone.

To define the insulin response element between nt –135 and nt –92, a series of 10-nucleotide scanning mutations was introduced in the wild-type nt –135/+79 promoter fragment. The effect of these mutations on the ability of insulin to inhibit promoter activity was studied in the presence of dexamethasone because of the low basal promoter activity (Fig. 3). Insulin inhibited promoter activity by 61—74% in the wild-type construct and in constructs containing the three upstream mutations, M1, M2 and M3. By contrast, no inhibition by insulin was seen in the constructs containing the M4 mutation (nt –108 to –99) or the M5 mutation (nt –96 to –87); in fact, in the experiment shown, insulin increased promoter activity. Loss of insulin inhibition in the M4 mutant has been consistently observed, although stimulation was not always seen. The effects of the M5 mutation have been more variable. These results suggest that the M4 region (and possibly M5) is important for the inhibition of rat IGFBP-1 promoter activity by insulin.

166

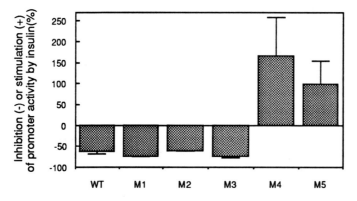

Fig. 3. Effect of scanning mutations between nt −135 and nt −87 on the inhibition of rat IGFBP-1 promoter activity by insulin. Scanning mutations were made in the nt −135/+79 fragment by substituting 10 bp of the wild-type (WT) sequence with 10 bp of a heterologous sequence that included an Xba I restriction site. The mutant constructs, designated M1, M2, M3, M4 and M5, contain substitutions of nt −135 to −126, −125 to −116, −119 to −110, −108 to −99 and −96 to −87, respectively. Promoter activity was determined in the presence of dexamethasone because of low basal promoter activity. The percent inhibition (−) or stimulation (+) of promoter activity after insulin treatment compared to untreated controls is shown for each construct. Adapted from [12].

The nucleotide sequence of the region containing the M4 and M5 mutations in the rat IGFBP-1 promoter, is identical in the human IGFBP-1 promoter [12,16]. Coupling this region of the human IGFBP-1 promoter to a heterologous thymidine kinase promoter made promoter activity inhibitable by insulin; the inhibition was abolished by mutations in two sites that correspond to M4 and M5 [16]. In other experiments, the human IGFBP-1 promoter fragment was coupled to a chloramphenicol acetyl transferase reporter gene and transfected into HepG2 cells. Mutation or deletion of the M4-equivalent region largely abolished the inhibition of promoter activity by insulin; mutation in the M5-equivalent region was much less effective. Thus, in the human IGFBP-1 promoter as in the rat promoter, the M4 region certainly is part of the insulin response element; the role of the M5 region remains to be established.

The rat phosphoenolpyruvate carboxykinase gene (PEPCK) contains an insulin response element on the complementary strand that is identical to the M4 region of the rat and human IGFBP-1 promoters at seven consecutive nucleotides and seven of 10 positions [17]. Ligation of four tandem copies of this sequence upstream from the thymidine kinase promoter made the promoter inhibitable by insulin [17]. These results suggest that the M4 region of the rat IGFBP-1 promoter, like its homologue in the PEPCK promoter, may be sufficient to confer insulin inhibition. The homologous insulin response elements in the PEPCK and IGFBP-1 genes may be recognized by the same or closely related transcription factors, possibly accounting for the similar rapid inhibition of both genes by insulin.

During the scanning mutagenesis experiments to identify the insulin response element, we noted that the stimulation of promoter activity by dexamethasone was decreased or abolished in nt −135 constructs that contained mutations in the M4

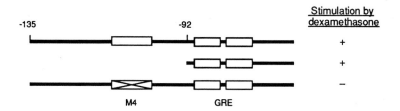

-135   -92

Stimulation by dexamethasone

M4   GRE

Fig. 4. Dexamethasone stimulation of the rat IGFBP-1 promoter is abolished in constructs containing a mutant M4 region and a wild-type GRE. Dexamethasone stimulates promoter activity in deletion constructs with 5′ ends at nt –135 (top) or nt –92 (middle). Both constructs contain a wild-type GRE (double open bar). Dexamethasone stimulation is lost, however, in a nt –135 construct that contains a mutant M4 region (indicated by an "X"), despite the presence of a wild-type GRE.

region. This result is illustrated schematically in Fig. 4. It was particularly surprising because the region between nt –135 and nt –92 could be deleted without abolishing dexamethasone stimulation. The fact that the GRE in the nt –92 deletion is sufficient for dexamethasone stimulation excludes the possibility that the GR needs to interact with essential accessory factors that bind to the M4 region (as described for the PEPCK promoter) [18].

A model to account for these results is presented in Fig. 5. According to this model, an inhibitor (Inh) of dexamethasone stimulation mediated by the GR binds to a region (other than M4) located between nt –135 and –92. When the Inh binds to the DNA, it interferes with binding or activation of the GRE by direct protein-protein interactions with the GR. Inhibition occurs, however, only when the M4 site has been mutated (top panel). We propose that a second factor (NT) that binds to wild type, but not mutant M4, neutralizes the Inh by binding to it or by stabilizing the GR against inhibition by Inh (bottom panel). Experiments to test this hypothesis are in progress.

Rat IGFBP-2 promoter

Rat IGFBP-2 gene expression is regulated in development and in fasting [19]. IGFBP-2 mRNA is abundant in fetal rat liver and decreases after birth. IGFBP-2 mRNA increases in adult rat liver after fasting. These changes in IGFBP-2 mRNA abundance result, at least in part, from changes in transcription.

A program was initiated to characterize the rat IGFBP-2 promoter in order to understand its transcriptional regulation. We cloned the rat IGFBP-2 gene and sequenced its promoter region [20]. It was GC-rich, but lacked a TATA box. Primer-extended reverse transcription and ribonuclease protection assays were performed to define the transcription initiation site, using total RNA from the BRL-3A cell line that expresses rat IGFBP-2 at a high level. Using different primers, primer extension gave conflicting results, namely, extended fragments whose size corresponded to the 5′

168

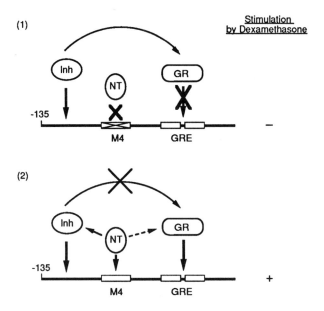

Fig. 5. Model to explain the effect of the M4 mutation on dexamethasone stimulation of rat IGFBP-1 promoter activity. GR, glucocorticoid receptor; Inh = inhibitor of the GR; NT = neutralizing factor that eliminates the inhibitory effect of Inh on the GR. (top panel) In the nt –135 construct that contains an M4 mutation, the Inh binds to the DNA (at an unspecified site in the nt –135 to nt -92 region, but not in M4 itself). This binding allows the Inh to interact with the GR, interfering with its ability to bind to the GRE. Accordingly, stimulation of promoter activity by dexamethasone is inhibited. Since the NT can not bind to the mutant M4 region, it is unable to overcome the inhibition by the Inh. (bottom panel) Dexamethasone stimulation occurs in the nt –135 construct containing a wild-type M4 region. In this case, the NT can bind to the wild-type (WT) M4 region, allowing it to overcome (neutralize) the Inh-induced inhibition of dexamethasone stimulation of promoter activity. The NT may act either by protein-protein interactions with the Inh (preventing it from complexing to the GR) or by interactions with the GR that stabilize it against inhibition by the Inh.

end of the mRNA being at nt –151 or nt –88 (with respect to the translation start site, ATG, +1). We favored nt –151, since BRL-3A RNA protected antisense riboprobe copies of genomic RNA beyond nt –88. We attributed the nt –88 extended transcript to premature termination of reverse transcription, probably related to the high GC content. Subsequently, Schwander and colleagues mapped the cap-site of human [21] and mouse [22] IGFBP-2 mRNAs to a unique site corresponding to a position near nt –88 of the rat IGFBP-2 promoter.

We have performed additional experiments to address these uncertainties. First, we determined the nucleotide sequence of the cDNA product obtained with a primer complementary to nt –76 to –99 of the rat IGFBP-2 gene whose length had suggested transcription initiation at nt –151. Unlike the nt –88 transcript [20], its sequence did not correspond to the sequence of the rat IGFBP-2 gene, indicating that the two primers used to obtain this extended fragment [20] had hybridized to RNAs other than IGFBP-2 RNA.

Next we used a new, sensitive, PCR-based method, tobacco acid pyrophosphatase (TAP) reverse ligation PCR [23], to definitively map the cap-site. In brief, total BRL-3A RNA is treated with DNase I (to remove residual DNA fragments), calf intestinal alkaline phosphatase (to eliminate pre-existing 5′-P from any partially degraded RNAs), then incubated with TAP to hydrolyze the 5′ cap structure of the mRNA (5′Gppp) to 5′-P. An RNA linker was added to the 5′-P of the mRNAs using T4 RNA ligase and cDNA copies of the elongated mRNAs prepared using AMV reverse transcriptase. IGFBP-2 cDNA originating at the cap-site, was selectively amplified by two rounds of PCR using a 5′ primer corresponding to the RNA linker and nested 3′ primers that were specific for the rat IGFBP-2 gene. By using a 5′ PCR primer specific for the RNA linker, amplification of a putative prematurely-terminated reverse transcript of the rat IGFBP-2 gene would not occur. Analysis of the PCR products on a sequencing gel revealed a single amplified DNA fragment whose size and sequence corresponded to a unique cap-site at nt –90 (Y. Boisclair, manuscript in preparation). Consistent with these results, Kutoh et al. [24] recently identified nt –90 as the site at which rat IGFBP-2 transcription is initiated using S1 protection and primer extension assays.

The occurrence of a unique transcription initiation site is somewhat surprising since the rat IGFBP-2 gene [20] contains neither a TATA box nor the loose consensus initiator sequence, $PyPyA_{+1}N(T/A)PyPy$ (Py = pyrimidine; N = any nucleotide; A_{+1} is the cap-site) that usually specifies the transcription start site [25]. In some natural TATA-less promoters, Sp1 binding sites near transcription initiation sites appeared to be involved in positioning the initiation complex [26]. Tjian and co-workers had proposed such a model [27] using TATA-less artificial promoters containing multiple GC boxes and an initiator. However, others have recently demonstrated that removing the initiator from such constructs resulted in weak and dispersed transcription [28]. Thus, the mechanism by which transcription of the rat IGFBP-2 gene initiates from a single start site at nt –90 remains to be elucidated.

Transient transfection of BRL-3A cells with constructs in which rat IGFBP-2 promoter fragments were coupled to a luciferase reporter gene, indicated that promoter activity is determined by both distal and proximal sites [29]. Promoter activity decreased 25-fold when the region between nt –581 and nt –189 was deleted. The nt –189 promoter deletion fragment, however, still had 20-fold higher activity than a promoterless luciferase construct [29]. Experiments were performed to characterize the responsible elements in the proximal promoter, in particular the role of the transcription factor Sp1 which binds to GC-rich sequences.

DNase I footprinting analysis was performed to locate the sites in the proximal promoter that bind proteins in BRL-3A nuclear extract [29] (Fig. 6). Incubation with BRL-3A nuclear extract protected a broad region of the DNA, from nt –125 to nt –189 and a smaller region from nt –215 to nt –234. Purified Sp1 protected the same two regions.

The size and sequence of the larger footprint suggested that it might contain three GC boxes that bind Sp1. This was demonstrated by introducing a block substitution mutation in the middle of the protected region. BRL-3A extract and Sp1 protected the

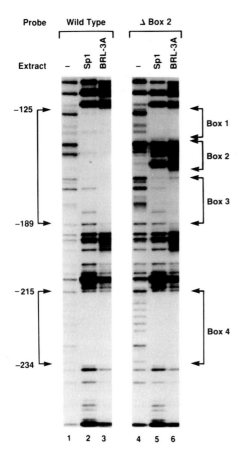

Fig. 6. DNase I footprinting analysis of the GC boxes in the proximal rat IGFBP-2 promoter. The DNA fragment (lanes 1-3) corresponding to nt −276 to −36 of the rat IGFBP-2 promoter was labeled on the noncoding strand and digested with DNase I in the absence of DNA binding proteins (lane 1) or in the presence of BRL-3A nuclear extract (lane 3) or purified human Sp1 (lane 2). The DNA fragments were resolved on a polyacrylamide-urea gel. A large protected sequence is seen between nt −189 and −125 (corresponding to GC boxes 1–3) and a smaller protected sequence between nt −234 and −215 (corresponding to GC box 4).

Lanes 4–6 differ from lanes 1–3 only in that nt −163 to −154 of the probe fragment in the middle of the longer protected sequence were replaced with a 10-bp Bgl II linker. This figure is adapted from [29].

5′ and 3′ ends of the original footprint, but did not protect the mutated internal region. Similar results were obtained using mutations in each of the other three GC boxes [29]. Each mutation affected binding only to the mutated region, but not to the other three GC boxes, indicating that binding to each box was independent of binding to the other three sites. Thus, the rat IGFBP-2 promoter contains three clustered proximal GC boxes and a fourth upstream GC box that bind Sp1 independently.

The nucleotide sequence of the rat IGFBP-2 promoter was examined to precisely locate the GC boxes. This was not a problem for boxes 1, 2 and 4, since their

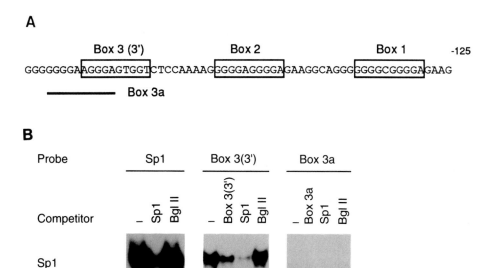

A

Box 3 (3')   Box 2   Box 1   -125

GGGGGGGA⌈AGGGAGTGGT⌉CTCCAAAAG⌈GGGGAGGGGA⌉GAAGGCAGGG⌈GGGGCGGGGA⌉GAAG

———————— Box 3a

B

Probe   Sp1   Box 3(3')   Box 3a

Competitor – Sp1 BglII   – Box3(3') Sp1 BglII   – Box3a Sp1 BglII

Sp1

Fig. 7. Gel retardation analysis showing the ability of oligonucleotides centered around candidates for GC box 3 to bind Sp1. Nucleotide sequence (bottom) of the rat IGFBP-2 promoter between nt –125 and nt –192. GC boxes 1, 2 and 3 (3') (nt –177 to –168) are enclosed. An alternative box 3 suggested by Schwander's group [21,24], box 3a (nt –184 to –173), is underlined below.

Oligonucleotide probes (top) containing an Sp1 consensus sequence, GC box 3 (3') (nt –187 to –160), or box 3a (nt –193 to –166) were incubated with purified Sp1 (1 ng). Each probe (20,000 cpm) was incubated alone (–) or together with a 100-fold molar excess of the unlabeled homologous oligonucleotide (Sp1, box 3 (3') or box 3a as indicated), or unrelated Bgl II oligonucleotide. Gel shift analysis was performed as previously described [29]. Only the region of the autoradiograms showing the protein: DNA complex is presented. Similar results were obtained using BRL-3A nuclear extract (results not shown).

nucleotide sequences corresponded closely with the Sp1 consensus sequence (GGGGCGGGGC) (Fig. 7) [29]. Two alternative assignments of GC box 3 were possible, however: box 3 (3'), corresponding to nt –177 to –168 [29], and box 3a, corresponding to nt –184 to –173 [21,24]. When oligonucleotides centered on these candidate GC boxes were prepared and used in gel retardation assays, probes containing box 3 (3'), but not those containing box 3a, formed the expected specific DNA: protein complexes with Sp1 (Fig. 7) and BRL-3A extract (not shown). These results establish that box 3 (3') is the correct assignment for GC box 3.

The nucleotide sequences of GC boxes 1–4 of the rat IGFBP-2 promoter retain the essential features of the Sp1 consensus sequence that are required for Sp1 binding (Fig. 7) [29]. Specifically nucleotides G2 and G3 contact zinc finger 3 and nucleotides G4 and G6 contact zinc finger 2 of Sp1 [30,31]. These four Gs are conserved in each of the four rat IGFBP-2 GC boxes. By contrast, the proposed GC box 3a [24] contains an A at position six and would not be expected to bind Sp1 according to this model.

The proteins in BRL-3A nuclear extracts that bind to GC boxes 1—4 have the same binding specificity as Sp1 and are immunologically related to it [29]. Two protein DNA complexes were formed in gel retardation assays with a double-stranded oligonucleotide probe containing the 10-bp Sp1 consensus sequence. Formation of both complexes was competitively inhibited by incubation with increasing concentrations of unlabeled Sp1 oligonucleotide, oligonucleotides corresponding to the four GC boxes of the rat IGFBP-2 promoter or antibodies directed against human Sp1 [29].

Sp1-dependent promoter activity was demonstrated using the SL2 *Drosophila* cell line. Like other insect cells, SL2 cells contain no endogenous Sp1. Cotransfection of an Sp1-expression plasmid with IGFBP-2 promoter luciferase constructs containing the proximal three GC boxes (nt –189 to –36) increased the promoter activity of IGFBP-2 promoter luciferase constructs 7—11-fold [29]. Thus, the three clustered GC boxes in the proximal rat IGFBP-2 promoter increased promoter activity in an Sp1-dependent fashion. Kutoh et al. [24] have also reported Sp1-dependent activation of the rat IGFBP-2 promoter in SL2 cells. Their results are perplexing, however, since the rat IGFBP-2 fragment used in their study (nt –195 to nt –105) lacked the

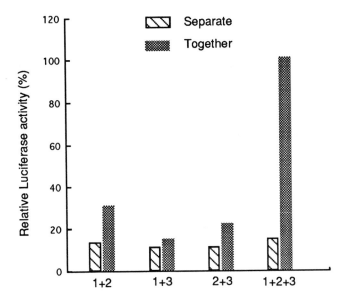

Fig. 8. The three clustered GC boxes activate the rat IGFBP-2 promoter synergistically. Double point mutations were generated in the proximal three GC boxes by site-directed mutagenesis of the nt –581 to nt –36 rat IGFBP-2 promoter fragment. (Specifically, the critical Gs at positions three and four were replaced by Ts). Plasmids containing the individual mutations in all possible combinations were coupled to a luciferase reporter gene and transfected by electroporation into BRL-3A cells. Luciferase activity for the wild type construct containing active boxes 1, 2 and 3 (1+2+3 together, solid bar), was taken as 100%. Promoter activity is 6-fold greater in this construct (containing three functional GC boxes) than in the sum of three separate transfections of constructs that each contained one functional GC box (1+2+3, separate, hatched bar). The relative luciferase activity of constructs containing two active GC boxes (1+2, 1+3, 2+3) present in the same construct (solid bar) was decreased to similar extents, 3—6 fold lower than the wild-type construct (1+2+3 together) and is slightly greater than the sum of the separate activities of the same two GC boxes.

transcription initiation site at nt −90, suggesting that the increased transcription efficiency must have occurred from an aberrant transcription initiation site. The cap-site was present in the constructs used in our experiments.

The three clustered GC boxes in the rat IGFBP-2 promoter are functionally equivalent (Fig. 8) [29]. This was demonstrated by the similar decrease in promoter activity that resulted from separate mutations in the individual GC boxes. This differs from the TATA-less promoter of the rat transforming growth factor α gene, in which the closest GC box of the cluster of three sites is functionally most important [32].

The three proximal, clustered GC boxes in the rat IGFBP-2 promoter act synergistically to stimulate promoter activity. Synergistic activation was demonstrated by introducing individual mutations in the three boxes by site-directed mutagenesis in all possible combinations (Fig. 8). Luciferase activity in cells transfected with wild-type promoters containing the three intact GC boxes was 6-fold greater than the activity predicted based on the sum of the activities in constructs containing each of the boxes separately.

Tjian and colleagues have proposed that synergistic activation results from the formation of Sp1 tetramers associated with each GC box, with the tetramers stacking to form multimeric complexes that provide a more effective activation surface for the transcription machinery and not from cooperative binding of Sp1 to the multiple clustered GC boxes [33,34]. In fact cooperative binding of Sp1 to a cluster of GC boxes has never been demonstrated despite being studied in arrangements similar to the one present in the IGFBP-2 promoter [29,34]. We have seen no indication of cooperative binding to the clustered GC boxes in the rat IGFBP-2 promoter, as mutation in any one GC box has little effect on the binding of Sp1 to the other three boxes in DNase I footprinting assays. Kutoh et al. [24] have presented results of gel retardation assays with DNA fragments containing rat IGFBP-2 GC boxes 1 and 2, or boxes 2 and 3, that they interpret as indicating positive cooperativity of binding: monomeric complexes form at lower concentrations of Sp1 than dimeric complexes. However, the interpretation of this experiment is not convincing. As Sp1 is added, the dimeric complex does not become the predominant form with either construct [35]. In addition, in the box 2 + box 3 experiment, free probe was depleted, so that dimer formation may have become a necessary rather than a favored event.

Future perspectives

These studies have begun to characterize the elements involved in the hormonal and metabolic regulation of the rat IGFBP-1 gene. It remains to identify the transcription factors that recognize the insulin response element and to understand the inhibitory and neutralizing factors that bind to the rat IGFBP-1 promoter and regulate its activation by the glucocorticoid receptor.

We also have described our first steps in defining the mechanisms by which basal transcription of the rat IGFBP-2 gene is regulated. Transcription begins at a unique site, 90 nt upstream from the translation initiation site. Transcription efficiency is

174

determined, at least in part, by three clustered Sp1 sites, 39—88 nt upstream from the cap-site, which act synergistically. These insights will enable us to study the molecular basis for the developmental and tissue-specific regulation of rat IGFBP-2 gene transcription.

References

1. Rechler MM. In: Weintraub BD (ed) Molecular Endocrinology: Basic Concepts and Clinical Correlations. New York: Raven, 1994 (in press).
2. Rechler MM. Vitam Horm 1993;47:1—114.
3. Lee PDK, Conover CA, Powell DR. Proc Soc Exp Biol Med 1993;204:4—29.
4. Hilding A, Brismar K, Thorén M et al. J Clin Endocrinol Metab 1993;77:1142—1147.
5. Ooi GT, Tseng LY-H, Tran MQ et al. Mol Endocrinol 1992;6:2219—2228.
6. Ooi GT, Tseng LY-H, Rechler MM. Biochem Biophys Res Commun 1992;189:1031—1037.
7. Pao C-1, Farmer PK, Begovic S et al. Mol Endocrinol 1992;6:969—977.
8. Unterman TG, Oehler DT, Murphy LJ et al. Endocrinology 1991;128:2693—2701.
9. Unterman TG, Lacson RG, Jentel JJ et al. Biochem Biophys Res Commun 1992;182:262—268.
10. Suwanichkul A, DePaolis LA, Lee PDK et al. J Biol Chem 1993;268:9730—9736.
11. Gong Y, Ballejo G, Alkhalaf B et al. Endocrinology 1992;131:2747—2754.
12. Suh D-S, Ooi GT, Rechler MM. Mol Endocrinol 1994;8:794—805.
13. Orlowski CC, Ooi GT, Brown DR et al. Mol Endocrinol 1991;5:1180—1187.
14. Roesler WJ, Vandenbark GR, Hanson RW. J Biol Chem 1988;263:9063—9066.
15. Truss M, Beato M. Endocrine Rev 1993;14:459—479.
16. Suwanickul A, Morris SL, Powell DR. J Biol Chem 1993;268:17063—17068.
17. O'Brien RM, Bonovich MT, Forest CD et al. Proc Natl Acad Sci USA 1991;88:6580—6584.
18. Lucas PC, Granner DK. Annu Rev Biochem 1992;61:1131—1173.
19. Tseng LY-H, Ooi GT, Brown AL et al. Mol Endocrinol 1992;6:1195—1201.
20. Brown AL, Rechler MM. Mol Endocrinol 1990;4:2039—2051.
21. Binkert C, Margot JB, Landwehr J et al. Mol Endocrinol 1992;6:826—836.
22. Landwehr J, Kaupmann K, Heinrich G et al. Gene 1993;124:281—286.
23. Fromont-Racine M, Bertrand E, Pictet R et al. Nucl Acid Res 1993;21:1683—1684.
24. Kutoh E, Margot JB, Schwander J. Mol Endocrinol 1993;7:1205—1216.
25. Javahery R, Khachi A, Lo K et al. Mol Cell Biol 1994;14:116—127.
26. Faber PW, van Rooij HCJ, Schipper HJ et al. J Biol Chem 1993;268:9296—9301.
27. Pugh BF, Tjian R. Cell 1990;61:1187—1197.
28. O'Shea-Greenfield A, Smale ST. J Biol Chem 1992;267:1391—1402.
29. Boisclair YR, Brown AL, Casola S et al. J Biol Chem 1993;268:24892—24901.
30. Kriwacki RW, Schultz SC, Steitz TA et al. Proc Natl Acad Sci USA 1992;89:9759—9763.
31. Kuwahara J, Yonezawa A, Futamura M et al. Biochemistry 1993;32:5994—6001.
32. Chen X, Azizkhan JC, Lee DC. Oncogene 1992;7:1805—1815.
33. Mastrangelo IA, Courey AJ, Wall JS et al. Proc Natl Acad Sci USA 1991;88:5670—5674.
34. Pascal E, Tjian R. Genes Devel 1991;5:1646—1656.
35. Tsai SY, Tsai M-J, O'Malley BW. Cell 1989;57:443—448.

Biological effects of IGF-regulated IGFBP in cultured human fibroblasts

Cheryl A. Conover, Jay T. Clarkson, Scott Wissink, Susan K. Durham and Laurie K. Bale

Endocrine Research Unit, Mayo Clinic and Mayo Foundation, Rochester, MN 55905, USA

The human fibroblast monolayer system has been defined and used extensively as a model for studying the various aspects of insulin-like growth factor (IGF) cellular physiology — peptides, receptors, receptor-mediated responses, and binding proteins. In this article, we focus on the complex interactions involving IGF binding protein-IV (IGFBP-4), a major secretory product and inhibitor of IGF action in these cells.

Under control serum-free culture conditions, normal adult human fibroblasts predominantly secrete 38/42-kDa IGFBP-3 and 24-kDa IGFBP-4, as assessed by Western ligand blotting with [^{125}I]IGF-I (Fig. 1A). Glycosylated IGFBP-4 was variably evident at 28-kDa. Treatment of human fibroblasts with IGF results in elevated levels of IGFBP-3 and an apparent loss of endogenous IGFBP-4. This IGF effect on IGFBP levels in culture medium was shown to be independent of specific receptor interaction [1–5], and was without influence on IGFBP-3 or IGFBP-4 mRNA transcript levels (Fig. 1B). Subsequently, we established that incubation of human fibroblast conditioned medium (HFCM) with IGF in the absence of cells resulted in the specific loss of IGFBP-4 [6]. IGFBP-4 in HFCM was decreased 80% within 2 h and was undetectable by 6 h of 37°C cell-free incubation with IGF-II; no loss of IGFBP-4 occurred when incubation was carried out at 4°C (Fig. 2). During cell-free incubation, there was no decrease in IGFBP-4 in the absence of IGF-II. Furthermore, IGF-II did not alter IGFBP-3 levels in HFCM. Our studies indicated that this decrease in secreted IGFBP-4 was due to a protease in HFCM, which cleaved the IGFBP-4 molecule into 18-kDa and 14-kDa IGFBP-4 fragments [6]. IGFBP-4 protease activity was inhibited by metalloproteinase inhibitors, EDTA and 1,10-phenanthroline [6]; it was not affected by conventional trypsin- or chymotrypsin-like serine proteinase inhibitors or aspartic proteinase inhibitors. Upon further characterization, this protease was found to be heat-labile (56°C, 60 min) and to have a broad pH activity profile (pH 5.5–9.0).

A unique feature of the IGFBP-4 protease is its strict dependence on IGFs for activation; addition of other peptides (insulin, growth hormone, epidermal growth factor, transforming growth factor-β) or steroid hormones (dexamethasone, β-estradiol, progesterone) to HFCM did not alter IGFBP-4 levels during incubation in a cell-free assay system. Fowlkes and Freemark [7] similarly reported on the IGF-dependence of IGFBP-4 proteolysis in human and sheep fibroblasts. IGF-II is more

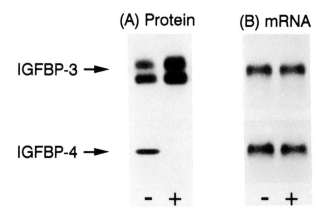

Fig. 1. Effect of IGF-II treatment on IGFBP expression in human fibroblasts. Human fibroblasts were treated without (–) or with (+) 5 nM IGF-II for 24 h. (A) Conditioned medium was analyzed by Western ligand blotting with [^{125}I]IGF-I. (B) Northern blots of total cellular RNA (20 μg/lane) were hybridized using ^{32}P-labeled human IGFBP-3 cDNA probe (Dr D. Powell, Baylor College of Medicine, Houston, Texas, USA) and human IGFBP-4 cDNA probe (Dr S. Shimasaki, The Whittier Institute, La Jolla, California, USA).

effective than IGF-I and can catalyze IGFBP-4 proteolysis to completion when incubated with recombinant human (rh)IGFBP-4 at a 0.25:1 (IGF-II:IGFBP-4) molar concentration [6]. This protease appears to be specific for IGFBP-4; no loss of exogenous IGFBP-1, IGFBP-2, IGFBP-3, IGFBP-5, or IGFBP-6 was observed during

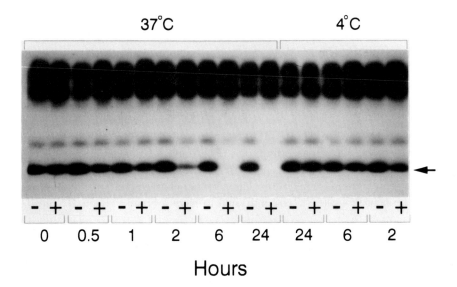

Fig. 2. Time and temperature dependence of IGF-II-induced IGFBP-4 proteolysis. HFCM was incubated under cell-free conditions without (–) or with (+) 10 nM IGF-II for the indicated times at 37°C or 4°C. The samples were then analyzed by Western ligand blot. The arrow indicates 24-kDa IGFBP-4.

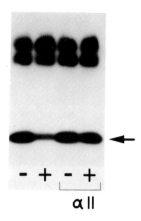

Fig. 3. Effect of an IGF-II immunoneutralizing antibody (αII) on IGF-II-induced IGFBP-4 proteolysis. HFCM was incubated under cell-free conditions without (–) or with (+) 5 nM IGF-II. After 1 h, 25 nM αIGF-II (AMANO) or equivalent volume of diluent was added and incubation continued for an additional hour. Then 10 nM rhIGFBP-4 was added and incubation continued for 6 h. Samples were analyzed by Western ligand blotting. The arrow indicates 24-kDa rhIGFBP-4.

cell-free incubation in HFCM with IGF-II.

A specific physical association between IGF-II and IGFBP-4 appears necessary for proteolysis to occur, since addition of an immunoneutralizing IGF-II antibody will halt IGFBP-4 proteolysis already initiated by IGF-II (Fig. 3). However, IGF binding affinity is not sufficient to explain IGF-dependent IGFBP-4 proteolysis [6], and other factors, as yet unidentified, are likely to be involved in the reaction.

Regulation of IGFBP-4 proteolysis

IGF-dependent IGFBP-4 proteolysis was evident in conditioned medium from all normal adult and fetal human fibroblasts tested, and did not appear to be altered by age of donor. HFCM derived from donors 14 to 96 years of age and from a subject with progeria, a syndrome of premature aging, were tested for IGF-dependent IGFBP-4 protease activity in cell-free assay. As shown in Fig. 4, there was no clear change in IGFBP-4 levels or ability to degrade IGFBP-4 in response to IGF-II in the HFCM samples from aged or progeric donors.

We also evaluated the effect of various fibroblast growth regulatory factors on IGFBP-4 and IGFBP-4 protease activity. Our most striking finding was that treatment of human fibroblasts with phorbol ester tumor promoters, which generally act through the protein kinase C pathway, blocked proteolysis of IGFBP-4 [8]. As indicated in Fig. 5, exposure of cells to β-phorbol 12,13-didecanoate (β-PDD) treatment effectively inhibited IGF-dependent IGFBP-4 proteolysis, whereas forskolin, which activates the protein kinase A pathway, did not. Interestingly, both agents increased IGFBP-4 6-fold to comparable levels in HFCM. Northern analysis of total RNA

178

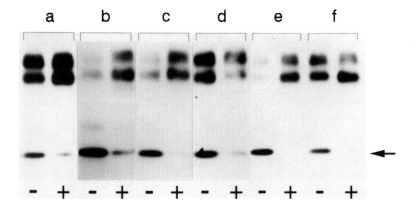

Fig. 4. The IGFBP-4/IGFBP-4 protease system in human fibroblasts: effect of in vivo age. Serum-free conditioned media were collected from early passage human fibroblasts cultured from the following donors: (a) M, 24 yrs; (b) M, 91 yrs; (c) M, 94 yrs; (d) M, 96 yrs; (e) F, 18 yrs; and (f) F, progeric 14 yrs. The HFCM samples were incubated for 6 h under cell-free conditions without (–) or with (+) 5 nM IGF-II and analyzed by Western ligand blot. The arrow indicates 24-kDa IGFBP-4.

extracted from β-PDD- and forskolin-treated fibroblasts (Fig. 6) demonstrated that forskolin increased steady-state levels of IGFBP-4 mRNA 4-fold at 6 h and 8-fold at 24 h. Beta-PDD had no effect on IGFBP-4 mRNA expression during this time. Clearly, regulators of intracellular metabolism can have profound effects on IGFBP-4 availability through transcriptional or posttranslational mechanisms.

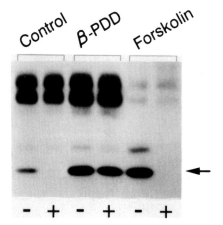

Fig. 5. The IGFBP-4/IGFBP-4 protease system in human fibroblasts: effect of phorbol esters and forskolin. Human fibroblasts were treated for 48 h with β-PDD (100 nM) or forskolin (10 μM). Conditioned media were collected and incubated for 6 h under cell-free conditions without (–) or with (+) 5 nM IGF-II, and samples analyzed by Western ligand blotting.

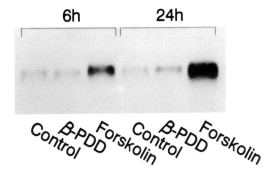

Fig. 6. IGFBP-4 mRNA expression in human fibroblasts: effect of phorbol esters and forskolin. Human fibroblasts were treated for the indicated times with β-PDD (100 nM) or forskolin (10 μM). Northern blots of total cellular RNA (20 μg/lane) were hybridized using a ^{32}P-labeled human IGFBP-4 cDNA probe.

Biological effects of IGFBP-4 proteolysis

Intact rhIGFBP-4 is a potent inhibitor of IGF-I-stimulated action in bone cells, rat B104 neuroblastoma cells, and bovine fibroblasts [6,9–11]. Since human fibroblast cultures rapidly hydrolyze endogenous and exogenous IGFBP-4 in the presence of IGF, experiments were designed to assess the biological consequence of IGF-induced IGFBP-4 proteolysis in these cells. Confluent human fibroblasts were washed and cultured in serum-free medium for 40 h to allow secretion and accumulation of IGFBP-4 and IGFBP-4 protease. IGF-II (4 nM) was added for 5 h, which resulted in the selective loss of ~80% of IGFBP-4 in the medium as assessed by Western ligand blot. Subsequently, IGF-I (5 nM) or insulin (100 nM) was added and [3H]thymidine incorporation measured. As shown in Fig. 7, IGF-II itself did not stimulate [3H]thymidine incorporation and did not affect insulin-stimulated [3H]thymidine incorporation (insulin binds to type I IGF receptor but does not bind to IGFBPs). However, pre-exposure to IGF-II enhanced IGF-I-stimulated [3H]thymidine incorporation in human fibroblasts 3-fold. Decreasing the volume of the medium (<0.5 ml) during the 40 h incubation resulted in decreased cell response to IGF-I alone and a magnification of the potentiating effect of low dose IGF-II (Table 1). Doubling the volume to 1 ml appeared to allow unrestricted IGF-I stimulation. Insulin action was not affected by these volume changes. These data suggest that pericellular IGFBP limits IGF-I access to cell receptors and that pretreatment with IGF-II can mitigate this barrier effect.

Significance

We propose that IGF-II increases fibroblast responsiveness to IGF-I partially through its ability to regulate IGFBP-4 protease activity. IGF-II is more effective than IGF-I in inducing IGFBP-4 proteolysis and IGF-I is more potent than IGF-II in activating

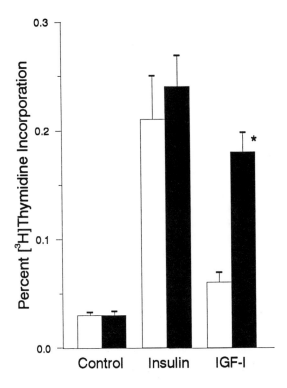

Fig. 7. IGF-I and insulin stimulation of DNA synthesis in human fibroblasts: effect of IGF-II. Human fibroblasts were washed and changed to 0.5 ml serum-free medium for 40 h. IGF-II (4 nM) was added to the medium and the incubation continued for 5 h. IGF-I (5 nM) or insulin (100 nM) was then added and [³H]thymidine incorporation measured at 22–26 h. Values are the mean ± SEM of 4 experiments. *Indicates a significant effect of IGF-II pretreatment at $p < 0.05$.

type I IGF receptor mediated signalling. Based on this information, we present a model of how IGFBP-4 proteolysis could play a role in focal hyperproliferation.

Table 1. Effect of media volume on fibroblast response to IGF-I and insulin

Media vol. (ml)	Fold stimulation[a]		% IGF-II potentiation of IGF-I effect[b]
	Insulin effect	IGF-I effect	
0.3	3.2	1.6	425%
0.4	4.2	1.9	381%
0.5	3.6	2.6	292%
1.0	3.6	6.3	105%

Human fibroblasts were washed and changed to various volumes of serum-free media for 40 h. IGF-II (4 nM) was added to the medium and the incubation continued for 5 h. IGF-I (5 nM) or insulin (100 nM) were then added and [³H]thymidine incorporation measured at 22–26 h.
[a]Insulin and IGF-I stimulated [³H]thymidine incorporation compared to Control.
[b]IGF-I stimulated [³H]thymidine incorporation with, compared to without, IGF-II pre-exposure.

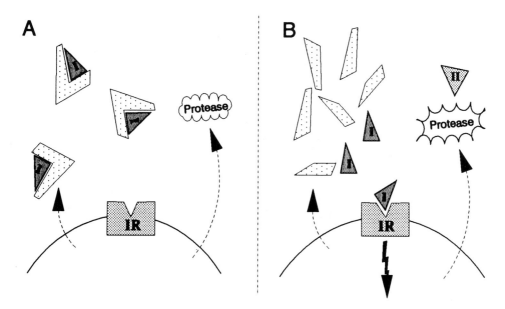

Fig. 8. Model of IGF-II regulation of fibroblast response to IGF-I via the IGFBP-4/IGFBP-4 protease system.

Under "basal" conditions (Fig. 8A), human fibroblasts secrete inhibitory IGFBP-4 and latent IGFBP-4 protease and are relatively unresponsive to IGF-I stimulation. Introduction of IGF-II (Fig. 8B) initiates rapid IGFBP-4 hydrolysis, increasing the local IGF-I available for type I IGF receptor interaction.

Of course, human fibroblasts secrete other IGFBPs, most notably IGFBP-3, the levels of which are up-regulated with IGFs by a receptor-independent mechanism [1–5]. In addition, prolonged incubation with IGF-I and especially IGF-I in combination with IGF-II will enhance IGFBP-5 mRNA expression (our unpublished data) and protein accumulation [12]. It is certain that these IGF-regulated IGFBPs also play an important, as yet undefined, role in human fibroblast biology.

Acknowledgements

This work was supported by NIH Grant DK-43258 (to CAC) and the Mayo Foundation.

References

1. Clemmons DR, Cascieri MA, Camacho-Hubner C, McCusker RH, Bayne ML. J Biol Chem 1990; 265:12210–12216.
2. Conover CA. J Clin Invest 1991;88:1354–1361.
3. Neely EI, Rosenfeld RG. Endocrinology 1992;130:985–993.

182

4. Martin JL, Ballesteros M, Baxter RC. Endocrinology 1992;131:1703—1710.
5. Bale LK, Conover CA. Endocrinology 1992;131:608—614.
6. Conover CA, Kiefer MC, Zapf J. J Clin Invest 1993;91:1129—1137.
7. Fowlkes J, Freemark M. Endocrinology 1992;131:2071—2076.
8. Conover CA, Clarkson JT, Bale LK. Endocrinology 1993;133:1347—1351.
9. Mohan S, Bautista CM, Wergedal J, Baylink DJ. Proc Natl Acad Sci USA 1989;86:8338—8342.
10. Kiefer MC, Schmid C, Waldvogel M, Schlapfer I, Futo E, Masiarz FR, Green K, Barr PJ, Zapf J. J Biol Chem 1992;267:12692—12699.
11. Cheung PT, Smith EP, Shimasaki S, Ling N, Chernausek SD. Endocrinology 1991;129:1006—1015.
12. Camacho-Hubner C, Busby WH Jr, McCusker RH, Wright G, Clemmons DR. J Biol Chem 1992; 167:11949—11956.

The insulin-like growth factors and their regulatory proteins
R.C. Baxter, P.D. Gluckman and R.G. Rosenfeld, editors

Modification of IGF action by insulin-like growth factor binding protein-5

D.R. Clemmons, T.J. Nam, W.H. Busby and A. Parker

Department of Medicine, CB #7170, University of North Carolina School of Medicine, Chapel Hill, NC 27599-7170, USA

Abstract. Insulin-like growth factor binding protein 5 (IGFBP-5) is an important regulator of IGF action in connective tissue cells. The ability of IGFBP-5 to modulate IGF action depends on its affinity for the ligand. Two important factors that have been shown to regulate IGFBP-5 affinity are proteolytic cleavage and binding to extracellular matrix. In these studies we have purified to homogeneity a protease that cleaves IGFBP-5 into a 23 kDa fragment. The protease is a calcium dependent, serine protease. Aprotinin and 3,4 dichlorisocoumarin (3,4 DCI) are potent inhibitors of its activity. A peptide containing the active site of α1 antichymotrypsin is a potent inhibitor of this protease, whereas α1 antitrypsin is not suggesting that it is in the chymotryptic-like serine protease family. The serpin family members antithrombin III and heparin cofactor II have some activity against the protease and coincubation with heparin results in complete inhibition. The protease has a high affinity for heparin since 2 M NaCl is required to elute it from heparin sepharose columns. IGFBP-5 contains a heparin binding domain in amino acid positions 201 to 218. A synthetic peptide containing this domain was also a potent inhibitor of proteolytic activity. Inhibition of the protease resulted in more intact IGFBP-5 being present in the conditioned medium and in the extracellular matrix (ECM). Because of the importance of ECM-binding the components of ECM that bound IGFBP-5 were determined. Treatment of ECM with heparinase resulted in a major reduction in IGFBP-5 binding and pure IGFBP-5 bound to immobilized heparin sepharose. Binding was determined to be specific since two peptides which contain the highly charged basic residue regions of IGFBP-5 competed specifically for binding to ECM and binding to heparin sepharose. Proteoglycans that contain heparan sulfate side chains, such as tenascin, and entactin both bound IGFBP-5 specifically and digestion with heparinase reduced their binding capacity. These findings indicate that glucosaminoglycans (GAGs) are important ECM binding moieties for IGFBP-5. Since IGFBP-5 is protected from proteolytic degradation when present in ECM the findings suggest that binding to ECM through heparin like sequences protects IGFBP-5 proteolysis and allows it to form a storage reservoir for IGF-I and II. Since IGFBP-5's affinity for IGF-I in ECM is reduced IGF-I is readily available to bind to receptors and through this interaction it can potentiate the effects of IGF-I on cell replication.

Introduction

Insulin-like growth factor binding protein 5 (IGFBP-5) is a high affinity form of IGFBP that is present in extremely low concentrations in serum, but is synthesized and secreted by connective tissue cells in culture [1,2]. The protein has several important properties including its capacity to bind IGF-I and II with extremely high affinity, its expression by osteoblasts [3] chondrocytes [4] and fibroblasts [5,6] and its ability to adhere tightly to extracellular matrix (ECM) [7]. Several recent studies have attempted to address the role of IGFBP-5 in modulating IGF action. Studies by

Ui and co-workers have demonstrated that IGFBP-5 can inhibit the capacity of IGF-I to stimulate ovarian steroidogenesis [8]. However, other investigations have shown that IGFBP-5 can potentiate IGF-I actions [7,9]. We have proposed a unifying hypothesis for understanding how IGFBP-5 controls IGF-I action that is based on its affinity for this ligand. Specifically if intact IGFBP-5 is in solution it either inhibits IGF-I actions [8] or it is neutral, as shown by Jones et al., in analyzing the effect of IGFBP-5 on human fibroblast replication [7]. However, if its affinity is significantly lowered, as when IGFBP-5 binds to ECM, then it is capable of potentiating the effects of IGF-I [7]. Andress and Birnbaum have shown that if its affinity is lowered significantly by proteolytic cleavage into a 23 kDa fragment, this fragment can also significantly potentiate the cell growth response to IGF-I both in cultured human fibroblasts and osteoblasts [9]. This suggests that factors that alter IGFBP-5 affinity for IGF-I will result in a major alteration in the way in which cells respond to this growth factor. Based on these differences we have been interested in the role of ECM binding and proteolytic cleavage of IGFBP-5 in controlling the cell growth response to IGF-I.

IGFBP-5 proteolysis

Our interest in IGFBP-5's functions began with the observation that when human skin fibroblasts are exposed to IGF-I in serum free medium there is an 8- to 10-fold increase in the amount of intact IGFBP-5 observed in the conditioned medium after 24 h [5]. However, when IGFBP-5 mRNA is analyzed there is no change in mRNA abundance even when multiple time points and multiple doses of IGF-I are examined. This suggests that the effect is entirely post-transcriptional. Likewise, further analysis failed to reveal a change in IGFBP-5 mRNA stability under these conditions. This suggested the possibility that IGFBP-5 might be proteolytically cleaved in the medium and incubation of the cells with IGF-I might result in inhibition of proteolysis. To that end we were able to show that when purified IGFBP-5 was added to conditioned medium it was degraded rapidly over a 14 h period. If IGF-I or IGF-II was added in the absence of cells no change in the rate of degradation was noted. However, if IGF-I or IGF-II was added with pure IGFBP-5 to fibroblast monolayers then incubated for 24 h, significant inhibition in the amount of IGFBP-5 that was degraded was noted suggesting that some cellular factor was necessary for the inhibitory effect of IGF-I or IGF-II to be manifest. However, IGF association with the IGFBP-5 seemed to be required since the addition of insulin or IGF analogs that did not bind to IGF binding proteins did not result in inhibition of proteolysis [10]. Conover has confirmed these results using transformed human fibroblasts [11].

To further understand this process we have purified and characterized the IGFBP-5 protease that is secreted into fibroblast media. As shown in Fig. 1, ligand blotting of fibroblast media results in no detectible intact IGFBP-5 if unconcentrated media is analyzed. In contrast, immunoblotting shows that media contain 23 kDa band that is easily visualized. Fibroblast ECM contains only intact IGFBP-5 and no fragment is

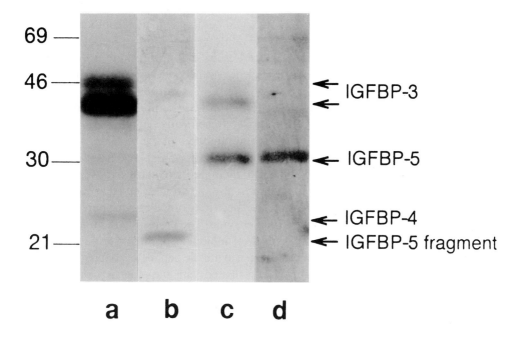

Fig. 1. IGFBP-5 in human fibroblast conditioned medium and ECM. Conditioned medium (lanes a and b) and ECM (lanes c and d) were prepared using normal dermal fibroblast cultures. Immunoblotting (lanes b and d) shows that medium contains only a 23-kDa fragment, whereas ECM contains only intact 31-kDa IGFBP-5. In contrast, ligand blotting (lanes a and c) shows predominately IGFBP-3 in media, but not ECM.

present. To purify the protease, four liters of conditioned media were obtained from GM-10 cells and further processed by heparin sepharose affinity chromatography. The choice of heparin sepharose was dictated by the fact that the heparin was shown to be a potent inhibitor of this protease. The conditioned medium was applied to the heparin sepharose column and two peaks of activity were eluted, one with 0.5 M NaCl and an additional one with 2.0 M NaCl. The 0.5 M NaCl peak contained mostly contaminant protein, whereas the 2.0 M NaCl peak contained substantially more protease activity and much less contaminant protein. The purified protease was then further processed by affinity chromatography using other peptides that have been shown to have inhibitory activity. A peptide termed PB145 which is a synthetic fragment antithrombin III, a known heparin cofactor, was linked to an affinity support and chromatography using this matrix resulted in a further 60-fold purification. Following elution from this column a final affinity purification step was completed using either an 18 amino acid peptide containing a heparin binding domain within IGFBP-5, or an affinity column that was prepared with a peptide containing the active site of α1 antichymotrypsin. These affinity purification steps resulted in substantial improvement in purity and the purified product was shown to be homogenous by SDS-PAGE with silver staining. The properties of the purified enzyme were analyzed

186

in detail. The enzyme was shown to be calcium dependent. Removal of calcium with EDTA showed that no proteolytic activity could be detected and readdition of 5 mM calcium was required to restore activity. However, it did not appear to be a metalloprotease since addition of 200 µM zinc did not restore activity. This characteristic is typical of calcium dependent, serine proteases such as the blood coagulation enzymes, and not of metalloproteases.

Further characterization studies with serine protease inhibitors showed that the protease was most likely a serine protease. Specifically aprotinin, 3,4 dichlorisocoumarin (3,4 DCI) and PMSF were potent inhibitors of the protease, whereas E-64, NEM, pepstatin and iodoacetic acid had no activity. EDTA and 1/10 phenanthroline were also inhibitory, probably due to their ability to chelate calcium (Fig. 2). These findings led us to conclude that this was a serine protease and that calcium was required for full activation. To determine the specificity of the enzyme pure IGFBP-1, -2, -3 and -4 were incubated with purified enzyme. The protease had no activity for these substrates. Because the protease had an inhibitor specificity profile that was similar to chymotryptic-like serine proteases, a synthetic peptide containing the active core region of α1 antichymotrypsin was incubated with the protease. This peptide showed potent inhibition of proteolysis and this effect was not mimicked by α1 antitrypsin suggesting this is a chymotryptic-like protease. To further characterize the inhibitor profile, serine protease inhibitors that occur naturally were tested for activity. Specifically antithrombin III (AT III) heparin cofactor II (HC II) and heparin were incubated with purified protease and IGFBP-5. HC II is a potent inhibitor of the protease and heparin alone had moderate activity (Fig. 3). AT III alone had very little activity. However, when AT III or HC II was combined with heparin total inhibition was noted. Several peptides containing the active site region of AT III were incubated with IGFBP-5 and the purified protease. The peptides termed PB-96, -98 and -145

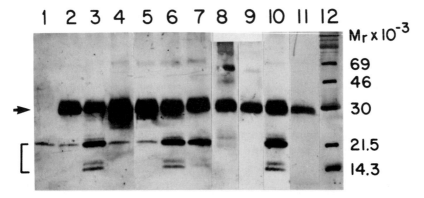

Fig. 2. Effect of protease inhibitors on IGFBP-5 proteolysis. Several protease inhibitors were incubated with purified IGFBP-5 protease and pure IGFBP-5 and the products of the reaction analyzed by SDS-PAGE. As shown in the results, the protease inhibitors 3,4 DCI (lane 8), PMSF (lane 9) and aprotinin (lane 11) were very active in inhibiting the protease. EDTA (lane 4) and 1/10 phenanthronine (lane 5) were also active, suggesting that this is a calcium dependent serine protease. E-64 (lane 6), iodoacetic acid (lane 7) and NEM (lane 10) had no effect compared to control (lane 3).

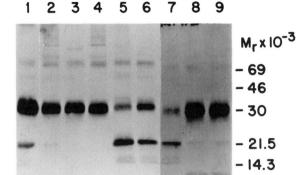

Fig. 3. Effects of serpins on IGFBP-5 protease activity. The serpin protease inhibitors, antithrombin III (lane 6) and heparin cofactor II (lane 2) were incubated with purified IGFBP-5 protease and IGFBP-5. Heparin alone (lane 1) was also tested, as well as combinations of HC-II (lane 3) and AT-III (lane 4) plus heparin. The combinations completely inhibited proteolytic activity and heparin cofactor II alone had significant inhibitory activity compared to control (lane 7); α1 antichymotrypsin (lanes 8 and 9) was also a potent inhibitor.

were potent inhibitors of proteolysis. A nonsense peptide 221 had minimal effects.

Since heparin was a potent inhibitor of proteolysis we wondered whether it might work by binding directly to IGFBP-5 and protecting it from proteolytic cleavage. A heparin binding domain was noted to be present at positions 201–218. Therefore a peptide encompassing this heparin binding domain was prepared. This peptide was shown to be a potent inhibitor of IGFBP-5 proteolysis, whereas a control IGFBP-5 peptide containing several basic amino acids but no heparin binding domain had no activity. This suggests that this heparin binding motif within IGFBP-5 is a potential site of proteolytic cleavage by the enzyme and that heparin binding to IGFBP-5 prevents this activity. Alternatively, heparin could act by binding the protease directly and the heparin binding domain of IGFBP-5 could be a competitive substrate. To determine the physiologic significance of IGFBP-5 proteolysis two types of experiments were carried out. A purified 23-kDa IGFBP-5 fragment was coincubated with increasing concentrations of IGF-I and cultured fibroblast monolayers. A 40% increase in the effect of IGF-I on the fibroblast replication was noted and the presence of IGFBP-5 fragment however concentrations as high as 5.0 µg/ml of peptide were required to see this degree of biologic effect. In contrast, incubation of peptide fragments of IGFBP-2 had no effect. Because of this observation we wondered whether inhibition of the generation of a physiologic amount of IGFBP-5 peptide might result in a change in the fibroblast DNA synthesis response. Therefore the peptide fragment that contains the heparin binding domain of IGFBP-5 was added with IGF-I to cultured fibroblast monolayers and the dose response to IGF-I assessed. In contrast to the predicted result, addition of the peptide resulted in further potentiation of the DNA synthesis response to IGF-I. Analysis of the conditioned medium showed that IGFBP-5 in the CM was protected from proteolysis.

A potential mechanism by which this might occur had been suggested in earlier studies [7]. These studies showed that increasing the concentration of IGFBP-5 in the medium resulted in an increase in the amount of IGFBP-5 in ECM and that increase in the IGFBP-5 concentration within the ECM resulted in potentiation of the IGF-I effect on cell growth. To determine the variables that regulated IGFBP-5 abundance in the ECM several studies were undertaken. To define the regions of IGFBP-5 that bind to ECM we added increasing concentrations of salt to ECM prepared from fibroblast cultures in the presence of exogenously added IGFBP-5. Salt concentrations above 0.15 M NaCl markedly decreased the amount of IGFBP-5 associated with ECM. This suggested that the ECM-IGFBP-5 interaction was at least partially dependent upon charged residues. For this reason we selected two highly charged regions within the IGFBP-5 molecule that contained several basic residues. The first, termed peptide A, had 10 out of 18 residues that were basic and the second, termed peptide B, had seven out of 11 basic residues. Increasing concentrations of each synthetic peptide were shown to inhibit IGFBP-5 association with ECM (Fig. 4). Peptide A was more active than peptide B in inhibiting IGFBP-5 association with ECM under these conditions. To further prove the physiologic relevance of this phenomenon these peptides were incubated with ECM that contained only IGFBP-5 that had been constitutively synthesized by fibroblasts. Again, both peptides inhibited IGFBP-5 binding to ECM.

During the course of these studies we noted the appearance of fragments of IGFBP-5 in ECM if peptide A was used for competition studies. Since in previous studies [7] we had never noted these two IGFBP-5 fragments (27 and 25 kDa) in

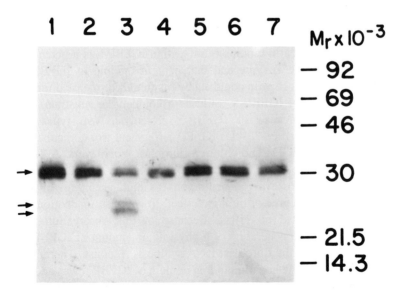

Fig. 4. Competition for IGFBP-5 binding to ECM with IGFBP-5 peptides. Two synthetic peptides that contained multiple basic amino acids, peptides A (lanes 2–4) and B (lanes 5–7) were incubated with pure IGFBP-5 and fibroblast ECM. Increasing concentrations of peptide A and peptide B competed for binding. However, peptide A was more active.

ECM, we were interested in the possibility that a protease was also present in the ECM that degraded IGFBP-5 and that its activity was enhanced in the presence of peptide A. To determine if a protease was released from the ECM, the supernatants from the experiments in which IGFBP-5 had been exposed to ECM were immuno-blotted. If peptide A was included in the incubation buffer the supernatant contained IGFBP-5 fragments. To classify the protease 3,4 DCI, α1 antichymotrypsin and EDTA were added to the incubation buffer with IGFBP-5 and incubated with intact ECM. 3,4 DCI markedly inhibited the appearance of IGFBP-5 fragments in the incubation buffer and in the ECM whereas EDTA and α1 antichymotrypsin had no effect (Fig. 5). Because EDTA and α1 antichymotrypsin are potent inhibitors of the IGFBP-5 protease released by the cells it appears that the protease that is present in ECM is not the same protease that is released into conditioned media. Since only those supernatants that contain peptide A have fragments, this suggests that peptide A caused release of the protease from ECM and that fragments that were generated in its presence had the capability of rebinding to ECM, whereas the 22 kDa fragment that is present in the medium does not have this capability. Since proteoglycans that contain heparin-like side chains are present in ECM and heparin is a potent inhibitor of the IGFBP-5 protease, we incubated heparin with IGFBP-5 and ECM. Heparin completely inhibited the ability of IGFBP-5 to bind to ECM and it prevented proteolysis of IGFBP-5 in the incubation buffer. These results suggested that heparin-like substances in ECM were inhibiting IGFBP-5 proteolysis. In further studies we showed that peptide A competed with IGFBP-5 binding to heparin sepharose beads, suggesting that heparan sulfate side chains of proteoglycans are important IGFBP-5 binding moieties. Therefore we incubated fibroblast ECM or purified ECM proteoglycans with heparinase and then determined their capacity to bind to IGFBP-5.

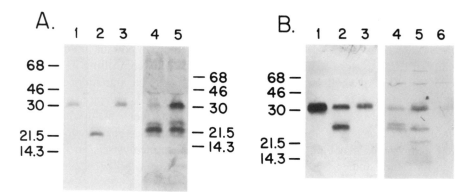

Fig. 5. Release of a protease from ECM into the assay buffer. Pure IGFBP-5 was bound to ECM then incubated with fresh assay buffer in the presence (lanes 2–5) and absence (lane 1) of increasing con-centrations of peptide A. In the presence of peptide A, two IGFBP-5 fragments (27 and 25 kDa) appeared in the incubation buffer (panel A, lanes 2, 4 and 5) and in the ECM (panel B, lanes 2, 4 and 5), whereas they were not detected if no peptide A was added. Their appearance in assay buffer or ECM could be inhibited by incubation with 3,4 DCI (lane 3), suggesting that their appearance was due to the presence of a serine protease. In contrast, EDTA (lane 4) had no effect on the activity of this protease. Heparin lane 6 completely prevented binding to ECM. PB-145 (lane 5), an AT III peptide, was partially inhibitory.

Heparinase digestion of ECM markedly reduced the amount of IGFBP-5 that was detected and, more importantly, peptide A could no longer compete for residual binding after heparinase digestion. Likewise the proteoglycans entactin and tenascin both of which are known to contain extensive glucosaminoglycan (GAG) side chains bound IGFBP-5. When these compounds were treated with heparinase their ability to bind IGFBP-5 was markedly reduced. These findings suggest that GAG-containing proteoglycans are an important IGFBP-5 binding components of ECM. However, they are not the only ECM proteins that bind IGFBP-5. Type IV collagen also binds IGFBP-5, but peptide A could not compete for binding to this ECM component suggesting that other matrix proteins that do not contain GAGs can bind to IGFBP-5. Therefore there are GAG-containing proteins in ECM that bind IGFBP-5 but some non-GAG-containing proteins also have this property.

The findings suggest that IGFBP-5 is an important regulator of connective tissue proliferation and that its storage in ECM provides a reservoir of IGFs that can act to potentiate cell growth under certain circumstances. More importantly, the abundance of IGFBP-5 and its ability to be sequestered in ECM are dependent upon the presence of GAGs in the ECM and proteases that are localized both in the cell culture media and ECM. Under basal conditions it appears that constitutively secreted IGFBP-5 is degraded if it is secreted into medium, whereas it remains intact if deposited into ECM. Substances in the ECM that contain GAG side chains inhibit protease activity and can act as enhancers of IGF action by increasing the IGFBP-5 reservoir. This situation is analogous to FGF where FGF is sequestered by GAGs in the extracellular matrix [12]. Activation during injury of plasminogen activator, plasmin and other serine proteases break down ECM proteins and release FGF, enabling it to bind to cell surface receptors [13]. Since components of the ECM inhibit the IGFBP-5 protease it appears that a similar mechanism may be operative. Future studies need to be directed to the possibility that during wound repair and following injury, release of proteases that are capable of degrading ECM proteins, or glycanases that are capable of degrading GAG side chains, could be extremely important in controlling the ability of ECM to store IGFBP-5 and therefore indirectly controlling its capacity to store IGF-I. Since the cell-secreted protease can determine the amount of IGFBP-5 that is present in the ECM and thereby influence the IGF-I, receptor, and ECM equilibrium, control of this protease may be an additional mechanism wherein the amount of IGF-I that is available to be presented to receptors is regulated. The role of ECM components that bind IGFBP-5 in controlling proteolysis is an important question for future studies.

Acknowledgements

The authors greatly acknowledge the contributions of Leigh Elliott who helped in preparation of this manuscript. We wish to thank Amy Gockerman and Alex Parker for their technical assistance in these studies. This work was supported by grants HL-36313 and AG-02331 from The National Institutes of Health.

References

1. Andress DL, Birnbaum RS. Biochem Biophys Res Commun 1991;176:213−218.
2. Bautista CM, Baylink DJ, Mohan S. Biochem Biophys Res Commun 1991;176:756−763.
3. Conover CA, Keifer MC. J Clin Endocrinol Metab 1993;76:1153−1159.
4. Roger-Gaillard D, Hossenlopp P, Adolphe M, Binoux M. Endocrinology 1989;124:2365−2372.
5. Camacho-Hübner C, Busby W, McCusker RH , Wright G , Clemmons DR. J Biol Chem 1992;267: 11949−11956.
6. Conover CA. Endocrinology 1992;130:3191−3200.
7. Jones JI, Busby WH, Gockerman A, Camacho-Hübner C, Clemmons DR. J Cell Biol 1993;121: 679−687.
8. Ui M, Shimonaka M, Shimasaki S, Ling N. Endocrinology 1989;125(2):912−916.
9. Andress DL, Birnbaum RS. J Biol Chem 1992;267:22467−22472.
10. Clemmons DR, Cascieri MA, Camacho-Hübner C, McCusker RH, Bayne ML. J Biol Chem 1990; 265:12210−12216.
11. Conover CA. J Clin Invest 1991;88:1354−1361.
12. Yayon A, Klagsbrun M, Esko JD, Leder P, Ornitz DM. Cell 1991;64:841−848.
13. Rifkin DB, Moscatelli D. J Cell Biol 1989;109:1−6.

Transcriptional and posttranscriptional regulation of IGFBP-4 and -5 in cultured rat granulosa cells

Shunichi Shimasaki[1], Hiroshi Tanahashi[1], Noritaka Onoda[1], Shoji Sumitomo[1], Gregory Mickey[1], Xin-Jun Liu[2], Nicholas Ling[2], Danmei Li[3] and Gregory Erickson[3]

[1]*The Whittier Institute, La Jolla, CA;* [2]*Neurocrine Biosciences Inc., San Diego, CA; and* [3]*University of California, San Diego, La Jolla, CA, USA*

Abstract. During folliculogenesis in the rat, granulosa cells from healthy dominant follicles do not express any of the six known IGFBP mRNAs, whereas IGFBP-4 and -5 mRNAs are present in granulosa cells of atretic follicles. This finding led us to postulate that IGFBP-4 and -5 might be involved in the atretic process and, therefore, regulated expression of the two IGFBPs could be crucial for follicle growth. Based on this hypothesis we have begun to explore the molecular mechanisms by which IGFBP-4 and -5 gene expression are regulated. Using an in vitro culture system of rat granulosa cells, we examined the effect of FSH on the expression of IGFBP-4 and -5 at the transcriptional and posttranscriptional levels. The effect of gonadotropin-releasing hormone on the expression of IGFBP-4 in the same cells was also studied.

Introduction

During the reproductive life span of female mammals, only a small number of follicles are selected by FSH to undergo the process of development, maturation and ovulation. A vast majority of the follicles become arrested during development and die by atresia [1,2]. A central question in reproductive biology relates to how these follicles are selected for either continual development or degenerative atresia. There is increasing evidence suggesting that follicular atresia may represent a natural process of apoptosis or programmed cell death [3]. Therefore it is tempting to propose that selection may constitute a rescue phenomenon requiring active intervention (perhaps by FSH) to prevent the programmed cell death mechanism. It has also been postulated that the follicular fluid in the atretic follicles contains factors which prevent the rescue phenomenon.

In 1989 we isolated a follicular fluid protein which specifically inhibited the action of FSH in granulosa cells (GCs) [4]. Upon further characterization by molecular cloning, this protein was shown to be an insulin-like growth factor binding protein-3 (IGFBP-3) [5,6]. The mechanisms by which IGFBP-3 antagonizes FSH-induced steroidogenesis was explained by its binding of the endogenous IGF-I produced by

---

Address for correspondence: Dr. Shunichi Shimasaki, Department of Molecular Endocrinology, The Whittier Institute, La Jolla, CA 92037, USA. Fax: +1-619-535-9473.

GCs [7]. In the course of this study we also found three novel IGFBPs and cloned their cDNAs in rat and human species [8—10], which are designated IGFBP-4, -5 and -6 (see review [11]). Our studies further yielded the findings that: A) GCs from the follicles which progress to ovulation do not express any IGFBPs, whereas those which are destined to die by atresia selectively express IGFBP-4 [12] and -5 [13]; and B) exogenous administration of either IGFBP-4 or -5 to the GC culture inhibits FSH-induced steroidogenesis [14,15]. These results suggest that regulated expression of IGFBP-4 and -5 may be crucial for the follicles to branch into two directions, growth or atresia. For this reason we have studied the regulation of IGFBP-4 and -5 gene expression in rat GCs at the transcriptional and posttranscriptional levels.

Materials and Methods

Materials

Androstenedione, diethylstilbestrol (DES) and bovine serum albumin (BSA) were from Sigma Chemical Co. (St. Louis, MO). McCoy's 5a medium, L-glutamine and antibiotics were from GIBCO (Santa Clara, CA). Ovine FSH (NIH-FSH-S17; activity 20 × NIH-FSH-S1 U/mg) and porcine FSH (USDA-pFSH-I-1; activity 81.6 × NIH-FSH-S1 U/mg) were obtained from the National Hormone and Pituitary Program, NIDDK (Baltimore, MD). GnRH-antagonist (D-pGlu,D-Phe^2,D-Trp^{3,6})GnRH and GnRH-agonist (des-Gly^{10},D-Trp^6,Pro^9-NHEt)GnRH were provided by Dr. Ling.

GC culture

Twenty-one to 23 day old female rats (Sprague-Dawley) were implanted (sc) with a 10 mm Silastic capsule containing approximately 10 mg DES. Four days later, the animals were killed using a carbon dioxide chamber and the ovaries collected. GCs were obtained from the ovaries by needle puncture and cultured in 60 × 15 mm tissue culture dishes which were precoated with serum ($5 × 10^6$ viable cells per dish) in 5 ml McCoy's 5a medium supplemented with 2 mM L-glutamine, 100 U/ml penicillin, 100 μg/ml streptomycin sulfate and 100 nM androstenedione in a humidified 95% air, 5% CO_2 incubator at 37°C. The rationale for serum-coating the dishes is to promote GC attachment which ensures that there will be no differential cell loss in the time course experiments [16]. We have ascertained that serum-coating had no significant effects on IGFBP-4 and -5 expression in control and hormone treated cultures when compared to nonserum coated dishes [17]. Cell viability was tested by trypan blue exclusion and cell number monitored by assaying the amount of DNA.

Cells were cultured in the presence or absence of FSH or GnRH-agonist alone or their combination for the appropriate time as described in each figures legends. For the experiments on nuclear run-on assay and the effects of transcription and translation inhibitors, porcine FSH was used because the ovine FSH was no longer available from NIDDK. Since porcine FSH is 4-fold more potent than ovine FSH on hCG-augmentation, we used 25 ng/ml porcine FSH instead of 100 ng/ml ovine FSH. All other experiments were performed using ovine FSH. At each time point of the cell culture, conditioned media were subjected to Western immunoblot analysis and the cells were used to prepare RNA for Northern analysis and/or to prepare nuclei for transcription run-on assay.

Western immunoblot analysis

Conditioned media were collected from the cell culture under the various experimental conditions and concentrated 10 times using Immersibles-CX10 ultrafilters (10,000 mol wt cut-off; Millipore). Samples were loaded onto 12% polyacrylamide gels (Tris-glycine percentage gel, Novex), electrophoresed at a constant voltage of 100 V for 1.5–2 h and then transferred to 0.45-μm nitrocellulose membranes (Bio-Rad) for 2 h at 150 milliamp using the Mini Blot module (Novex). The mol wt of the IGFBPs were estimated by comparison with prestained mol wt standards (Bio-Rad). Immunostaining was performed by first treating the nitrocellulose membranes with casein/TBST buffer for 1 h at room temperature. This was followed by incubation with diluted antisera in casein/TBST buffer overnight at 4°C. The IGFBP-4 antiserum was used at 1:400 dilution and the IGFBP-5 antiserum at 1:200 dilution. The membranes were washed three times with TBST buffer and then incubated for 2 h at 23°C with peroxidase-conjugated goat antirabbit IgG (Calbiochem, San Diego, CA) diluted 1:5,000 in casein/TBST buffer. The membranes were washed three times with TBST buffer and incubated with ECL Western blotting reagents (Amersham, Arlington Heights, IL) for 1 min and then covered with Saran Wrap for exposure to Hyperfilm-ECL (Amersham) for 30 sec to 30 min.

Northern analyses

Total RNA prepared by the conventional method was electrophoresed on a 0.66 M formaldehyde-agarose gel and then transferred onto nylon membrane filters (Hybond N, Amersham). Hybridization was performed at 68°C for 15 h with a ^{32}P-labeled cRNA probe in a solution of 50% formamide, 6 × SSPE (60 mM NaPO$_4$, pH 7.0, 1.08 M NaCl, 6 mM EDTA), 0.5% SDS, 5 × Denhardt's solution (0.1% Ficoll, 0.1% polyvinylpyrrolidone, 0.1% bovine serum albumin), 0.2 mg/ml yeast tRNA and 0.2 mg/ml denatured salmon sperm DNA. Probes for hybridization were prepared by in vitro transcription using rat IGFBP-4 [8], -5 [9] and cyclophilin [18] cDNAs. The filters were washed with vigorous agitation in 300 mM NaCl/30 mM sodium citrate/0.1% SDS for 30 min at room temperature and then incubated in 15 mM NaCl/1.5 mM sodium citrate/0.1% SDS for 30 min at 68°C. Autoradiography was performed on an X-ray film with a DuPont Cronex intensifying screen (Wilmington, DE) at −80°C. The same filter was used for either IGFBP-4 or -5 and cyclophilin Northern analyses. The density of the specific bands was determined by scanning on an LKB Ultrascan XL densitometer.

196

Nuclear transcription assays

Nuclei were prepared from the cultured cells by a conventional method [19] and nuclear transcripts were elongated using [α-^{32}P]UTP (3000 Ci/mmol, 10 mCi/ml). The labeled RNA probe in one ml TES solution was mixed with one ml of TES/NaCl solution and used for hybridizing to DNA immobilized on strips of nylon membrane filters (Zeta Probe, Bio-Rad, Richmond, CA). Target DNAs were prepared by PCR; the rat IGFBP-4 DNA, nucleotide 275~769 [8]; the rat IGFBP-5 DNA, nucleotide 53~811 [9]; the rat inhibin α subunit DNA, nucleotide 1~1076 [20]; the rat cyclophilin DNA, nucleotide –8~833 [18] (based on the published cDNA relative to the translation start site).

Hybridization was performed for 36 h at 65°C. After hybridization, filters were washed twice with 50 ml 2 × SSC for 30 min at room temperature, followed by 2 × SSC for 1 h at 65°C. Filters were treated with 50 ml 2 × SSC containing 10 µg/ml RNase A and incubated for 30 min at 37°C. The filters were washed once more in 50 ml 2 × SSC at 37°C for 1 h, dried on Whatman 3 MM paper and then exposed to X-ray film.

Densitometric analyses

Each band on the X-ray films for Western, Northern and transcription analyses was scanned using a laser densitometer (Ultra Scan XL, LKB, Bromma, Sweden). The relative densities of the bands were expressed as arbitrary absorbance units per mm.

Results and Discussion

Dose-response effects of FSH on IGFBP-4 and -5 protein expression

The GCs prepared from DES-primed immature rat ovaries were cultured in serum free medium for 48 h with or without an increasing dosage of ovine FSH from 1 to 100 ng/ml. Conditioned media from the cells were concentrated 10-fold and analyzed by Western immunoblot. As shown in Fig. 1A, the intensities of the bands corresponding to a nonglycosylated (24 kDa) and a glycosylated form of IGFBP-4 (28 kDa) were increased at doses of FSH up to 10 ng/ml. In contrast, the band intensities were markedly decreased at 30 ng/ml or higher FSH concentrations and in addition two lower molecular mass bands of 21.5 and 17.5 kDa for IGFBP-4 were noted at 30 ng/ml and higher concentrations of FSH. On the contrary Fig. 1B showed that the intensities of two distinct bands of IGFBP-5 at 30 kDa (O-glycosylated, Sumitomo & Shimasaki, unpublished data) and 29 kDa (nonglycosylated) decreased in a dose-dependent manner and one lower band of 21 kDa was noted at 30 ng/ml and higher concentrations of FSH. These findings indicate that FSH induced the production of a protease from the GCs that degraded IGFBP-4 and -5 in the culture medium.

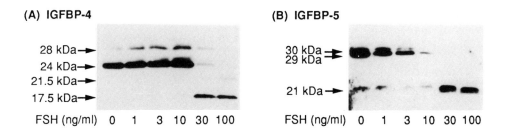

Fig. 1. Dose-response effects of FSH on IGFBP-4 (panel A) and IGFBP-5 (panel B) protein accumulation in 48 h culture of rat GCs.

Specificity of FSH-induced protease

In order to examine the specificity of the FSH-induced protease which degraded IGFBP-4 and -5, we incubated 3 ng of each IGFBP with 10 μl of 10-times concentrated FSH-conditioned medium in 10 μl HEPES buffer, pH 7.4 for 0 and 8 h at 37° C. As shown in Fig. 2, incubation of intact IGFBP-4 for 8 h caused degradation of the intact protein resulting in decreased intensity of the 24 kDa band and increased intensity of the cleaved 17.5 kDa band in comparison with the control which was not incubated. In contrast, incubation of intact IGFBP-2, -3 and -6 for 8 h did not result in any decrease in intensity of the respective intact protein bands at 30.5, 42.0–45.0 and 26.5 kDa in comparison with control. Thus, the granulosa derived protease is very specific towards IGFBP-4. IGFBP-5 is also cleaved by protease present in the conditioned media from the 100 ng/ml FSH treated cells, as shown in Fig. 1.

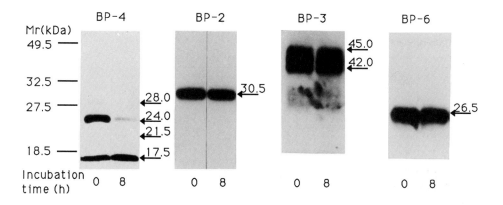

Fig. 2. Specificity of the FSH-induced protease activity. IGFBP-2, -3, -4 and -6 (3 ng per treatment) was incubated for 8 h with conditioned medium from GCs which had been cultured with 100 ng/ml ovine FSH for 72 h and then subjected to Western immunoblot analysis.

198

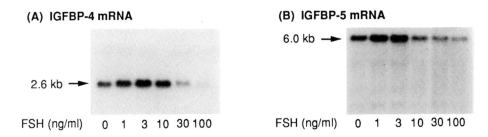

Fig. 3. Dose-response effects of FSH on IGFBP-4 (panel A) and IGFBP-5 (panel B) mRNA levels in 48 h culture of rat GCs.

Dose-response effects of FSH on IGFBP-4 and -5 mRNA levels

Total RNA was prepared from the same GCs used for the protein analysis shown in Fig. 1 and the mRNA accumulation levels of IGFBP-4 and -5 were analyzed. At low

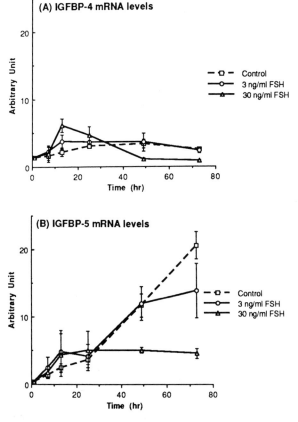

Fig. 4. Time course effects of FSH on IGFBP-4 mRNA levels (panel A) and IGFBP-5 mRNA levels (panel B) in cultured rat GCs.

doses of FSH (<3 ng/ml) there was a slight stimulation of IGFBP-4 and -5 mRNA accumulation in comparison with the control (Figs. 3A and 3B). However, higher concentrations of FSH were able to inhibit the expression of both IGFBP-4 and -5 mRNAs in a dose-dependent manner, with inhibition of IGFBP-5 mRNA noticeable at 10 ng/ml, while IGFBP-4 mRNA required 30 ng/ml to show inhibition.

Time-course effects of FSH on IGFBP-4 and -5 mRNA levels

Time-course effects of FSH on IGFBP-4 and -5 mRNA levels in GCs were also examined. Treatment of the cells with both the low (3 ng/ml) and high (30 ng/ml) doses of FSH caused an initial increased accumulation of IGFBP-4 mRNA in comparison with the control up to 24 h (Fig. 4A). Thereafter, the levels of IGFBP-4 mRNA under the high dose of FSH started to decrease and reached minimum levels after 48 h, whereas at the low dose of FSH after 24 h, the IGFBP-4 mRNA levels were similar to the control. In contrast, IGFBP-5 mRNA levels in the control cells were continuously accumulated up to 72 h (Fig. 4B). At the high-dose of FSH the mRNA levels were maintained for up to 72 h at the same level as it was at 24 h, whereas the low-dose of FSH was not able to suppress the mRNA levels resulting in a steady increase of the mRNA levels similar to control.

Effect of FSH on the transcription rate of IGFBP-4 and -5 genes

In order to determine whether the steady state levels of BP-4 and -5 mRNAs in the control and FSH treated cells at a time point of 72 h incubation are under transcriptional or posttranscriptional control, we performed a nuclear run-on assay using the nuclei from GCs cultured with or without 25 ng/ml porcine FSH (equivalent to 100 ng/ml of ovine FSH, see materials and methods) for 72 h.

As shown in Fig. 5, it was not possible to differentiate the transcription rate of the

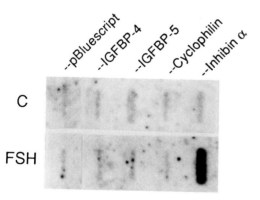

Fig. 5. Nuclear run-on assay. GCs from DES-treated immature rat ovaries were cultured with or without 25 ng/ml porcine FSH in serum free medium. Nuclei were collected and subjected to the nuclear run-on assay as described above. Nylon membrane dotted with 10 μg each of indicated PCR-amplified DNA fragments were used for hybridization.

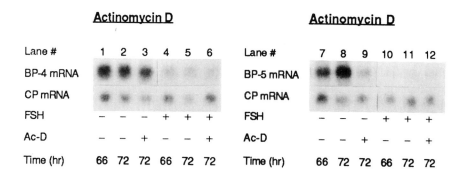

Fig. 6. Effect of actinomycin D on IGFBP-4 and -5 mRNA levels. During a 6 h period after a 66 h preculture in the presence or absence of 25 ng/ml of porcine FSH, cells were treated with or without actinomycin D (5 μg/ml). Northern analysis was performed using either the IGFBP-4 or -5 probe. The same filter was used for hybridization with a cyclophilin probe. BP-4: IGFBP-4; BP-5: IGFBP-5; CP: cyclophilin; Ac-D: actinomycin D.

IGFBP-4 gene between the control and FSH-treated cells, because the intensity of their signals was the same as those of the control (pBluescript). However, the transcription rate of the IGFBP-5 gene appeared to be significantly higher for the control cells than that of the FSH treated cells. The transcription rate of a reference gene, inhibin α subunit, was activated by FSH in accord with a previous report showing that FSH stimulated inhibin α subunit mRNA accumulation in similar experiments [21].

Effect of actinomycin D and cycloheximide on IGFBP-4 and -5 mRNA levels

Further attempts to explore the mechanism responsible for the different steady state levels of IGFBP-4 and -5 mRNA at a time point of 72 h incubation, were employed by using a transcription and a translation inhibitor (actinomycin D and cycloheximide, respectively). The GCs were precultured with or without 25 ng/ml porcine FSH (equivalent to 100 ng/ml of ovine FSH, see materials and methods) for 66 h and without changing the medium, the cells were further cultured in the presence or absence of actinomycin D (5 μg/ml) or cycloheximide (10 μg/ml) for 6 h. As presented in Fig. 6, there was little effect of actinomycin D on the mRNA levels of IGFBP-4, regardless of the FSH treatment, indicating that the IGFBP-4 gene transcription rate during the 6 h incubation from 66 to 72 h after the preculture is extremely low, if any at all, in both control and FSH treated cells (compare lanes 1, 2 and 3 as well as lanes 4, 5 and 6 in Fig. 6). In addition, it seems that the IGFBP-4 mRNAs in both control and FSH treated cells were not degraded (compare lanes 1 and 3 as well as lanes 4 and 6) during the 6 h incubation.

In the case of IGFBP-5, the mRNA level in the control cells was spontaneously increased (lanes 7 and 8), whereas actinomycin D treatment lowered the mRNA level during the 6 h period (lanes 7 and 9). Although more detailed experiments, including

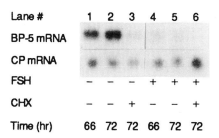

Cycloheximide

Lane #	1	2	3	4	5	6
BP-5 mRNA						
CP mRNA						
FSH	−	−	−	+	+	+
CHX	−	−	+	−	−	+
Time (hr)	66	72	72	66	72	72

Fig. 7. Effect of cycloheximide on IGFBP-5 mRNA level. The same experiments as shown in Fig. 6 were performed using cycloheximide (10 µg/ml) instead of actinomycin D. BP-5: IGFBP-5; CP: cyclophilin; CHX: cycloheximide.

the time-course effects of actinomycin D, are necessary to determine the stability of the IGFBP-5 mRNA, the present finding indicates that the high mRNA levels in the control at 72 h (lane 8) is likely due to active transcription, supporting the results of the nuclear run-on assay (Fig. 5). In contrast, the IGFBP-5 mRNA levels in the FSH treated cells did not change during the 6 h incubation, regardless of the actinomycin D treatment (lanes 10, 11 and 12). All of the mRNA levels remained remarkably low, indicating that the IGFBP-5 gene transcription in these cells is greatly suppressed by FSH.

Similar experiments were performed using cycloheximide (10 µg/ml) instead of actinomycin D as shown in Fig. 7. Treatment with cycloheximide for 6 h resulted in a marked decrease of the IGFBP-5 mRNA level in the control cells, suggesting that the high level of IGFBP-5 mRNA accumulation required on-going protein synthesis. In contrast, the mRNA levels of the FSH treated cells were not altered by the cycloheximide treatment and remained very low.

Taken together, these results suggest that at the time point of 72 h after starting the culture with or without FSH, both: A) IGFBP-4 and -5 transcription is suppressed by FSH; B) IGFBP-4 transcription in the control cells is ceased but IGFBP-5 transcription is still highly active. Therefore, in addition to the suppression of IGFBP-4 and -5 gene expression by FSH, an important new finding is the remarkable induction of spontaneous transcription of the IGFBP-5 gene in the control cells even after a relatively long (>48 h) incubation. This behavior of the IGFBP-5 gene might be involved in the mechanisms of the atretic process.

Dose-response effects of GnRH on IGFBP-4 protein expression

Since GnRH and GnRH-agonist are known to act directly on rat ovary cells to modulate FSH action in the GCs through cell surface receptors [22], we have also examined the effect of a GnRH-agonist on IGFBP gene expression [17]. Figure 8 shows that a GnRH-agonist caused a dose-dependent increase in the accumulation of

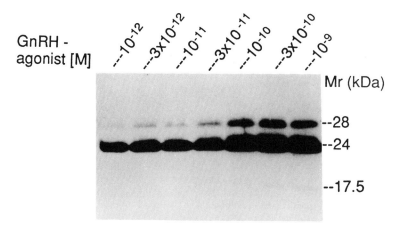

Fig. 8. Dose response effect of GnRH-agonist on IGFBP-4 protein accumulation in the conditioned media. GCs were cultured for 48 h with the indicated concentrations of GnRH-agonist. The media were removed and analyzed by Western immunoblot using a rat IGFBP-4 antibody.

the 24 and 28 kDa bands. The ED_{50} is approximately 1×10^{-10} M. It is noteworthy that the GnRH-agonist treatment did not cause degradation of IGFBP-4 as the case with FSH.

Since the antagonistic effect of GnRH on FSH action in the GCs is mediated by the lowering of intracellular cAMP levels and elevation of phosphodiesterase activity [23–25], we examined the effect of FSH on the GnRH-agonist induced expression of IGFBP-4 (Fig. 9). In the presence of a saturating dose of ovine FSH (100 ng/ml),

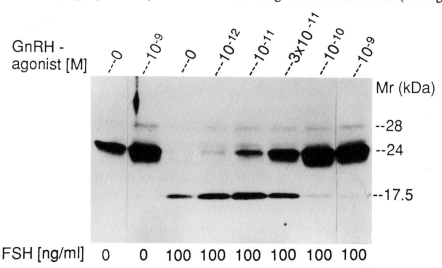

Fig. 9. Effect of FSH on the GnRH-agonist induced IGFBP-4 protein levels. GCs were cultured for 48 h as controls (no hormones) or together with or without a constant amount of FSH (100 ng/ml) and increasing concentrations of a GnRH-agonist. The media were removed and analyzed by Western immunoblot using rat IGFBP-4 antibody.

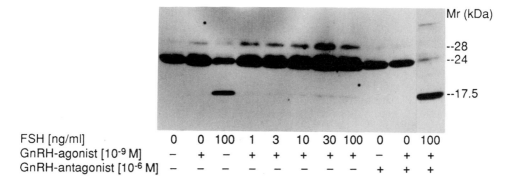

FSH [ng/ml]	0	0	100	1	3	10	30	100	0	0	100
GnRH-agonist [10^{-9} M]	–	+	–	+	+	+	+	+	–	+	+
GnRH-antagonist [10^{-6} M]	–	–	–	–	–	–	–	–	+	+	+

Fig. 10. Effect of GnRH-agonist on FSH suppression of IGFBP-4 protein levels. GCs were cultured for 48 h on serum-coated dishes with the indicated concentrations of FSH, GnRH-agonist, and GnRH-antagonist. The media were removed and analyzed by Western immunoblot using a rat IGFBP-4 antibody.

concentrations of GnRH-agonist as low as 10^{-11} M appeared to induce detectable increase of the 24 kDa band, with a maximal effect at 10^{-10} M. Our present data also indicate that degradation of IGFBP-4 induced by FSH was almost entirely abolished by coincubation with GnRH at a concentration of 10^{-10} M or higher.

We have also examined the effect of a GnRH-agonist on the FSH response by coincubating the GCs with a saturating dose of GnRH-agonist (10^{-9} M) with increasing concentrations of FSH. As seen in Fig. 10, the GnRH-agonist stimulation of IGFBP-4 was essentially unaffected by FSH (1–100 ng/ml). The effect of a potent GnRH-antagonist was also investigated and the results showed that the GnRH-antagonist (10^{-6} M) alone did not significantly alter IGFBP-4 accumulation in the control cells, but it completely blocked the stimulation of IGFBP-4 accumulation by the GnRH-agonist (10^{-9} M). Further, in the presence of the GnRH-antagonist (10^{-6} M), FSH (100 ng/ml) decreased the 24 kDa band intensity and stimulated protease activity, despite the presence of the GnRH-agonist (10^{-9} M).

Taken together, these results showed that GnRH-agonist stimulated IGFBP-4 production in GCs and blocked the effects of FSH on IGFBP-4 expression. In regard to our working hypothesis that IGFBP-4 and -5 gene expression is a physiological marker for atresia in rat ovaries [12,13], our present findings may imply that the inhibitory action of GnRH in steroidogenesis of rat GCs is mediated by mechanisms involving induction of the antigonadotropin, IGFBP-4. Similar experiments to examine the effect of GnRH on IGFBP-5 expression in rat GCs are in progress.

Acknowledgements

This work was supported by NICHD Program Project Grant HD-09690, NICHD contract NO1-HD-0-2902, NICHD Research Grant HD-24585, and NICHD Public Health Service Grant R1HD29008.

References

1. Ingram DL. In: Zuckerman S, Mandly AM, Eckstein P (eds) The Ovary 1. New York: Academic Press, 1962;247—268.
2. Erickson GF, Magoffin DA, Dyer CA, Hofeditz C. Endocrine Rev 1985;6:371—399.
3. Tilly J. Endocrine J 1993;1:67—72.
4. Ui M, Shimonaka M, Shimasaki S, Ling N. Endocrinology 1989;125:912—916.
5. Shimasaki S, Shimonaka M, Ui M, Inouye S, Shibata F, Ling N. J Biol Chem 1990;265:2198—2202.
6. Shimasaki S, Koba A, Mercado M, Shimonaka M, Ling N. Biochem Biophys Res Commun 1989; 165:907—912.
7. Bicsak TA, Shimonaka M, Malkowski M, Ling N. Endocrinology 1990;126:2184—2189.
8. Shimasaki S, Uchiyama F, Shimonaka M, Ling N. Mol Endocrinol 1990;4:1451—1458.
9. Shimasaki S, Shimonaka M, Zhang H-P, Ling N. J Biol Chem 1991;266:10646—10653.
10. Shimasaki S, Gao L, Shimonaka M, Ling N. Mol Endocrinol 1991;4:938—948.
11. Shimasaki S, Ling N. Prog Growth Factor Res 1991;3:243—266.
12. Erickson GF, Nakatani A, Ling N, Shimasaki S. Endocrinology 1992;130:625—636.
13. Erickson GF, Nakatani A, Ling N, Shimasaki S. Endocrinology 1992;130:1867—1878.
14. Ling NC, Liu X-J, Malkowski M, Guo Y-L, Erickson GF, Shimasaki S. Growth Reg 1993;3:70—74.
15. Liu X-J, Malkowski M, Guo Y, Erickson GF, Shimasaki S, Ling N. Endocrinology 1993;132:1176—1183.
16. Orly J, Sato G, Erickson GF. Cell 1980;20:817—827.
17. Erickson GF, Li D, Sadrkhanloo R, Liu X-J, Shimasaki S, Ling N. Endocrinology 1994;134:1365—1372.
18. Danielson PE, Forss-Petter S, Brow MA, Calavetta L, Douglass J, Milner RJ, Sutcliffe JG. DNA 1988;7:261—267.
19. Groundine M, Peretz M, Weintraub H. Mol Cell Biol 1981;1:281—288.
20. Esch FS, Shimasaki S, Cooksey K, Mercado M, Mason AJ, Ying S-Y, Ueno N, Ling N. Mol Endocrinol 1987;1:388—396.
21. Turner IM, Saunders PTK, Shimasaki S, Hillier SG. Endocrinology 1989;2790—2792.
22. Clayton R. J Endocrinol 1987;120:11—19.
23. Knechet M, Catt KJ. Science 1981;214:1346—1348.
24. Knechet M, Renta T, Katz MS, Catt KJ. J Biol Chem 1981;256:34—36.
25. Magoffin DA, Erickson GF. Mol Cell Endocrinol 1982;27:191—198.

Regulation and actions of insulin-like growth factor binding protein (IGFBP)-4 and IGFBP-5 in bone: physiological and clinical implications

Subburaman Mohan[1,2,4], Donna D. Strong[1,2,3], Thomas A. Linkhart[2,5] and David J. Baylink[1,2,5]

Departments of [1]Medicine, [2]Biochemistry, [3]Microbiology, [4]Physiology and [5]Pediatrics, Loma Linda University and Pettis VA Medical Center, Loma Linda, CA 92357, USA

Abstract. The regenerative potential of bone which is reflected in fracture healing may be dependent on the activities of growth factors stored in bone and produced by bone cells. IGF-II, the most abundant growth factor in human bone, appears to be incorporated into the bone matrix by means of IGFBP-5, which binds avidly to both hydroxyapatite and to IGFs. Unlike other IGFBPs, IGFBP-5 increases IGF actions on bone cells. Upon release from the bone matrix storage depot during bone resorption, IGFs and IGFBP-5 are thought to act in a delayed paracrine manner to mediate, in part, the coupling of bone formation to bone resorption. In addition to IGFBP-5, bone cells produce IGFBP-4 and other IGFBPs. Several findings suggest that IGFBP-4 and IGFBP-5 may function in the bone cell microenvironment to regulate IGF activities and thus regulate bone formation. In contrast to IGFBP-5, IGFBP-4 is not bound in bone matrix, and is a potent inhibitor of IGF actions. Studies on regulation of IGFBP-4 and IGFBP-5 production reveal that agents which increase osteoblastic cell proliferation (progesterone and IGFs) stimulate IGFBP-5 production and inhibit IGFBP-4 production, while agents which inhibit cell proliferation have opposite effects. Studies of underlying mechanisms of regulation suggest that IGFBP-4 and IGFBP-5 activities in the bone microenvironment are regulated at multiple levels of both synthesis and degradation. Because IGFBP-4 and IGFBP-5 significantly affect IGF actions on bone cells and because the production of these IGFBPs is regulated by local and systemic effectors of bone metabolism, we speculate that IGFBP-4 and IGFBP-5 have important functions in the local regulation of bone formation.

Introduction

The remarkable regenerative potential of the bone enables it to remodel itself in response to changing physical demands and to repair itself after injury. Bone formation is essential for these adaptive and regenerative properties. In the adult skeleton, bone formation is confined to specific remodeling sites and the net bone gained or lost depends on the extent of bone formation in each one of these sites. Studies to understand the mechanism by which bone is able to regenerate itself after injury led to the important discoveries that bone is a store house for growth factors, and that growth factors stored in bone and growth factors released by osteoblasts and other bone cells could play an important role in regulating bone formation locally [1—4]. Considerable evidence suggested that of the various growth factors present in bone (IGF-I, IGF-II, transforming growth factor (TGF)-β, platelet-derived growth factor, fibroblast growth factor and bone morphogenetic proteins), the IGFs are important local regulators of bone formation: 1) IGFs are the most abundant growth factors stored in bone and produced by bone cells; 2) the production of IGFs is regulated by both systemic and local effectors of bone metabolism; 3) IGFs stimulate both bone cell proliferation and collagen synthesis, two essential components of bone formation; 4) the amounts of IGFs stored in bone are not invariant (for example, IGF levels were increased in bones from osteoarthritic subjects with elevated bone density and decreased in bones from aged females with decreased bone density); and 5) about 50% of basal osteoblastic cell proliferation in serum-free cultures could be blocked by inhibiting the actions of endogenously produced IGFs by bone cells [1,2,5—7].

Of the two major IGFs present in bone, IGF-II appears to be an important mitogen for adult human bone while IGF-I is more important in rat and mouse bone. This conclusion is based on the findings that in contrast to rats and mice, human bones contain 10—15-fold more IGF-II than IGF-I, and human bone cells in culture produce 50—100-fold more IGF-II than IGF-I [1,8,9]. Because, a number of systemic factors (PTH, 1,25-dihydroxyvitamin D_3, progesterone) and local growth factors (BMP-7 and TGF-β) modulate their effects on human bone cells in part by regulating the actions of IGF-II, we and others have proposed that IGF-II could play an important role in the local regulation of bone formation [1,2,10].

IGF-II and other growth factors produced by osteoblasts are either incorporated into bone matrix or diffuse through the extracellular fluid. Based on data that IGF-II by itself exhibits no binding affinity for hydroxyapatite or collagen while IGFBP-5 binds with high affinity to both IGF-II and hydroxyapatite, we propose that IGF-II is fixed in bone by means of IGFBP-5 [9,11]. Thus, the amount of IGF-II stored in bone may be determined not only by the amount of IGF-II produced but also by the amount of IGFBP-5 produced by bone cells. Similarly, studies have shown that TGF-β, the second most abundant growth factor in human bone, is fixed in matrix by binding to a specific proteoglycan called beta glycan [12]. In regard to the functional significance of growth factors such as IGF-II and TGF-β stored in bone, we propose that growth factors are fixed in bone for future actions. IGF-II fixed in bone by means of IGFBP-5 may be released eventually during bone resorption in a bioactive form to act on osteoblast precursor cells and mature osteoblasts. By this delayed paracrine mechanism, IGF-II and IGFBP-5 released from bone could mediate in part the coupling of bone formation to resorption [11]. In addition to delayed paracrine actions, IGF-II secreted into extracellular fluid can act immediately in an autocrine manner on the same cell type that produces it or it can act immediately in a paracrine manner on cells of different stages of the osteoblast lineage (such as osteoblast precursor cells). The acute actions of IGFs in the bone microenvironment are regulated by several components of the IGF system including IGF-I, IGF-II, IGF variants, IGF-I receptors, IGF-II receptors, IGFBPs and IGFBP proteases [1,2,9]. Of these components of the IGF system, IGFBPs and IGFBP proteases appear to have important regulatory roles in bone formation, and hence these two components will be described here in detail.

IGFBPs produced by bone cells

Osteoblast-like human bone cells in serum-free culture produce a number of IGFBPs (25, 29—31, 32—34 and 38.5—41.5 kDa forms) [13—17]. Osteoblast-like cells obtained from fetal mouse and rat calvaria have also been shown to secrete multiple IGFBPs [18—20]. Although we and others have observed differences in the amounts and types of IGFBPs secreted by untransformed normal human bone cells derived from various skeletal sites, and by various human osteosarcoma cell lines (U2, MG63, TE85, TE89, SaOS-2), the physiological and genetic factors contributing to these differences in IGFBP production between various osteoblastic cell types have not been determined. IGFBPs of several apparent molecular weights are observed in western ligand blots of conditioned media from different osteoblastic cells. Characterization of these various IGFBPs produced by various bone cell types by immunologic, purification and sequencing studies has shown that the 25 and 29—31 kDa IGFBPs represent IGFBP-4 and IGFBP-5, respectively (a 29 kDa IGFBP-4 form is also produced); 32—34 kDa IGFBPs represent IGFBP-2 and IGFBP-6 and 38.5—41.5 kDa IGFBPs represent glycosylated forms of IGFBP-3. Of these various IGFBPs, the 25 kDa IGFBP-4 and 38.5—41.5 kDa IGFBP-3 appear to be the most abundant IGFBPs produced by human bone cells in vitro.

Regulation of IGFBP production in bone cells

Recent studies have shown that the concentrations of IGFBPs in the bone cell microenvironment can be regulated at multiple levels including transcriptional, posttranscriptional, translational and posttranslational (Fig. 1). In this regard, we and others have shown that the production of IGFs by bone cells is regulated by both local and systemic effectors of bone metabolism (Table 1). Treatment of normal human bone cells and UMR 106-01 rat osteosarcoma cells with PTH increased production of IGFBP-4 both at the protein and mRNA level with no significant effect on IGFBP-3 production. Consistent with the interpretation that the PTH effect on IGFBP-4 production in bone cells is mediated by the cAMP second messenger signaling system, we found that dibutyryl cAMP (DBcAMP) and agents which increased cAMP production also increased IGFBP-4 production. In addition, DBcAMP increased IGFBP-4 gene transcription rates 3—5-fold in both TE85 and SaOS-2 human osteosarcoma cells [21]. Consistent with these findings, studies on the characterization of the rat and human IGFBP-4 promoter regions have revealed that both rat and human IGFBP-4 genes contain cyclic AMP response elements (CRE). These findings together suggest that cAMP is a major regulator of the IGFBP-4 gene and that PTH and other agents which increase intracellular cAMP may modulate IGFBP-4 gene transcription by a pathway involving protein kinase-A [22,23].

In addition to PTH, 1,25-dihydroxyvitamin D_3, another major systemic calcium regulating hormone, stimulated IGFBP-4 production both at the protein and mRNA levels in MC3T3-E1 mouse osteoblasts, in normal human osteoblasts and in MG63

208

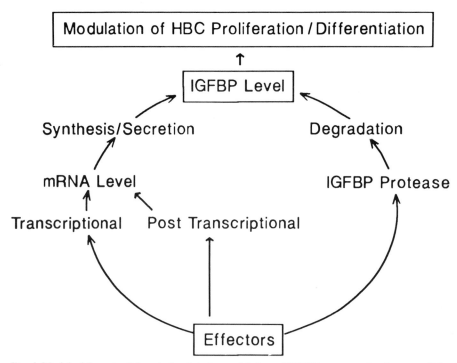

Fig. 1. Model of the potential control points for modulation of IGFBP concentration in extracellular fluid by systemic and local factors. The effect of a given IGFBP on IGF action will depend on its concentration or level which is determined by 1) the synthesis/secretion rate of IGFBP, and 2) the extracellular degradation of the IGFBP. A given effector may modulate the synthesis/secretion at multiple regulatory sites including transcriptional as well as posttranscriptional mechanisms. In addition, the given effector may modulate degradation by influencing the production and/or activity of the corresponding IGFBP protease (e.g., concentration of activators or inhibitors).

human osteosarcoma cells [24,25]. In addition, the serum IGFBP-4 concentrations in psoriasis patients treated orally with 1,25-dihydroxyvitamin D_3 were significantly higher than pretreatment levels [25]. These findings suggest that 1,25-dihydroxyvitamin D_3 plays a major role in regulating IGFBP-4 secretion both in vitro and in

Table 1. Effects of systemic and local agents on HBC proliferation and IGFBP production in HBCs

Effector	HBC proliferation	IGFBP-4 level	IGFBP-5 level
Progesterone	Increase	Decrease	Increase
BMP-7	Increase	Decrease	Increase
IGFs	Increase	Decrease	Increase
1,25-$(OH)_2D_3$	Decrease	Increase	ND
Dexamethasone	Decrease	No change	Decrease

ND = Not determined.

vivo.

Several studies suggest that bone cell expression of various IGFBPs are differentially regulated by physiological agents which affect bone cell proliferation. For example, dexamethasone decreased human bone cell proliferation, had no significant effect on IGFBP-4 production but decreased IGFBP-5 production in several osteoblastic cell types [26]. In contrast, progesterone increased human bone cell proliferation, decreased the IGFBP-4 mRNA level and increased the IGFBP-5 mRNA level but had no effect on IGFBP-3 or IGFBP-6 mRNA abundance. IGF-I and IGF-II increased bone cell proliferation, decreased the amount of IGFBP-4 in the culture medium but increased the amount of IGFBP-3 and IGFBP-5. Finally, in TE85 and SaOS-2 human osteosarcoma cells, osteogenic protein-1 (BMP-7) increased DNA synthesis, decreased IGFBP-4 mRNA levels by more than 50% as well as increased IGFBP-3 and IGFBP-5 mRNA levels by 5–10-fold after 24 h of treatment [10]. Based on this evidence, we propose that the production of each of the various IGFBPs is modulated independently, and effects of local and systemic effectors on bone cell proliferation may, to a large extent, be determined by the resulting balance between IGFs, inhibitory IGFBPs and stimulatory IGFBPs.

Regulation of IGFBP levels in bone cells by proteases

Subsequent to the discovery of IGFBP-3 proteases in the serum of pregnant women and rats, additional studies suggested that the degradation of IGFBPs by specific proteases may be as important as synthesis in determining IGFBP abundance in the local extracellular fluid [27]. We and others have shown that human bone cells in culture produce proteases that are relatively specific to IGFBP-4 and IGFBP-5 [28,29]. In this regard, Campbell et al. [30] have proposed that the serine protease plasmin selectively destroys the IGFBP moiety of IGF-IGFBP complexes in bone. However, IGFBP proteases produced by U2 osteosarcoma cells and normal human bone cells appear to be different from that of plasmin since plasmin is not inhibited by EDTA and plasmin activity is not specific for distinct IGFBPs.

The recent findings that the proteolytic degradation of IGFBPs by bone derived proteases is modulated by IGFs suggest that local factors could modulate local IGFBP concentrations and thus activities of IGFBPs by regulating the protease activities. In this regard, Fowlkes and Freemark [31] and Conover et al. [32] reported evidence for the presence of IGF dependent proteases regulating IGFBP-4 levels in the conditioned medium of fibroblasts. Camacho-Hübner et al. [33] also showed evidence for the presence of an IGF dependent IGFBP-5 protease regulating IGFBP-5 in the conditioned medium of human fibroblasts. Consistent with these findings, we and others have shown that exogenous addition of IGF-II to cell-free conditioned medium of human bone cells increased IGFBP-4 proteolysis. Since IGFBP-4 proteolysis is not induced by the addition of insulin, des(1-3)IGF-I or des(1-6)IGF-II which bind IGFBP-4 at extremely low affinity, we propose that the binding of IGF-II to IGFBP-4 may enhance the susceptibility of IGFBP-4 to proteolytic degradation (Fig. 2). In

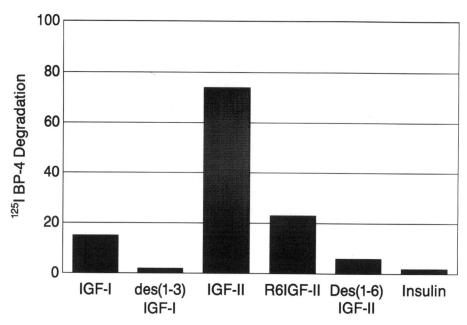

Fig. 2. Effect of IGF analogs on IGFBP-4 proteolytic activity of cell-free conditioned medium from U2 cells. Cell-free U2 conditioned medium was incubated with [^{125}I]IGFBP-4 (50,000 cpm) in the presence of vehicle, IGF-I, des(1-3)IGF-I, IGF-II, R6 IGF-II, des(1-6)IGF-II and insulin at 37°C for 24 h. The samples were then subjected to polyacrylamide gel electrophoresis in the presence of sodium dodecyl sulfate prior to autoradiography. % IGFBP-4 proteolytic degradation was determined by determining the intensity of bands by laser densitometry (Biomed Instruments, Fullerton, CA).

contrast to effects of IGF-II to increase IGFBP-4 proteolysis, treatment of U2 cells and normal human bone cells with IGF-II decreased IGFBP-5 proteolysis. We also found that exogenous addition of IGF-II to cell free U2 conditioned medium had no significant effect on IGFBP-5 proteolysis. In contrast to these latter findings, Fielder et al. [34] and Conover et al. [35] recently reported that exogenous addition of IGF-II to conditioned medium of rat granulosa cells and U2 osteosarcoma cells decreased IGFBP-5 proteolysis. Thus, further studies are needed to determine the mechanisms by which IGFs modulate IGFBP-5 proteolysis in the conditioned medium of human bone cells.

Based on the findings that bone cells as well as several other cell types in culture produce proteases capable of degrading IGFBP-4 and IGFBP-5 into fragments that bind IGFs with much lower affinity, and that IGF-II is an important modulator of IGFBP-4 and IGFBP-5 proteolysis, it can be speculated that systemic and local factors could regulate local IGF actions by modulating the proteolysis of IGFBPs. Future studies on the regulation and mechanism of action of proteases will help in elucidating the role of IGFBP proteases in bone cell physiology.

Molecular mechanism of IGFBP actions in bone cells

In order for the IGFBPs to be an important component of the IGF system in bone, it is essential for IGFBPs to have significant biological actions in bone cells. In this regard, there is now ample evidence which demonstrates that IGFBPs are important modulators of IGF actions in bone cells. We have found that the biological actions of IGFBP-3 vary depending on the culture conditions. Under acute conditions, addition of IGFBP-3 inhibited both basal and IGF induced MC3T3-E1 mouse bone cell proliferation. Upon preincubation of MC3T3-E1 cells with IGFBP-3 prior to the addition of IGFs, this IGFBP had a biphasic effect on IGF induced MC3T3-E1 cell proliferation [9]. In contrast to IGFBP-3, IGFBP-4 inhibited IGF induced cell proliferation in chick calvaria cells, MC3T3-E1 mouse osteoblasts, TE85 human osteosarcoma cells and neuroblastoma cells under a variety of culture conditions [9,13]. These findings, together with the findings that addition of antisense oligomer to IGFBP-4 stimulated bone cell proliferation demonstrate that IGFBP-4 is an important negative regulator of bone cell proliferation [36].

IGFBP-5 stimulates IGF-II actions in MC3T3-E1 mouse osteoblasts when IGFBP-5 was added simultaneously with IGFs [9,11]. Similar potentiating effects of IGFBP-5 purified from U2 cell conditioned medium were reported by Andress and Birnbaum [37] although Kiefer et al. [38] have reported that recombinant IGFBP-5 produced in yeast inhibited IGF-I and IGF-II induced glycolysis in human osteoblasts. The findings that IGFBPs can modulate IGF actions either positively or negatively and that the production of IGFBPs is regulated by various physiological agents support the conclusion that the balance between the stimulatory and inhibitory classes of IGFBPs will determine the degree and extent of IGF induced cellular responses in target tissues.

There have been very few studies on the molecular mechanisms by which different IGFBPs modulate IGF actions in any cell type. We investigated the effects of IGFBP-4 and IGFBP-5 on the binding of IGF-I and IGF-II to bone cells since the affinity with which IGFs bind to their receptors is an important determinant of IGF action. We found that inhibitory IGFBP-4 decreased the binding of $[^{125}I]IGF$-II while the stimulatory IGFBP-5 increased the binding of $[^{125}I]IGF$-II to bone cells. To determine if IGFBP-4 and IGFBP-5 modulated binding of labeled IGF binding to IGF receptors rather than to some other binding sites, purified IGF-I receptor was incubated with labeled IGF-I in the presence of varying concentrations of IGFBP-4 and IGFBP-5. Binding of labeled IGF-I to receptors was assessed by affinity cross linking, gel electrophoresis and autoradiography. IGFBP-4 completely blocked the binding of labeled IGF-I to receptors. In contrast, IGFBP-5 had no significant effect on labeled IGF-I binding to purified receptors. Subsequent studies on the mechanism by which IGFBP-5 increased IGF binding revealed that IGFBP-5 binds to bone cells independent of IGF receptors and thus increases IGF binding to bone cells [39].

Based on our in vitro findings, we have developed models as shown in Fig. 3 to explain the potential mechanisms by which IGFBP-4 and IGFBP-5 may modulate IGF actions in bone cells. Accordingly, IGFBP-4 inhibits IGF binding to the receptor by

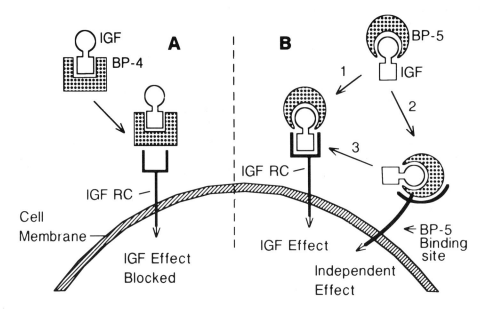

Fig. 3. Potential mechanisms by which IGFBP-4 and IGFBP-5 may modulate their actions acutely on bone cells. According to this model, IGFBP-4 inhibits IGF binding to IGF receptors by binding to IGFs near or at the receptor binding site. With regard to IGFBP-5, three alternate models are proposed. In model 1, IGFBP-5 binds to a site distant from that of IGFBP-4 and the complex of IGFBP-5 + IGF binds to IGF receptors with higher affinity than IGFs alone. In model 2, IGFBP-5 binds to bone cell surface independent of IGF receptors. Such IGFBP-5 binding sites may recruit IGFs at the surface of IGF responsive cells, enabling the ligand to be easily captured by the IGF receptors.

binding to IGFs near or at the receptor binding site. IGFBP-4 may thus act like soluble interleukin-1 receptors which inhibit IL-1 action [12]. With regard to IGFBP-5, three alternate models are proposed:

— Model 1, IGFBP-5 binds to a site distant from that of IGFBP-4 and the complex of IGFBP-5 + IGF binds to IGF receptors with higher affinity than IGFs alone. This would be analogous to a mechanism whereby the affinity of basic FGF to its receptor is increased upon binding to heparin sulfate.

— Model 2, IGFBP-5 has binding sites on the bone cell surface independent of IGF receptors. IGFBP-5 upon binding to its receptors may stimulate signal transduction pathways which may modulate some of its effects.

— Model 3, IGFBP-5 binding sites may recruit IGFs to the surface of IGF responsive cells, enabling the ligand to be easily captured by the IGF receptors. A similar function has been proposed for FGF binding protein, heparin, which may shuttle FGF as well as TGF-β binding protein, β glycan, which may shuttle TGF-β.

Further studies are needed to sort out whether any of these mechanisms are responsible for mediating IGFBP actions in bone cells.

Evidence that systemic effectors may modulate multiple components of the IGF regulatory system in bone

Since the IGF system in bone is made up of multiple components, for a given hormone to produce a maximal effect on cell proliferation, it must regulate the components of the IGF regulatory system in a coordinated manner [9]. Progesterone seems to operate in this manner. Accordingly, we found that treatment of human bone cells with progesterone caused a decrease in IGFBP-4 synthesis and an increase in IGFBP-5 synthesis. Progesterone caused an increase in IGF-II production which increases IGFBP-4 proteolysis and decreases IGFBP-5 proteolysis. In addition, progesterone has also been shown to increase mRNA levels for both type I and type II IGF receptors. These changes in IGFBP synthesis and degradation along with an increase in IGF receptor synthesis should lead to an increase in the activity of IGF-II and thus an increase in bone cell proliferation. However, it is not known whether all hormones which stimulate IGF production also produce this entire cascade of responses or whether some hormones influence only certain components of the IGF cascade.

Physiological significance of IGFBPs in bone

The bone disease, osteoporosis, has been shown to result in part because bone formation is inadequate. In the adult skeleton, bone formation is confined to specific remodeling sites and the net bone loss or gain will depend on the formation of new bone at each one of these sites. In regard to the mechanisms by which local bone formation is controlled in these bone remodeling sites, studies in our laboratory and other laboratories have shown that the amount of new bone formed at these remodeling sites may be regulated by both local and systemic factors. In regard to local mechanisms, both the amount of growth factors such as IGF-II released from bone during resorption as well as the rate of growth factor production by nearby bone cells may play a role. Systemic factors also modulate the IGF system. Accordingly, systemic hormones such as PTH and progesterone may regulate local bone formation in part by regulating the production of IGFBPs by bone cells [9,40]. Consistent with this concept, serum IGFBP-4 levels were increased in elderly subjects with hip fractures who had elevated PTH levels [41]. In addition, serum IGFBP-4 levels were also increased during oral 1,25-dihydroxyvitamin D_3 therapy in psoriasis patients [25]. These findings suggest that during calcium deficiency, the increase in serum PTH and 1,25-dihydroxyvitamin D_3 may, in addition to stimulating bone resorption, inhibit bone formation in part by increasing the production of IGFBP-4 by bone cells. Perhaps as a consequence bone is lost during calcium deficiency. Further studies are needed to establish the cause and effect relationship between PTH and 1,25-dihydroxyvitamin D_3 induced changes in IGFBP production and decreased bone formation seen in osteoporotic patients.

214

Acknowledgements

We thank Jerry L. Pettis Veterans Hospital Medical Media Department for illustrations. This work was supported by funds from NIH (AR31062), the Veterans Administration and Department of Medicine, Loma Linda University.

References

1. Mohan S, Baylink DJ. Clin Orthoped Rel Res 1991;263:30—48.
2. Mohan S, Baylink DJ. In: Spencer EM (ed) Modern concepts of insulin-like growth factors. New York: Elsevier, 1991;169—184.
3. Canalis E, McCarthy T, Centrella M. J Clin Invest 1988;81:277—281.
4. Hauschka PV, Mavrakos AE, Iafrati MD, Doleman SE, Klagsbrun M. J Biol Chem 1986;261:12665—12674.
5. Mohan S, Jennings JC, Linkhart TA, Baylink DJ. Biochim Biophys Acta 1988;966:44—55.
6. Dequeker J, Mohan S, Finkelman RD, Aerssens J, Baylink DJ. Br J Rheumatol 1993;36:1702—1708.
7. Nicolas V, Prewett A, Bettica P, Mohan S, Finkelman RD, Baylink DJ, Farley JR. J Clin Endocrinol Metab 1994;78:1011—1016.
8. Mohan S, Bautista CM, Herring SJ, Linkhart TA, Baylink DJ. Endocrinology 1990;126:2534—2542.
9. Mohan S. Growth Reg 1993;3:65—68.
10. Knutsen R, Sampath K, Baylink DJ, Mohan S. J Bone Min Res 1992;7(suppl 1):S104 (abstract).
11. Bautista C, Baylink DJ, Mohan S. Biochem Biophys Res Commun 1991;176:756—763.
12. Taga T, Kishimoto T. FASEB J 1992;7:3387—3396.
13. Mohan S, Bautista CM, Wergedal J, Baylink DJ. Proc Natl Acad Sci USA 1989;86:8338—8342.
14. Mohan S, Strong DD, Lempert UG, Tremollieres F, Wergedal JE, Baylink DJ. Acta Endocrinol (Copenh) 1992;127:555—564.
15. Mohan S, Baylink DJ. J Bone Min Res 1991;6(suppl 1):S141 (abstract).
16. Mohan S, Baylink DJ. Growth Reg 1991;1:110—118.
17. Hassager C, Fitzpatrick LA, Spencer EM, Riggs BL, Conover CA. J Clin Endocrinol Metab 1992; 75:228—233.
18. Chen TL, Chang LY, DiGregorio DA, Perlman AJ, Huang Y-F. Endocrinology 1993;133:1382—1389.
19. Schmid C, Ernst M, Zapf J, Froesch ER. Biochim Biophys Res Commun 1989;160:788—794.
20. Slootweg MC, Hoogerbrugge CM, De Poorter TL, Duursma SA, van Buul-Offers SC. J Endocrinol 1990;125:271—277.
21. Lee K, Mohan S, Baylink DJ. J Bone and Mineral Res 1992;7(suppl 1):S232 (abstract).
22. Strong DD, Morales S, Lee K-W, Mohan S, Baylink D. J Bone Min Res 1993;8(suppl 1):S305 (abstract).
23. Gao L, Ling N, Shimasaki S. Biochem Biophys Res Commun 1993;190:1053—1059.
24. Scharla SH, Strong DD, Mohan S, Baylink DJ, Linkhart TA. Endocrinology 1991;129:3139—3146.
25. Scharla SH, Strong DD, Rosen C, Mohan S, Holick M, Baylink DJ, Linkhart TA. J Clin Endocrinol Metab 1993;77:1190—1197.
26. Chevalley T, Strong DD, Mohan S, Baylink DJ, Linkhart TA. J Bone Min Res 1993;8(suppl 1):S158 (abstract).
27. Lalou C, Binoux M. Reg Peptides 1993;48:179—188.
28. Kanzaki S, Hilliker S, Baylink DJ, Mohan S. Endocrinology 1994;134:383—392.
29. Conover C, Kiefer MC. J Clin Endocrinol Metab 76;1153—1159.
30. Campbell PG, Novak JF, Yanosick TB, McMaster JH. Endocrinology 1992;130:1401—1412.
31. Fowlkes J, Freemark M. Endocrinology 1992;131:2071—2076.
32. Conover CA, Kiefer MC, Zapf J. J Clin Invest 1993;91:1129—1137.

33. Camacho-Hübner C, Busby WH Jr, McCusker RH, Wright G, Clemmons DR. J Biol Chem 1992; 267:11949–11956.
34. Fielder PJ, Pham H, Adashi EY, Rosenfeld RG. Endocrinology 1993;133:415–418.
35. Conover CA, Kiefer MC. J Clin Endocrinol Metab 1993;76:1153–1159.
36. Malpe R, Strong DD, Baylink DJ, Mohan S. J Bone Min Res 1992;7(suppl 1):S125 (abstract).
37. Andress DL, Birnbaum RS. Biochem Biophys Res Commun 1991;176:213–218.
38. Kiefer MC, Schmid C, Waldvogel M, Schläpfer I, Futo E, Masiarz FR, Green K, Barr PJ, Zapf J. J Biol Chem 1992;267:12692–12699.
39. Mohan S, Nakao Y, Honda Y, Baylink DJ. 75th Annual Meeting of the Endocrine Society. Las Vegas, Nevada, 1993;56 (abstract).
40. LaTour D, Mohan S, Linkhart TA, Baylink DJ, Strong DD. Mol Endocrinol 1990;4:1806–1814.
41. Rosen C, Donahue LR, Hunter S, Holick M, Kavookjian H, Kirschenbaum A, Mohan S, Baylink DJ. J Clin Endocrinol Metab 1992;74:24–27.

The insulin-like growth factors and their regulatory proteins
R.C. Baxter, P.D. Gluckman and R.G. Rosenfeld, editors

Regulation of IGF bioavailabilty by IGFBP proteases

Michel Binoux, Claude Lalou, Claudine Lassarre and Berta Segovia
Unité de Recherches sur la Régulation de la Croissance, INSERM U.142, Hôpital Saint Antoine, 75571 Paris Cedex 12, France

Abstract. Limited proteolysis of IGFBPs by serine proteases in vivo, initially observed during pregnancy, structurally alters them, especially IGFBP-3. Studies of patients with GH secretion abnormalities suggest GH/IGF-I regulation of the IGFBP-3 proteolytic balance.

In pregnancy serum, the alteration of IGFBP-3 diminishes its affinity for IGFs, facilitating their dissociation from IGF-IGFBP complexes, thus increasing free IGF-I.

The biological activity of IGFs studied in cultured chick embryo fibroblasts (CEF) is significantly greater in pregnancy serum than in normal serum.

Fragments generated by in vitro proteolysis of rhIGFBP-3 have been purified, one of which IGF-independently inhibits CEF cell growth.

Introduction

The discovery which took place in our laboratory [1,2] and independently by other groups [3,4] that limited proteolysis of serum IGFBPs (IGFBP-3 in particular) occurs under the influence of one or more serine proteases during pregnancy opened up new lines of research in IGF physiology. Over the past few years, extensive work by several teams has thrown some light on the conditions for proteolysis to occur, its origins, the nature of the proteases involved, and the functional repercussions on IGF bioavailability.

In this report, we summarize some of our laboratory's more recent findings in this field.

Occurrence and regulation of serum IGFBP proteolysis

The initial observations had been based on Western ligand blot analysis of serum IGFBPs and proteolysis experiments in which samples under study were incubated with normal serum as source of IGFBP-3 substrate. However, with this methodology, proteolysis could be detected only in circumstances where it was abundant, such as during pregnancy and under pathological conditions such as severe illness [5] or after elective surgery [6]. More efficient analytical techniques then considerably broadened the scope of research. A proteolysis assay was developed using ^{125}I-recombinant IGFBP-3 as substrate [7] and, with the ECL Western blotting detection system (Amersham, UK) based on luminol oxidation, the sensitivity of immunoblot revelation was increased 100-fold over the classical colorimetric techniques. Using laser densitometry scanning, estimations could be made from the proteolysis assay of the residual IGFBP-3 protease activity in a biological sample and, from the immunoblots, the proportions of IGFBP-3 (or other IGFBP) that had been proteolysed in vivo or in a cell culture system.

Thus, it could be shown that IGFBP-3 proteolysis occurs in the normal state [8,9], and we have detected it in all tested serum samples [9]. In Fig. 1, the electrophoretic profiles of normal serum IGFBPs in Western ligand- and immunoblotting are compared with those of pregnancy serum IGFBPs. In the latter, the 39—42-kDa doublet which is characteristic of intact IGFBP-3 had practically disappeared. Immunoblotting revealed a major proteolytic fragment of 30 kDa and smaller fragments of 20 and 16 kDa. The 30-kDa fragment was also visible in normal serum, but in smaller quantities.

Since serum concentrations of IGF-I and IGFBP-3 reflect their production by the liver under the control of growth hormone (GH), it seemed logical to investigate the changes in IGFBP-3 proteolysis in relation to different levels of GH secretion and serum IGF-I concentration. An inverse relationship was found between GH/IGF-I status and the extent of IGFBP-3 proteolysis. On average, the proportions of proteolysed IGFBP-3 were estimated to be 37% in normal subjects, more than 50% in GH-deficient patients, and only 15% in acromegalic patients [10]. This would suggest that the regulation of proteolytic activity is adapted to circulating levels of IGF-I, increasing bioavailability when its concentrations are low and decreasing

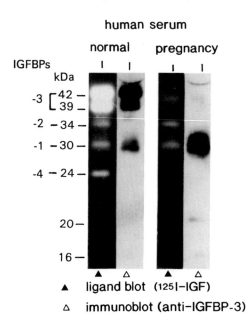

Fig. 1. Western ligand blot (▲) and immunoblot analysis (Δ) of serum IGFBPs in normal and pregnancy serum (3 µl per slot). The same nitrocellulose sheet was used first to detect IGFBPs using ^{125}I-IGF-I and -II, then to detect IGFBP-3 and its fragments using anti-IGFBP-3 antibody.

bioavailability when they are high. We had the opportunity to analyse serum IGFBPs in two patients with Laron-type GH-insensitivity, before and during a therapeutic test with IGF-I (Fig. 2). Before treatment, IGFBP-3 was at the limit of detection in ligand blotting, but unexpectedly an abundant 30-kDa fragment was detected by immuno-blotting, indicating IGFBP-3 proteolysis at a level similar to that in pregnancy. During IGF-I treatment, the intact form of IGFBP-3 reappeared and the proteolytic fragment either remained unchanged or decreased slightly.

We also examined IGFBP profiles in children with constitutionally variant stature, where the existence of GH secretion abnormalities remains controversial. In the series of prepubertal subjects studied, IGF-I levels in controls of the same age were 216 ± 22 ng/ml, in the short children they were 144 ± 13 ng/ml, and in the tall children 388 ± 25 ng/ml. The ligand blot profiles for serum IGFBPs in short children and in about half of the tall children were similar to those in controls, but in the other half, IGFBP-3 was reduced. IGFBP-3 proteolysis, as estimated by immunoblotting, was similar in short children and controls, but it was very marked in the tall children whose IGFBP-3 had appeared reduced in ligand blotting. These findings suggest that, in addition to inappropriate IGF-I levels for age, some dysregulation of the synthesis and/or degradation of IGFBP-3 may contribute towards abnormal growth.

Sources and specificity of IGFBP proteases

It is likely that during pregnancy the placenta, which is a known source of proteases,

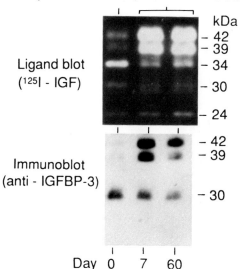

Fig. 2. Western ligand and immunoblot analysis of serum IGFBPs in a patient with Laron's syndrome, before and during a therapeutic test with IGF-I.

220

releases larger quantities into the serum, where they would be responsible for the specific degradation of IGFBP-3 and -4 and, to a lesser extent, of IGFBP-2; this accounts for the marked protease activity observed in pregnancy serum [11]. With a view to determining the original sites of IGFBP-3 proteolysis, we compared serum and lymph (which reflects the interstitial compartment) from the same subjects. Greater proportions of IGFBP-3 were proteolysed in lymph than in serum, and incubations with ^{125}I-IGFBP-3 showed that proteolytic activity in lymph was almost 8-fold that in serum where it was minimum. Like that in pregnancy serum, the activity was calcium-dependent and inhibited by aprotinin [9]. These findings suggest that the initial sites of proteolysis are in the tissues, and that the same types of serine protease are involved. They also suggest that limited proteolysis of IGFBP-3 may be an essential mechanism in controlling the bioavailability of the IGFs, not only in the bloodstream, but also at cellular level. Direct evidence has been provided by Conover et al. who showed that the IGFBP-3 associated with the cell surface of cultured bovine fibroblasts was processed to smaller forms when cell responsiveness to IGF-I was enhanced [12].

Gargosky et al., who analysed different biological fluids (peritoneal, follicular, amniotic, seminal, cerebrospinal), found that all of them displayed the same proteolytic activity towards IGFBP-3 [8]. Frost et al. reported that the sera of pregnant women, postoperative patients and patients with cancer contain proteases which cause fragmentation of IGFBP-3, but have little effect on IGFBP-1 [13]. However, we have noted that in amniotic fluid IGFBP-1 is extensively proteolysed and that in cerebrospinal fluid, IGFBP-2 is proteolysed, but IGFBP-6 is intact (Fig. 3).

It would therefore seem that there are several proteases, each with specificity for an IGFBP. Nevertheless, in the tissues, proteases with less restricted specificity may degrade several IGFBP species. Campbell et al. have noted that in osteosarcoma cells

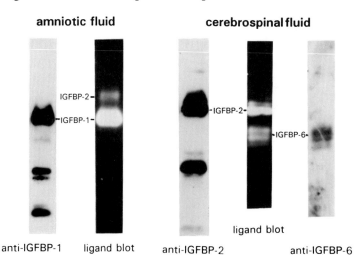

Fig. 3. Western ligand blot and immunoblot analysis of IGFBPs in amniotic fluid (1 μl) and cerebrospinal fluid (100 μl). The anti-IGFBP-1, -IGFBP-2 and -IGFBP-6 antibodies were gifts from Kabi Pharmacia, J. Schwander (Basel) and Chiron Corporation, respectively.

plasminogen is activated by cell surface urokinase and that the resulting plasmin proteolyses either free or IGF-complexed IGFBPs found in the pericellular environment [14].

Functional repercussions of IGFBP proteolysis

Serum IGFBP-3

In normal adults, IGFBP-3 carries in the 140-kDa complexes at least 80% of the IGFs in the circulation. It can therefore be expected that proteolysis of IGFBP-3 would increase IGF bioavailability. Although the structural alteration of IGFBP-3 and its loss of affinity for the IGFs have been clearly demonstrated by Western ligand- and immunoblotting, some authors have expressed doubt as to its physiological significance, since both IGFBP-3 and the acid-labile (α) subunit are found in the 140-kDa material and ternary complex formation is possible with acidified pregnancy serum in the presence of α subunit [15]. In fact, in our initial work on pregnancy serum, we showed that the 140-kDa complex was not disrupted in pregnancy serum analysed by neutral pH gel filtration, although there were also small IGFBP-3 fragments in the fractions containing low molecular mass proteins [2]. It therefore seemed possible that the stability of the 140-kDa complex would be diminished and the IGFBP-3 functionally altered, even if proteolysis remained limited.

Using partially purified preparations of plasma IGFBP-3, we investigated the different parameters for IGF binding. In competitive binding studies at equilibrium at 4°C, Scatchard analysis of the radio-competition curves showed that the affinity of pregnancy plasma IGFBP-3 for IGF-I was 10 times weaker than that of normal plasma IGFBP-3, and for IGF-II, twice. In terms of relative affinities for IGF-I and IGF-II, normal plasma IGFBP-3 had 3 times less affinity for IGF-I than for IGF-II, and pregnancy plasma IGFBP-3, 10 times less for IGF-I than for IGF-II (Table 1). In studies at 37°C of the kinetics of dissociation of ^{125}I-IGF-I and -II bound to IGFBP-3, IGF-II was dissociated approximately 6 times faster, and IGF-I, 10 times faster from pregnancy plasma IGFBP-3 than from normal plasma IGFBP-3 (Table 2).

Considering the changes in the structure-to-affinity relations of proteolysed IGFBP-3 and, in addition, the fact that in pregnancy plasma IGFBP-1 is increased, and IGFBP-4, and to a lesser extent, IGFBP-2, altered, one would expect the IGFs to be redistributed among the three circulating pools: the 140-kDa complexes, the 40-kDa complexes and free IGFs. We therefore chromatographed individual normal and

Table 1. Equilibrium association constants (K) of normal and pregnancy plasma IGFBP-3 calculated from Scatchard analysis of results of competitive binding experiments performed at 4°C

Equilibrium association constants (K)	IGF-I	IGF-II
Normal IGFBP-3	1.5 x 10^{10} M^{-1}	4.4 x 10^{10} M^{-1}
Pregnancy IGFBP-3	0.2 x 10^{10} M^{-1}	1.9 x 10^{10} M^{-1}

222

Table 2. Kinetics of dissociation at 37°C of ^{125}I-IGF-I and -II bound to IGFBP-3 from normal plasma and pregnancy plasma. Times for dissociation of half the bound IGFs

	IGF-I	IGF-II
Normal plasma IGFBP-3	6 h	20 h
Pregnancy plasma IGFBP-3	0.5 h	3 h

pregnancy plasmas so as to isolate each of the three pools and to measure their IGF-I and IGF-II contents. A first series done at 4°C did not reveal significant differences in IGF distribution between the two types of plasma. However, following preincubation of the samples in the presence of EDTA at 37°C so as to allow the pools to re-equilibrate in closer-to-physiological conditions and then chromatography at room temperature, the differences became quite marked (Tables 3 and 4). The proportion of total IGF-I in free form was nearly 3 times greater in pregnancy than in normal plasma, whereas that of free IGF-II was slightly smaller. The mean ratios of the molar concentrations of IGF-I/IGF-II were 0.43 in normal plasma and 2.23 in pregnancy plasma. Relative to total IGF-I, the proportion in the 140-kDa complexes was significantly smaller in pregnancy than in normal plasma, whereas the relative proportion of IGF-II was greater. In the 40-kDa complexes, the IGF-I proportions were similar in pregnancy and normal plasmas, whereas the IGF-II proportions were significantly smaller in pregnancy plasma. This means that in pregnancy plasma free IGF-I is enriched at the expense of the fraction in the 140-kDa complex, whereas relatively, IGF-II is concentrated in the 140-kDa complex at the expense of the 40-kDa complex.

Table 3. Distribution of IGF-I and IGF-II among their bound and free forms in plasmas from normal adults and pregnant (3rd trimester) women

Plasma levels	IGF-I (% of total)		IGF-II (% of total)	
	Normal	Pregnant	Normal	Pregnant
140 kDa	78.08 ± 1.57	68.99 ± 2.19[a]	77.18 ± 1.04	84.67 ± 1.93[b]
40 kDa	17.78 ± 1.25	19.62 ± 2.51	20.82 ± 1.07	13.79 ± 1.66[a]
Free	4.14 ± 0.51	11.38 ± 1.42[c]	2.00 ± 0.21	1.54 ± 0.31

[a]$p < 0.02$; [b]$p < 0.04$; [c]$p < 0.005$ (pregnancy (n = 7) vs. normal (n = 5)).

Table 4. Free IGF-I and IGF-II levels in plasmas from normal adults and pregnant (3rd trimester) women

	Normal	Pregnancy
IGF-I (mol/l)	1.32 ± 0.16	5.13 ± 1.05[a]
IGF-II (mol/l)	3.20 ± 0.49	2.42 ± 0.47
IGF-I/IGF-II ratio	0.43 ± 0.06	2.23 ± 0.25[a]

[a]$p < 0.005$ (pregnancy vs. normal plasma).

All these observations support the conclusion that IGFBP-3 is structurally and functionally altered by pregnancy-associated protease(s), resulting in depressed affinity for the IGFs, particularly IGF-I, hence accelerated kinetics of dissociation, and redistribution of the IGFs among the three circulating pools, with increased IGF in free form. From data on the half-lives of IGFs in man [16], our calculations indicate that the production rate of free IGF-I would be almost quadrupled in pregnant women.

It is therefore evident that the bioavailability of IGF-I is increased during pregnancy, in response to the enhanced metabolic and growth requirements accompanying placental and foetal development. This increased availability of IGF-I would also account for certain acromegalic features sometimes observed in pregnant women.

With a view to demonstrating this increased IGF availability to the cells as related to IGFBP-3 proteolysis, we compared the stimulatory activity of pregnancy and normal sera on chick embryo fibroblasts which are particularly sensitive to IGFs. Two pools were made up, one of pregnancy serum and one of normal serum, from samples in which the IGFBPs had been analysed by ligand blotting and the IGF-I and IGF-II contents measured. The samples were then mixed in proportions to yield identical IGF concentrations in the two pools.

Both pools dose-dependently stimulated DNA synthesis in cultured chick embryo fibroblasts. Stimulation by pregnancy serum was twice that by normal serum at 0.05–0.2% concentrations ($p < 0.001$). An addition of excess monoclonal anti-IGF-I and -II antibodies reduced the stimulatory activity of both pools and to the same degree. The greater potency of pregnancy serum was therefore dependent on IGFs. In order to show that this effect reflected greater availability of IGF to the cells, experiments were performed in the presence of increasing concentrations of rhIGFBP-3 (Fig. 4). Stimulation by both pools was dose-dependently reduced, more so for normal serum at lower concentrations, but equally for each at 100 ng/ml IGFBP-3. These results indicate that IGFs are released more readily from pregnancy serum, accounting for the weaker inhibitory effect of low IGFBP-3 concentrations. The study therefore demonstrates the functional consequences at cellular level of serum IGFBP-3 proteolysis.

Recombinant human IGFBP-3

As previously reported, the system comprising plasminogen and its activators, which is normally involved in the process of bone remodelling, also plays a role in the proteolysis of IGFBPs secreted by human osteoblast-like cells [14]. In a preliminary study, we investigated the IGFBPs released into the culture medium by these cells and found that the immunoblot profile of IGFBP-3 proteolysed by plasmin was the same as that of IGFBP-3 in pregnancy serum [17].

We then determined the conditions for proteolysis of recombinant nonglycosylated IGFBP-3 by plasmin, with a view to isolating the resulting fragments and studying their activities. A major proteolytic fragment of about 20 kDa (equivalent to the 30-

224

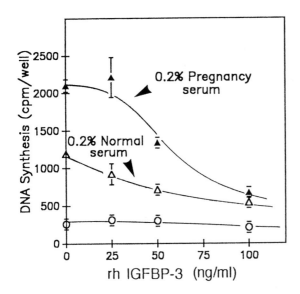

Fig. 4. Dose-dependent inhibition by IGFBP-3 of the stimulation of DNA synthesis in chick embryo fibroblasts by pregnancy (▲–▲) and normal (Δ–Δ) serum. Control without serum (O–O).

kDa fragment of glycosylated IGFBP-3 in serum) and a minor fragment of 11 kDa were separated by HPLC in an acetonitrile gradient. In ligand blotting, the 20-kDa fragment weakly bound radio-iodinated IGFs, whereas with the 11-kDa fragment there was a total lack of binding (Fig. 5). Competitive binding experiments confirmed the considerably reduced affinity of the larger fragment for the IGFs, and particularly IGF-I, and the complete loss of affinity of the smaller fragment.

In the chick embryo fibroblast assay, as expected, intact IGFBP-3 inhibited the stimulation of DNA synthesis by 15 ng/ml IGF-I, but had no effect on that induced by 1 µg/ml insulin. The 20-kDa fragment weakly inhibited the action of IGF-I, which agrees with its weak affinity for IGF-I and with our findings for pregnancy serum IGFBP-3. However, it unexpectedly also inhibited the action of insulin. Even more unexpectedly, the 11-kDa fragment, which fails to bind IGFs, totally inhibited the action of both IGF-I and insulin. This activity may account for the recently reported inhibitory effects attributed to an intrinsic action of IGFBP-3 [18,19].

Several points arise from this work:
1. Limited proteolysis of IGFBP-3 emerges as an essential mechanism in controlling the bioavailability of IGFs both from the 140-kDa complexes in the blood and at cellular level.
2. The physiological significance of IGFBP-3 (and other IGFBP) proteolysis fit in with more general systems of activation, or release from the extracellular matrix, of a variety of growth factors, like the FGFs and TGFβ.
3. Generation by plasmin of fragments with biological activity despite their loss of affinity for IGFs, although unexpected, fits in with known mechanisms of protein

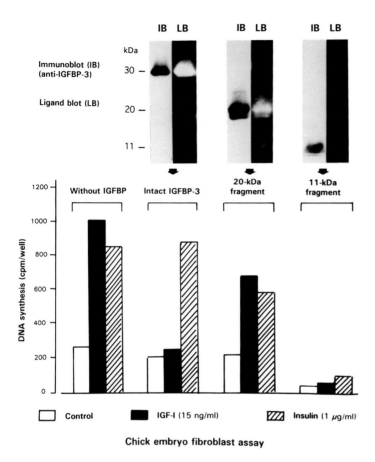

Fig. 5. Biological activity of intact rh (nonglycosylated) IGFBP-3 and its proteolytic fragments. IGFBP-3 was proteolysed by plasmin and the resulting fragments isolated by HPLC. The upper section shows Western ligand and immunoblot analysis. The lower section shows biological activity on chick embryo fibroblasts.

or polypeptide processing from their precursors. Moreover, it adds a further degree of complexity to the remarkable variety of combinations afforded by the system of the IGFs, their receptors and the IGFBPs, together with other factors, to regulate cell metabolism and growth.

Acknowledgements

This work was supported by the Institut National de la Santé et de la Recherche Médicale. Clinical investigations were done in collaboration with Dr. Micheline Gourmelen and the Laboratoire d'Explorations Endocriniennes at Hôpital Trousseau (Paris). We thank Jacqueline Villaudy (Institut Curie, Paris) for her technical assistance. We are particularly indebted to Christopher Maack of Celtrix Pharmaceuticals, Inc. for repeated donations of recombinant human IGFBP-3.

References

1. Hossenlopp P, Bredon M, Frankenne F, Binoux M. Ann Endocrinol (Paris) 1988;49:18C.
2. Hossenlopp P, Segovia B, Lassarre C, Roghani M, Bredon M, Binoux M. J Clin Endocrinol Metab 1990;71:797–805.
3. Giudice LC, Farrell EM, Pham H, Lamson G, Rosenfeld RG. J Clin Endocrinol Metab 1990;71:806–816.
4. Davenport ML, Clemmons DR, Miles MV, Camacho-Hübner C, D'Ercole AJ, Underwood LE. Endocrinology 1990;127:1278–1286.
5. Davies SC, Wass JA, Ross RJ, Cotterill AM, Buchanan CR, Coulson VJ, Holly JM. J. Endocrinol 1991;130:469–473.
6. Davenport ML, Isley WL, Pucilowska JB, Beaty Pemberton L, Lyman B, Underwood LE, Clemmons DR. J Clin Endocrinol Metab 1992;75:590–595.
7. Lamson G, Giudice LC, Rosenfeld RG. J Clin Endocrinol Metab 1991;72:1391–1393.
8. Gargosky SE, Pham HM, Wilson KF, Liu F, Giudice LC, Rosenfeld RG. Endocrinology 1992;131:3051–3060.
9. Lalou C, Binoux M. Regulatory Peptides 1993;48:179–188.
10. Lassarre C, Lalou C, Perin L, Binoux M. Growth Regulation 1994;(in press).
11. Davenport ML, Pucilowska J, Clemmons DR, Lundblad R, Spencer JA, Underwood LE. Endocrinology 1992;130:2505–2512.
12. Conover CA. Endocrinology 1992;130:3191–3199.
13. Frost VJ, Macaulay VM, Wass JAH, Holly JMP. J Endocrinol 1993;138:545–554.
14. Campbell PG, Novak JF, Wines K, Walton PE. In: Binoux M and Zapf J (eds) Proc 2nd Int Workshop on IGF binding proteins. Growth Regulation 1993;3:95–98.
15. Suikkari AM, Baxter RC. J Clin Endocrinol Metab 1992;74:177–183.
16. Guler HP, Zapf J, Schmid C, Froesch ER. Acta Endocrinol (Copenh) 1989;121:753–758.
17. Lalou C, Silve C, Segovia B, Binoux M. 2nd Int Workshop on IGF Binding Proteins, Opio (France), Aug 27–30, 1992 (abstract).
18. Liu L, Delbé J, Blat C, Zapf J, Harel L. J Cell Physiol 1992;153:15–21.
19. Oh Y, Müller HL, Lamson G, Rosenfeld RG. J Biol Chem 1993;268:14964–14971.

Determinants of complex formation between IGFBP-3 and the acid-labile subunit

Robert C. Baxter[1], Jin Dai[2], Sara Holman[2] and Moira S. Lewitt[2]

[1]Kolling Institute of Medical Research, Royal North Shore Hospital; and [2]Department of Endocrinology, Royal Prince Alfred Hospital, Sydney, NSW, Australia

Introduction

Insulin-like growth factor binding protein-3 (IGFBP-3), a glycoprotein of 40—45 kDa, differs from the other IGFBPs by being able to combine with the α subunit (acid-labile subunit, ALS), in the presence of IGF-I or IGF-II, to form a ternary complex [1]. ALS is an 85-kDa glycoprotein, a member of a family of hydrophobic proteins containing a well-conserved leucine-rich motif which recurs many times in the protein structure. Members of this family are characterized by their participation in protein-protein interactions [2].

Many subforms of IGFBP-3 exist, due to a variety of possible posttranslational modifications. These include glycosylation, phosphorylation, and limited proteolysis, all of which can affect the ability of the protein to form binary and ternary complexes by altering the affinity for its two ligands [1]. ALS may also exist in natural variant forms, of which glycosylation variants and a variable N-terminus have been identified to date [3,4]. The two IGFs themselves have several different subforms, arising by both pre- and posttranslational mechanisms, including recognized charge variants, C-terminally extended precursors (with glycosylation variants), and variants derived from alternative mRNA splicing [5—7].

Insulin-like growth factors (IGFs) and IGFBP-3 in the ternary complex have similar mobility on gel permeation chromatography to the serum IgG peak, so that the complex is commonly described as having a molecular mass of 150 kDa [8]. However, since each component of the complex can exist in a multiplicity of forms, many of which retain their ability to interact with the other component proteins, it is clear that the "complex" is in fact a multiplicity of complexes, which probably mainly fall within the size range of 100—140 kDa.

In addition to the biochemical factors regulating complex formation, several physiological factors will dictate the concentration of ternary complex in vivo: the relative sites of synthesis of the component proteins, and their concentrations, stability and processing in the circulation. In this paper, recent progress in the study of these biochemical and physiological factors will be discussed.

Sites of synthesis of IGFBP-3 and ALS

As recently reviewed, IGFBP-3 is secreted by many normal and malignant cell types, including osteoblasts, Sertoli cells, granulosa cells, fibroblasts, endothelial cells, and mammary cancer cells [1]. This is reflected in the broad tissue distribution of IGFBP-3 mRNA [9]. However, primary rat hepatocyte monolayers do not secrete IGFBP-3 into the culture medium [10,11], and in the liver IGFBP-3 mRNA expression appears confined to nonparenchymal cells, rather than hepatocytes [12]. IGF-I, in contrast, is produced by rat hepatocytes at a rate which can account for circulating levels [13].

We initially reported wide tissue distribution of ALS mRNA in the rat, in studies using a 1.8 kb cDNA probe [14]. The predominant hybridizing band appeared ~4.4 kb long. However, by using a shorter, more specific cDNA probe, it has now become apparent that the major stable transcript is only ~2 kb, and ALS expression is confined predominantly or exclusively to the liver. Fig. 1 shows a Northern blot of total RNA extracted from various tissues, fractionated on a formaldehyde agarose gel, and probed with a ^{32}P-labeled, 0.35 kb rALS cDNA fragment. Only the liver shows positive hybridization. Primary rat hepatocytes have therefore been used as a model system to study the regulation of ALS synthesis. Using a newly developed RIA for rat ALS [4], we have shown ALS secretion to be under growth hormone (GH) regulation in hepatocyte cultures; similarly, ALS mRNA expression shows marked GH-dependence (unpublished data).

Since IGF-I and ALS originate in one hepatic cell type, and IGFBP-3 in another, it is clear that ternary complex formation cannot occur until the secreted products of these different cells enter a common compartment, presumably the circulation.

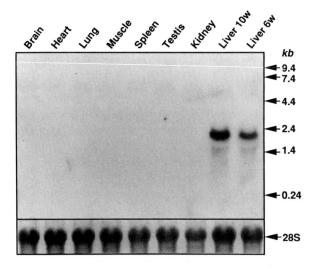

Fig. 1. Northern analysis of ALS mRNA in various tissues from adult male rats. Total RNA was extracted from the tissues shown, and 20 μg aliquots were fractionated on a 2.2 M formaldehyde-agarose gel, and probed with a ^{32}P-labeled 0.35 kb fragment of previously-described rALS cDNA [14]. Lower panel: Ethidium bromide-stained 28S ribosomal RNA. Size markers are indicated on the right.

Although IGFBP-3 has been identified in human lymphatic fluid [15], almost none of it is found in the 150 kDa form; similarly, IGFs in rat lymph are predominantly in the 50 kDa form [16]. These observations again suggest that, in man and the rat, ALS and the ternary complex are entirely confined to the circulation.

Stability of the complex in the circulation

Human IGFBP-3, injected into normal rats in an amount similar to that of endogenous rat IGFBP-3, is immediately distributed between two major molecular forms, the 50 kDa form which may or may not contain bound IGFs, and the 150 kDa complex. More than 50% of injected hIGFBP-3 complexes within 2 min, indicating a highly accessible pool of free, or weakly bound, IGF-I [17]. The source of this unexpectedly large supply of free IGF-I, or the proteins to which it might be bound with relatively low affinity, have not been identified. However, it is clear that the available IGF-I does not arise by dissociation from endogenous IGFBP-3, since little change in the rat IGFBP-3 ternary complex is observed [17]. In states of partial IGF-I deficiency, due either to diabetes [17] or GH-deficiency [18], formation of the ternary complex in vivo is impaired, but restored when IGF-I is coinjected, confirming the observation in vitro that ALS association with IGFBP-3 requires the presence of IGFs.

IGFBP-3 in the 50-kDa form leaves the circulation within minutes, whereas complexed protein circulates stably for many hours. Fig. 2 shows that IGFBP-3

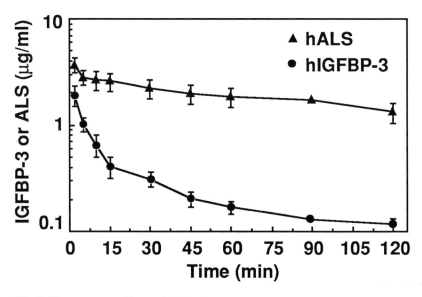

Fig. 2. Disappearence of human IGFBP-3 and human ALS from rat serum. Either natural IGFBP-3 (90 µg/kg) or natural ALS (180 µg/kg) was injected as a bolus into GH-deficient (*dw/dw*) rats, blood was sampled from an indwelling cannula at the times indicated, and IGFBP-3 and ALS were measured in each sample by primate specific RIAs. Mean values ± SE, three animals per group. Experimental details are as previously described [18].

injected into GH-deficient rats, which have insufficient available IGF-I to complex most of the exogenous IGFBP-3, is 90% cleared within 60 min. This stability of the residual IGFBP-3 is apparently conferred by association with ALS. Human ALS, injected into GH-deficient rats, has an apparent half-life of over 3 h, as illustrated in Fig. 2. In this experiment, subsequent examination of the size distribution of the hALS in rat serum, using a human-specific RIA, indicated that almost none of the exogenous protein was ternary complexed, indicating that endogenous rALS was present in excess of the ternary complex even in GH-deficiency [18]. ALS in the ternary complex is likely to have an even more prolonged half-life, like that of complexed IGFs and IGFBP-3 (at least 16 h).

Natural variants of ALS

Little is currently known about the important structural determinants on ALS. Enzymatic deglycosylation of human ALS indicates that the doublet band observed on SDS-PAGE at approximately 84–86 kDa is due to N-linked glycosylation [3], the deglycosylated form appearing close to the predicted size of 63 kDa [2]. Although six potential N-glycosylation sites are conserved between human and rat ALS [2,14], no functional studies have yet been reported from this or any other laboratory on unglycosylated ALS, so the importance of carbohydrate in ALS function remains to be determined.

As noted above, ALS belongs to a group of proteins which contain multiple highly conserved repeating units rich in leucine and other aliphatic amino acids. In human and rat ALS these repeating units are 24 amino acids long [2,14]. The abundance of hydrophobic residues in proteins of this type is believed to contribute to their propensity for forming protein-protein interactions. In the case of the complex between ALS and IGFBP-3, however, it appears that charge-charge interactions play an important role. Both polyanionic (e.g., glycosaminoglycans) and polycationic (e.g., protamine) substances are able to block ternary complex formation, and even moderate salt concentrations (e.g., 0.15 M NaCl) severely inhibit ALS binding [19]. ALS possesses a strong negative charge at physiological pH, since a high salt concentration is required to remove it from anion-exchange columns [3]. Although a conserved cluster of acidic amino acids is found near the N-terminus of ALS [2,14], it is also possible that acidic groups on its carbohydrate chains contribute to its negative charge. The possibility of sulfation, in particular, is raised by the observation that decorin, biglycan and fibromodulin, other members of the leucine-rich family of proteins, contain sulfated carbohydrates [20].

Variants in the primary sequence of ALS have also been identified recently, with the purification of rat serum ALS [4]. Two N-terminal sequences were obtained, one corresponding to the N-terminus of human serum ALS, and the other extended by four residues into the region previously believed to be part of the secretion signal peptide. These sequences are compared in Fig. 3. Since the signal peptide should be cleaved before ALS is secreted from the hepatocyte, it appears that the processing site

HUMAN ALS

M-A-L-R-K̲-G̲-G-L̲-A-L-A̲-L̲-L-L-L̲-S̲-W-V-A-L-G-P-
R̲-S̲-L-E̲-G-A̲|-D-P-G-T̲-P̲-G̲-E̲-A-E-G-P-A̲-C-P-A̲-A-

RAT ALS (predicted)

M-A-L-R-T-G-G-P-A-L-V-V-L-L-A-F-W-V-A-L-G-P-
C-H-L-Q-G-|T̲|-D-P-G-A-S-A-D-A-E-G-P-Q-C-P-V-A-

RAT ALS (found)

A : H-L-Q-G-T-D-P-G-A-S-A-D-A-E-G-P-Q-C-P-V-A-

B : T-D-P-G-A-S-A-D-A-E-G-P-Q-X-P-V-A-

Fig. 3. Comparison of the amino-terminal sequence of human and rat ALS. Underlined residues indicate differences between the two species. The boxed residues indicate the amino-terminus of hALS extracted from serum, and the corresponding predicted rALS amino-terminus. Preceding residues are assumed to constitute the signal peptide. The two sequences obtained from rat serum ALS (A and B) were found in a relative abundance of 3:1. Redrawn from Baxter and Dai [4], with permission. © The Endocrine Society.

has been incorrectly identified, and that at least some of rat, and presumably also human, ALS circulates in a slightly truncated form. It is at present unknown whether N-terminal truncation has any effect on ALS activity, although removal of a short peptide might alter activity significantly, as seen in the case of des(1−3)IGF-I.

Natural variants of IGFBP-3 — studies with IGF-I analogs

Although IGFBP-3 has at least two natural glycosylation variants and is also subject to phosphorylation [1], the best-described variants are those resulting from limited proteolysis. The proteolysis of IGFBP-3 was first observed in pregnancy serum, where it was found to render the protein undetectable by ligand blotting, and led to the appearance of an immunoreactive IGFBP-3 fragment of approximately 30 kDa [21]. Subsequently, IGFBP-3 proteolytic activity has been described in serum from patients with a variety of conditions [22], as well as in various other biological fluids.

The functional lesion induced by pregnancy-associated serum proteolysis of IGFBP-3 has not been fully defined. A reduced affinity for IGF binding is apparent in proteolyzed IGFBP-3 depleted of its IGFs by acid-chromatography or SDS-PAGE [21]. The physiological interpretation of this is complicated, however, by the observations that such proteolyzed IGFBP-3 still circulates in a ternary complex

232

which is normal both in apparent molecular weight and IGF-carrying capacity [23], remains indistinguishable in size from nonpregnancy IGFBP-3 (as determined by gel chromatography) after destruction of the ternary complex by transient acidification [23], and rebinds ALS with normal affinity even after purification by immunoaffinity chromatography [24].

The low binding of radioiodinated IGF tracers by proteolyzed IGFBP-3 appears to be due in part to the modification of tyrosine residues 24 and 60 of IGF-I caused by the iodination [24,25]. Using IGF-I analogs in which each of the three tyrosines was substituted for another residue [26], it has been possible to show in competitive binding studies that proteolyzed IGFBP-3 binds [Ser[24]]IGF-I and [Leu[60]]IGF-I at least 10 times less potently than normal-sequence IGF-I or [Ala[31]]IGF-I, whereas intact IGFBP-3 shows little discrimination between the four analogs [25]. This phenomenon is illustrated in Fig. 4. To perform these studies it was necessary to use [Tyr[31]]mono-iodoIGF-I as tracer, since tracers iodinated on the other tyrosines showed more severely inhibited binding to proteolyzed IGFBP-3 [25].

Because of its poor binding to proteolyzed IGFBP-3, [Leu[60]]IGF-I appears useful as a biochemical marker of proteolysis. Binary complexes of intact IGFBP-3 and [Leu[60]]IGF-I bind [^{125}I]ALS somewhat better than complexes with normal IGF-I (in contrast to those with [Ser[24]]IGF-I, which bind ALS poorly [27]); yet in the presence of [Leu[60]]IGF-I, proteolyzed IGFBP-3 shows almost no ALS binding [24]. Thus the ability of IGFBP-3 in patient serum to form ternary complexes in the presence of [Leu[60]]IGF-I will provide information about the extent of proteolysis.

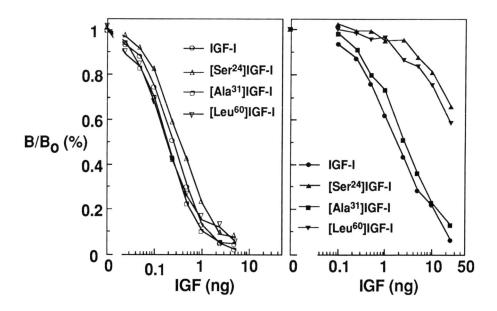

Fig. 4. Displacement of [Tyr[31]]monoiodoIGF-I tracer from intact (left) or proteolyzed (right) IGFBP-3 by IGF-I, [Ser[24]]IGF-I, [Ala[31]]IGF-I and [Leu[60]]IGF-I, as indicated. Reproduced from Baxter and Skriver [25] with permission.

IGFBP-3 proteolysis in healthy subjects and in chronic renal failure

In the serum of healthy subjects, fractionation by gel permeation chromatography indicates that approximately 90% of IGFBP-3 is present in 150-kDa complexes, and 10% in the ~50-kDa form. If sufficient IGFs and ALS are readily available to complex exogenous IGFBP-3, as indicated by studies in rats [17], it is not immediately clear why some 10% of endogenous IGFBP-3 fails to complex.

To examine this question, serum samples from healthy subjects have been fractionated on Superose-12 (Pharmacia), and separate pools containing ~150-kDa and ~50-kDa IGFBP-3 prepared and depleted of ALS by transient acidification. [^{125}I]ALS-binding studies on these fractions show that IGFBP-3 in the ~50-kDa pool is much poorer at forming the ternary complex than that in the ~150-kDa pool. Further, after depletion of endogenous IGFs and replacement with either natural-sequence IGF-I or [Leu^{60}]IGF-I, ~150-kDa IGFBP-3 shows normal to enhanced complex formation in the presence of the analog, whereas the low ALS-binding activity of the ~50-kDa preparation is decreased further. These observations indicate that the 10% of IGFBP-3 in the serum of healthy subjects which appears in the 50-kDa form is not in simple equilibrium with ternary-complexed IGFBP-3, but has been modified in a way which inhibits its ability to bind [^{125}I]ALS. The study with [Leu^{60}]IGF-I suggests that the modification is a form of limited proteolysis.

This phenomenon is exacerbated in the serum of patients with chronic renal failure (CRF). Recent studies indicate that such patients may have increased immunoreactive serum IGFBP-3, but that much of it is of a size smaller than the ternary complex [28,29]. Fig. 5 (left) compares the IGFBP-3 size distribution of CRF serum,

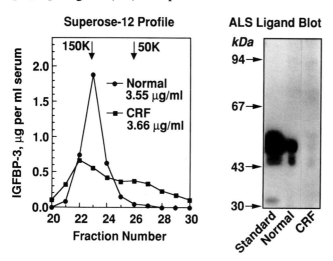

Fig. 5. Left: Normal and chronic renal failure (CRF) sera fractionated by Superose-12 chromatography. The total immunoreactive IGFBP-3 content of each sample is similar, but the CRF sample has a much higher proportion of noncomplexed IGFBP-3. Right: ALS ligand blot of the same serum samples. Pure plasma IGFBP-3 (standard, 250 ng) and normal and CRF serum samples (2.5 µl) were run on 10% SDS-PAGE, transferred to nitrocellulose, and incubated 16 h at 22°C with [^{125}I]ALS tracer (~20,000 cpm/ml) plus 100 ng/ml IGF-I. The nitrocellulose was autoradiographed for 7 days at –70°C.

234

fractionated on Superose-12, to that of normal serum with a similar total IGFBP-3 content. Almost 50% of the immunoreactivity appears in the ~50-kDa region, with a small proportion of even smaller size (presumably fragments). ALS binding studies similar to those described above for normal serum samples indicate that IGFBP-3 in the ~50-kDa peak of CRF sera binds ALS very poorly, and even worse in the presence of [Leu[60]]IGF-I, again suggestive of limited proteolysis. In contrast, IGFBP-3 in the relatively small 150-kDa pool from CRF serum binds [^{125}I]ALS virtually as well as that in the corresponding pool from healthy subjects (data not shown).

The inability of much of the IGFBP-3 in CRF sera to form a ternary complex can also be seen by ALS ligand blot (Fig. 5, right). When subjected to SDS-PAGE, blotted onto nitrocellulose and probed with [^{125}I]ALS in the presence of excess IGF-I, IGFBP-3 in the CRF sample binds much less ALS than a sample of normal serum with the same immunoreactive IGFBP-3 content. In summary, IGFBP-3 in CRF serum may not be qualitatively very different from that in normal serum, containing both complexing and non-complexing forms, but the proportion of IGFBP-3 in noncomplexing (proteolyzed) forms is greatly increased, presumably due to impaired clearance.

Conclusion

It has been the purpose of this review to discuss recent studies which shed light on the regulation of IGFBP-3 ternary complex formation at both physiological and biochemical levels. Physiological constraints include the compartmentalization of IGFBP-3 and ALS biosynthesis in different cell types, ensuring that the complex only forms in the circulation, and the relative production rates and stability of the component proteins. Biochemical constraints might be imposed by posttranslational modifications, of which variable glycosylation and limited proteolysis are examples.

There is abundant evidence that incorporation into the ternary complex limits the bioavailability of IGFs. This appears equally true for exogenous IGFs and for those entering the circulation from their many endogenous sites of synthesis, and has implications for both the growth-promoting and insulin-like activities of the IGFs. An understanding of the factors which regulate the ternary complex will thus lead to a better understanding of the regulation of body growth and of glucose homeostasis, and should allow optimization of administration regimes for recombinant IGF-I in the treatment of growth and metabolic disorders.

Acknowledgements

The gifts of [Tyr[31]]monoiodoIGF-I tracer (L. Skriver, Novo-Nordisk, Copenhagen) and IGF-I analogs with tyrosine substitutions (M.A. Cascieri, Merck, Sharp & Dohme, NJ) are gratefully acknowledged. The authors' studies are supported by grants from the National Health and Medical Research Council, Australia.

References

1. Martin JL, Baxter RC. Growth Reg 1992;2:88–99.
2. Leong SR, Baxter RC, Camerato T, Dai J, Wood WI. Mol Endocrinol 1992;6:870–876.
3. Baxter RC, Martin JL, Beniac VA. J Biol Chem 1989;264:11843–11848.
4. Baxter RC, Dai J. Endocrinology 1994;134:848–852.
5. Hampton B, Burgess WH, Marshak DR, Cullen K, Perdue JF. J Biol Chem 1989;264:19155–19160
6. Van den Brande JL, Hoogerbrugge CM, Beyreuther K, Roepstorff P, Jansen J, Van Buul-Offers SC. Acta Endocrinol 1990;122:683–695.
7. Daughaday WH, Trivedi B, Baxter RC. Proc Natl Acad Sci USA 1993;90:5823–5827.
8. Hintz RL, Liu F, Rosenfeld RG, Kemp SF. J Clin Endocrinol Metab 1981;53:100–104.
9. Albiston AL, Herington AC. Endocrinology 1992;130:497–502.
10. Schmid C, Zapf J, Meier P, Böni M, Ernst M, Froesch ER. In: Drop SLS, Hintz RL (eds) Insulin-like growth factor binding proteins. Amsterdam: Elsevier, 1989;267–272.
11. Scott CD, Baxter RC. Biochem J 1991;275:441–446.
12. Takenaka A, Miura Y, Mori M, Hirosawa M, Kato H, Noguchi T. Agric Biol Chem 1991;55:1191–1193.
13. Scott CD, Martin JL, Baxter RC. Endocrinology 1985;116:1094–1101.
14. Dai J, Baxter RC. Biochem Biophys Res Commun 1992;188:304–309.
15. Binoux M, Hossenlopp P. J Clin Endocrinol Metab 1988;67:509–514.
16. Cohen KL, Nissley SP. Endocrinology 1975;97:654–664.
17. Lewitt MS, Saunders H, Baxter RC. Endocrinology 1993;133:1797–1802.
18. Lewitt MS, Saunders H, Phuyal JL, Baxter RC. Endocrinology 1994 (in press).
19. Baxter RC. Biochem J 1990;271:773–777.
20. Kreis T, Vale R (eds) Guidebook to the extracellular matrix and adhesion proteins. Oxford: Oxford University Press, 1993.
21. Hossenlopp P, Segovia B, Lassarre C, Roghani M, Bredon M, Binoux M. J Clin Endocrinol Metab 1990;71:797–805.
22. Davies SC, Wass JAH, Ross RJM, Cotterill AM, Buchanan CR, Coulson VJ, Holly JMP. J Endocrinol 1991;130:469–473.
23. Suikkari A-M, Baxter RC. J Clin Endocrinol Metab 1992;74:177–183.
24. Baxter RC, Suikkari A-M, Martin JL. Biochem J 1993;294:847–852.
25. Baxter RC, Skriver L. Biochem Biophys Res Commun 1993;196:1267–1273.
26. Bayne ML, Applebaum J, Chicchi GG, Miller RE, Cascieri MA. J Biol Chem 1990;265:15648–15652.
27. Baxter RC, Bayne ML, Cascieri MA. J Biol Chem 1992;267:60–65.
28. Blum WF, Ranke MB, Kietzmann K, Tönshoff, Mehls O. In: Drop SLS, Hintz RL (eds) Insulin-like growth factor binding proteins. Amsterdam: Elsevier, 1989;93–99.
29. Powell DR, Liu F, Baker B, Lee PDK, Belsha CW, Brewer ED, Hintz RL. Pediatr Res 1993;33:136–143.

Vascular endothelium, IGFs and IGF binding proteins

Robert S. Bar, Mary Boes, Barbara A. Booth, Brian L. Dake, David R. Moser and
Ngozi E. Erondu

The University of Iowa, Diabetes Endocrinology Research Center, Department of Internal Medicine, 3E19 VA Medical Center, Iowa City, IA 52246, USA

Abstract. In the past decade, several findings have indicated a diversified interaction between the vascular endothelium and the insulin-like growth factors (IGFs). Specific type 1 and type 2 IGF receptors are present in cultured endothelial cells as well as in endothelium of intact blood vessels. The IGFs stimulate several metabolic functions in cultured microvessel endothelial cells and increase production of sulfated glycosaminoglycans and proteoglycans in both microvascular and large vessel cells. Most recently, endothelial cells in culture have been found to have mRNAs specific for IGF binding proteins (IGFBPs) 2–6 and to secrete large quantities of IGFBP-2, -3 and -4 into the culture media. IGFBP-3 and -5, but not IGFBP-1, -2, -4 and -6, specifically bind to the endothelial cell surface as well as the extracellular matrix secreted by the cells. The affinity of IGFBP-3 and -5 for the endothelial cell surface is dependent on a C-terminal region of the binding protein, which is highly enriched in basic amino acids. Synthetic 18 amino acid peptides corresponding to this portion of IGFBP-3 and -5 compete for IGFBP-3 and -5 binding, directly bind to the cell monolayer and stimulate acute metabolic processes in endothelial cells, a property not shared by intact IGFBP-3 or -5. Finally, IGFBP 1–6 can cross endothelial barriers in vivo. The transendothelial transport of the IGFBPs can be hormonally modulated and the subendothelial distribution of the binding protein is influenced by its association with IGFs. These findings suggest that the vascular endothelium can influence or determine endocrine and autocrine functions of the insulin-like growth factors by several mechanisms.

The vascular endothelium is composed of a single layer of cells that forms the intimal lining of all blood vessels. Once thought to be an inert barrier to the transfer of blood-borne macromolecules, the vascular endothelium is now recognized as a highly specialized tissue with multidimensional responses to normal and pathological conditions. In vivo, the endothelium is bathed by circulating IGFs and IGF binding proteins (IGFBPs) and presumably plays a role in the egress of IGFs from the circulation. This report will review the interactions of the IGFs with the vascular endothelium, then focus on more recent studies of the potential interplay between the vascular endothelium and the IGFBPs.

Address for correspondence: Robert S. Bar, The University of Iowa, Diabetes Endocrinology Research Center, Department of Internal Medicine, 3E19 VA Medical Center, Iowa City, IA 52246, USA.

238

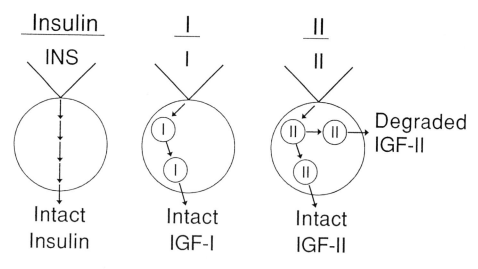

Fig. 1. Processing of receptor-bound insulin (Ins), IGF-I and IGF-II by endothelial cells.

IGF receptors, bioactivity and degradation by endothelial cells

Specific type 1 and type 2 IGF receptors are present in cultured endothelial cells as well as in the endothelium of intact blood vessels [1–4]. The receptor concentration is particularly high in microvessel (capillary) endothelial cells where the binding capacity for IGF-I and II is 4–8-fold greater than for insulin[1]. After binding to their respective receptors, IGF-I and II are internalized by the cell where IGF-I is retained for several hours as an unchanged, bioactive molecule while IGF-II is slowly degraded, with the degraded fragments secreted from the cell [5]. The endothelial cell processing of IGF-I and IGF-II differs from the cell's handling of insulin (Fig. 1). Insulin binds to the endothelial cell surface insulin receptor, the insulin internalized, then rapidly (<30 min) extruded from the cell as intact, biologically active insulin. Similar cell processing of insulin apparently occurs in vivo (perfused heart), where insulin binding to its capillary insulin receptor is necessary for biologically active insulin to reach its subendothelial site of action (cardiac muscle) [6,7]. For the IGFs, if such properties of IGF processing were retained in vivo, the vascular endothelium would have the ability to concentrate IGFs, provide a storage compartment for IGF and/or transport IGF from the circulation to tissue sites of action. However, such functions for capillary endothelium have not yet been demonstrated.

The IGFs affect several metabolic processes in cultured endothelial cells [1,2,8]. In microvessel endothelial cells, IGF-I/II are potent stimulators of glucose and α aminoisobutyric acid (AIB) uptake as well as thymidine incorporation into DNA. Although these processes are similarly affected by insulin, the IGF effects are

---

[1]Classical insulin receptors have also been characterized on endothelium both in cultured cells and in vivo.

mediated through their own receptors and not via IGF interacting with the insulin receptors of the endothelial cell [8]. In addition to their effects on acute metabolic processes in microvessel cells, IGF-I and II stimulate the synthesis and release of sulfate-containing proteoglycans in both microvessel and large vessel endothelial cells, a property that is not shared by insulin [9].

IGFBPs

In initial studies of ^{125}I-IGF binding to endothelial cell monolayers, it was noted that not all IGF binding was to type 1 and 2 IGF receptors, but that some IGF associated with a loosely-bound surface component of ~40 kDa. These low-molecular weight binding sites were subsequently identified as IGFBPs, predominantly IGFBP-3. When studying cells that secreted larger amounts of IGFBP-3, such as microvessel endothelial cells, as much as 35% of total monolayer IGF binding was to surface IGFBP, whereas in cells which produced little IGFBP-3, e.g., human umbilical vein endothelial cells, <5% of IGF binding was to surface IGFBP. These early binding studies led to a more in-depth evaluation of IGFBP production, regulation and function in vascular endothelium. The following section will review several studies of IGFBPs and vascular endothelium performed in cultured endothelial cells, isolated perfused hearts and intact animals.

Cultured endothelial cells

Cultured endothelial cells contained mRNA specific for IGFBP-2 through IGFBP-6 and secreted substantial quantities of IGFBP-2, IGFBP-3 and IGFBP-4 into the culture medium [10]. Endothelial cells derived from larger vessels, particularly bovine pulmonary artery cells, predominantly secreted IGFBP-4 and lesser amounts of IGFBP-3 while microvessel cells primarily secreted IGFBP-2 and IGFBP-3.

IGFBP-3 and -5 specifically bound to endothelial cell monolayers [11]. This property was not shared by IGFBP-1, -2, -4, and -6. IGFBP-3 (glycosylated and nonglycosylated) and -5 binding was to both the endothelial cell surface and to the extracellular matrix secreted by the cell, with the majority of binding to the endothelial cell surface. Homologous binding protein and several charged compounds (heparin, heparan sulfate and protamine) effectively competed for IGFBP-3 and IGFBP-5 binding to the monolayer. In addition to their binding to endothelial cells, IGFBP-3 and -5 also had significant affinity for the glycosaminoglycan, heparin. When comparing the primary structure of IGFBP-3 and -5 to other known heparin-binding proteins, both IGF binding proteins had a similar "consensus" basic sequence near the C-terminus that was also present in other known heparin binding proteins[2]

---

[2]The Cardin-Weintraub "consensus" sequences for heparin binding proteins are XBBXBX and XBBBXXBX where B is a basic amino acid and X is usually a hydropathic amino acid.

240

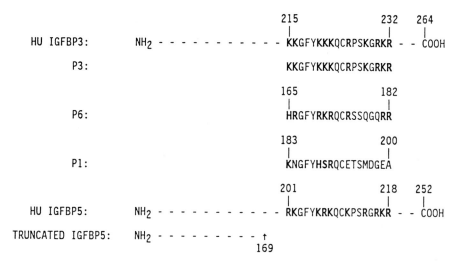

Fig. 2. Synthetic peptides corresponding to amino acid positions 215–232 of IGFBP-3 and position 165–182 of IGFBP-6. P1 is the homologous location (relative to the C-terminus) 18 amino acid segment of IGFBP-1, P3 of IGFBP-3 and P6 of IGFBP-6. The truncated IGFBP-5 represents IGFBP-5 with deletion of amino acids 170–252. Basic amino acids lysine (K), arginine (R) and histidine (H) are highlighted in bold letters.

[12] (Fig. 2). A similar sequence was also found in IGFBP-6, a binding protein which does not bind to endothelial cell monolayers and has a lower affinity for heparin. Eighteen amino acid peptides corresponding to a C-terminal portion of IGFBP-3 (P3) and IGFBP-6 (P6) and containing the consensus Cardin-Weintraub heparin-binding sequence were synthesized (Fig. 2). The ability of P3 and P6 to compete for IGFBP-3/-5 binding and to directly bind to endothelial cell monolayers was tested. P3 and P6 competed for IGFBP-3/-5 binding to monolayers, with P3 being more effective than P6. ^{125}I-labeled P3 and ^{125}I-P6 also bound directly to the endothelial cell monolayer. In contrast to intact IGFBP-3 and IGFBP-5, which had 30–40% of monolayer binding to the extracellular matrix and 60–70% to the endothelial cell surface, ~90% of P3 and P6 binding was to the extracellular matrix, with minimal binding to the endothelial cell surface.

Peptides P3 and P6 also possessed intrinsic biological activity in microvessel endothelial cells, stimulating 2-deoxyglucose uptake to 150–225% of control. This bioactivity was not shared by intact IGFBP-3, -5 or -6. The homologous 18 amino acid sequence of IGFBP-1 (P1) did not compete for IGFBP-3/-5 binding, did not bind to the monolayer and had no bioactivity, suggesting specificity of the P3 and P6 activities. Furthermore, a C-terminal truncated form of IGFBP-5, which did not contain the C-terminal basic portion of the molecule (tBP5) (Fig. 2), did not bind to the endothelial cell monolayer and did not compete for ^{125}I-IGFBP-3 or ^{125}I-IGFBP-5 binding to the cell monolayer. The nature of the endothelial cell binding site for IGFBP-3 and IGFBP-5 is uncertain. Treatment of the monolayer or extracellular matrix with heparinases or chondroitinase ABC caused minimal reduction in IGFBP-

3, -5 or P3 binding suggesting that heparin, heparan-sulfate, dermatan sulfate- or chondroitin sulfate-proteoglycans are unlikely primary contributors to the IGFBP binding, despite the fact that the IGFBP had significant affinity for heparin.

In summary, these data indicate that: 1) IGFBP-3 and -5 specifically bind to the endothelial cell surface and extracellular matrix secreted by the cells; 2) a region of IGFBP-3 and IGFBP-5 near the C-terminus, which is enriched with basic amino acids, may be necessary for the binding protein to associate with the endothelial cell monolayer; 3) synthetic 18 amino acid peptides corresponding to this basic C-terminal region of IGFBP-3 and -6 compete for IGFBP-3 and -5 binding, bind directly to the extracellular matrix and have intrinsic biological activity in microvessel endothelial cells, the latter property not shared by the intact IGFBPs; 4) although the 18 amino acid basic sequence may be necessary for an IGFBP to bind to endothelial cell monolayers, this sequence, by itself, is not sufficient for binding since P6, the 18 amino acid C-terminal basic sequence of IGFBP-6, can bind to the monolayer, but the intact IGFBP-6 has no affinity for the cultured cell or its extracellular matrix. This suggests that structure in other regions of the binding protein can either inhibit or potentiate the association of the binding protein with the endothelial cell monolayer; 5) fragments of the intact binding protein, such as peptides P3 and P6, can have properties that are not present in the intact binding protein. If such fragments of binding proteins are generated in vivo, then the intact IGFBP would serve as a precursor for more bioactive proteolytic products. The physiologic/pathologic relevance of these findings will be dependent on a) the demonstration that such IGFBP proteolysis occurs in vivo and b) the spectrum of processes affected by the generated IGFBP fragments.

Perfused heart and intact animal

The isolated, perfused, beating rat heart preparation has been utilized to study the transcapillary transport and subendothelial tissue distribution of perfused IGFI/II, IGFBP 1—4 and each IGFBP complexed with IGF-I [13—15]. This heart preparation has previously been shown to retain most properties of the heart in situ, including retention of several IGF and insulin mediated functions. Rat hearts have been perfused with ^{125}I-IGF-I/II, ^{125}I-IGFBP-1, -2, -3, -4 and IGFBP complexed with IGF-I. With one exception, each of the perfused substances crossed the capillary endothelium and distributed in subendothelial muscle and connective tissue (C.T.) elements in a ratio of ~2—3:1 (muscle:C.T. elements). When IGF-I was crosslinked to the IGFBP the complex also crossed the capillary endothelium with ~70—90% the efficiency of the free binding protein. Tissue distribution of the [IGFBP/IGF] complex was similar to that of the free IGFBP. The one exception to the common tissue distribution of perfused IGFBPs was IGFBP-4, studied as preparations of both recombinant IGFBP-4 (nonglycosylated) and IGFBP-4 that had been purified from endothelial cell conditioned media and separated into glycosylated and nonglycosylated IGFBP-4. All three IGFBP-4 preparations behaved in a similar manner. Each crossed the capillary boundary, but had a subendothelial tissue distribution that was strikingly different than the other IGFBPs. Instead of being primarily localized to cardiac muscle, as observed for the other three binding proteins, IGFBP-4 had much less affinity for cardiac muscle, being concentrated in C.T. elements in a ratio ~1:20 (muscle:C.T.) vs. the 3:1 muscle:C.T. ratio of IGFI/II and IGFBP-1, -2 and -3. However, when IGFBP-4 was crosslinked to IGF-I and the [IGFBP-4/IGF-I] complex perfused through the heart, it had a tissue distribution of muscle:C.T. of 3:1, i.e., the tissue localization appeared to be dictated by the IGF, not the IGFBP-4. Essentially identical findings were obtained when the different IGFBP-4 preparations were injected into the circulation of intact rats followed by removal and analysis of the heart.

The isolated beating heart preparation has also been utilized to determine whether growth hormone or insulin could alter the transcapillary movement of IGFBP-1, IGFBP-2 and endothelial cell-derived IGFBPs (a mixture of IGFBP-3 and IGFBP-4). Human growth hormone did not affect the transcapillary movement of any of the IGFBPs. However, insulin had a major effect [16] (Fig. 3). In these studies, IGFBPs were individually perfused through isolated beating rat hearts in the absence and

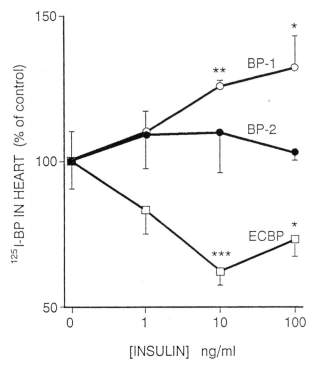

Fig. 3. ^{125}I-BP retained in hearts perfused with 0, 1, 10 or 100 ng/ml insulin. Isolated, beating rat hearts were perfused with buffer or insulin (1, 10 or 100 ng/ml) for 20 min, then perfused with ^{125}I-IGFBP-1, ^{125}I-IGFBP-2 or ^{125}I-ECBP (~500,000 cpm/ml) with the appropriate insulin concentration for 1 min. The hearts were rapidly perfused with 0.1 M cacodylate buffer for 1 min and counted for radioactivity. Data are expressed as the mean ± SEM of several individual heart preparations. For IGFBP-1 (BP-1) n = 3, 5 and 7 hearts at 1, 10 and 100 ng/ml, for IGFBP-2 (BP-2) n = 3 at all insulin concentrations and for endothelial cell binding proteins (ECBP) n = 5–6 hearts at each insulin concentration. * = p < 0.05, ** = p < 0.01, *** = p < 0.005.

Blood

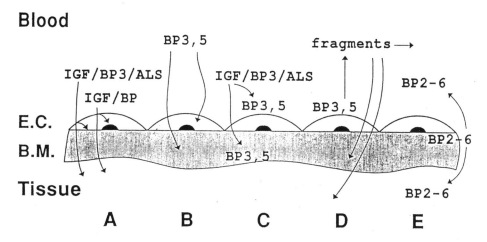

Fig. 4. Schematic model of the potential interactions of the vascular endothelium with the IGFBPs. E.C. = endothelial cell, B.M. = basement membrane, BP3 = IGFBP-3, ALS = acid-labile subunit.

presence of insulin. The subendothelial content of the ^{125}I-IGFBP was determined in hearts perfused with 0, 1, 10 and 100 ng/ml insulin (Fig. 3). Insulin increased the transcapillary movement of IGFBP-1, decreased the transcapillary movement of endothelial-derived IGFBPs (mixture of IGFBP-3 and -4) and had no effect on the transport of IGFBP-2, indicating that the transcapillary movement of circulating IGFBPs is likely to be under selective hormonal regulation.

Conclusions

These studies suggest several levels of interaction of the vascular endothelium with IGF binding proteins. In the model presented in Fig. 4, IGF-I/II could dissociate from either the dominant, circulating 140 kDa complex (IGF/IGFBP-3/Acid labile subunit) or other IGF/IGFBP complexes in the circulation (Fig. 4A). The free IGF then interacts with the endothelium and/or is transported to subendothelial tissues. Blood-bourne IGFBP-3 and -5 (or IGFBP/IGF complex), with their affinity for the endothelial cell surface and basement membrane, might localize to the endothelium (Fig. 4B) and concentrate IGF-I/II at these sites (Fig. 4C). The endothelial-associated IGFBP-3 and -5 could also be cleaved into bioactive fragments that are released into the circulation, reassociate with the endothelium or are transported to subendothelial tissue (Fig. 4D). Finally, the vascular endothelial cell is capable of synthesizing IGFBP-2—IGFBP-6, giving the endothelium the potential to change regional blood and tissue levels of IGFBP-2—IGFBP-6 (Fig. 4E). If indeed present in vivo, each of these interactions has the potential for complex regulation, which would result in an extremely sensitive, highly regulated control system that impacts on the autocrine, paracrine and endocrine effects of the IGF.

244

Acknowledgements

This work was supported by NIH grants DK25421, DK25295 and VA research funds.

References

1. Bar RS, Boes M, Dake BL, Booth BA, Henley SA, Sandra A. Am J Med 1988;85(suppl 5A):59−70.
2. King GL, Goodman AD, Buzney S et al. J Clin Invest 1985;75:1028−1036.
3. Bar RS, Boes M. Biochem Biophys Res Commun 1984;124:203−209.
4. Bar RS, Boes M, Sandra A. Biochem Biophys Res Commun 1988;152:93−98.
5. Bar RS, Boes M, Yorek M. Endocrinology 1986;118:1072−1080.
6. Bar RS, Boes M, Sandra A. J Clin Invest 1988;81:1225−1233.
7. King GL, Johnson SM. Science 1986;227:1583−1586.
8. Bar RS, Siddle K, Dolash S, Boes M, Dake B. Metabolism 1988;37:714−720.
9. Bar RS, Dake BL, Stueck S. Am J Physiol 1987;253:E21−E27.
10. Moser DR, Lowe WL Jr, Dake BL, Booth BA, Boes M, Clemmons DR, Bar RS. Mol Endocrinol 1992;6:1805−1814.
11. Booth BA, Boes M, Andress DL, Dake BL, Kiefer MC, Maack C, Linhardt RJ, Bar RS. IGFBP-3 and IGFBP-5 binding to vascular endothelium. Submitted.
12. Cardin A, Weintraub B. Arteriosclerosis 1989;9:21−32.
13. Bar RS, Clemmons DR, Boes M, Busby WH, Booth BA, Dake BL, Sandra A. Endocrinolgoy 1990; 127:1078−1086.
14. Boes M, Booth BA, Sandra A, Dake BL, Bergold A, Bar RS. Endocrinology 1992;131:327−330.
15. Bar RS, Boes M, Dake BL, Sandra A. Bayne M, Cascieri M, Booth BA. Endocrinology 1990;127: 3243−3245.
16. Bar RS, Boes M, Clemmons DR, Busby WH, Sandra A, Dake BL, Booth BA. Endocrinology 1990; 127:497−499.

Growth, development and differentiation

©1994 Elsevier Science B.V. All rights reserved
The insulin-like growth factors and their regulatory proteins
R.C. Baxter, P.D. Gluckman and R.G. Rosenfeld, editors

Genetically engineered IGF-I deficient mice

Lyn Powell-Braxton, Cara Warburton and Nancy Gillett[1]
Department of Endocrine Research and [1]Department of Pathology, Genentech Inc., 460 Pt. San Bruno Blvd., South San Francisco, CA 94080-4990, USA

Introduction

Insulin like growth factors (IGF-I and IGF-II) are involved in many aspects of growth and development. For many years much of the study of IGF action has been carried out in vitro or by administration of synthesized factor to animals by injection or mini-pump. Transgenic technology addresses the question of overproduction or atypical expression of protein throughout development in the context of an otherwise normal animal. Transgenic mice overexpressing IGF-I have demonstrated that high levels of IGF-I can enhance body growth [1], although this was not as dramatic as that seen in GH transgenic mice [2]. The more recently developed embryonal stem (ES) cell technology enables us to study the effects of removing gene expression from the animal and is an invaluable tool for studying the role of growth factors in pre- and postnatal development. Mice lacking a functional IGF-II gene are viable, demonstrating that the IGF-II protein is not essential for development and survival although they are significantly smaller than normal [3].

We have used ES cell technology to derive several strains of mice deficient in IGF-I. Mice with one functional IGF-I (IGF-I$^{+/-}$) allele are 10—20% smaller than their wild-type littermates and have lower circulating IGF-I levels showing a significant gene dosage effect. Mice totally lacking a functional IGF-I gene (IGF-I$^{-/-}$) progress through prenatal development, but greater than 95% die at birth. These IGF-I knockout mice are just over half the size of their normal littermates, they have a severe muscle dystrophy affecting both cardiac and skeletal muscle. One strain of mice expresses IGF-I at low level (IGF-I$^{m/m}$). Homozygous animals of this strain have circulating IGF-I levels <25% of normal. These mice are viable, but are approximately 60% of normal adult size.

Generation of IGF-I deficient mice [4]

Briefly a 18 kb genomic clone encompassing the 5' end of the murine IGF-I locus was isolated and sequences were identified corresponding to exon 3 of the rat gene [5]. This was used to create an insertion vector in which a phosphoglycerate kinase (PGK)-neomycin resistance gene expression cassette [6] interrupted amino acid 15 of the mature protein. The targeting vector contained 10 kb of homology to the endogenous mouse gene, including exons 1, 2 and the disrupted exon 3. This construct introduced multiple stop codons in all reading frames in IGF-I. A CMV driven thymidine kinase cassette was placed next to the 5' end of the IGF-I homologous sequences to permit negative selection against nonhomologous integration events [7]. AB.1 embryonal stem cells were transfected with this construct and clones were isolated based on resistance to G418. DNA extracted from these clones were screened for homologous recombination by Southern blot analysis. DNA from clones with a disrupted IGF-I allele were hybridized with a probe external to the targeting vector. The presence of a new Bgl II restriction site introduced by the neomycin cassette results in a novel 6.5 kb Bgl II band in addition to the 9 kb wild-type band. One in 82 G418 resistant colonies contained homologously recombined sequences. This frequency increased to 1:11 when additional selection with FIAU was used to select against thymidine kinase expression. Five clones were injected into C57BL/6J blastocysts and the embryos reimplanted into pseudopregnant recipient females. Chimeric mice derived from three independent clones had incorporated the ES cells into their germ line and transmitted the mutated DNA to offspring. Two of the clones (# s 220 and 432) were found to be complete disruptions of the IGF-I gene. Heterozygous animals were identified by southern blot analysis using tail DNA and interbred so as to produce animals in which both IGF-I alleles were inactivated. The absence of a product derived from the wild-type allele identified homozygous mutant mice (IGF-I$^{-/-}$). No IGF-I was detectable in serum from homozygous mice from these two lines. Reverse transcription and PCR amplification of IGF-I message from wild-type and IGF-I$^{-/-}$ mice showed no detectable mRNA from the IGF-I allele in the mutant mice. One of the ES cell clones, #200, showed an identical restriction pattern at the 5' end of the IGF-I gene, but was different 3' of the neomycin cassette. Homozygous mice derived from this clone still contain sequences corresponding to uninterrupted exon 3. IGF-I levels were detectable in serum from these mice, but at levels much lower than wild-types or heterozygous mice. Mice derived from this strain which have reduced IGF-I levels were intermediate in size between wild-type and those totally lacking IGF-I and have been christened "midi" mice (IGF-I$^{m/m}$).

Phenotype of IGF-I heterozygous mice

Heterozygous mice from all three lines were found to be smaller than their wild-type littermates. The size difference was detectable at birth and continued throughout the growth of the mice (Fig. 1).

Upon necropsy there was a corresponding reduction in the wet weights of most of the organs of both heterozygous males (5) and females (3) at 10 weeks of age. No abnormalities or obvious differences were detected in a complete set of tissues from all eight animals on histological examination. Serum IGF-I levels were determined and found to be approximately 65% of wild-type levels. There were no significant

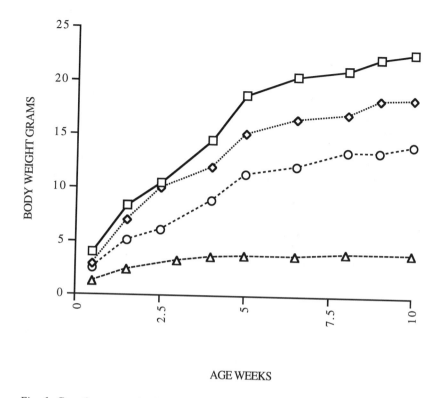

Fig. 1. Growth curves of wild type (□), heterozygous IGF-I$^{+/-}$ (◊), homozygous IGF-I$^{m/m}$ (O) and homozygous IGF-I$^{-/-}$ (Δ) female mice. The mean of at least eight animals in each group is represented with the exception of the IGF-I$^{-/-}$ mice in which only three surviving females have been obtained.

differences in serum components or blood cell profiles. Tetracycline labeling of the growth plate showed no significant differences between heterozygous and wild-type mice in 129/Sv × C57BL/6J Fls. Male and female heterozygous mice were fertile and healthy and were intercrossed to generate homozygous IGF-I$^{-/-}$ mice. Litter sizes tended to be smaller (6—>8 pups) than those found with wild-type 129/Sv × C57BL/6J crosses (8—>10 pups).

Phenotype of homozygous IGF-I$^{-/-}$ mice

Greater than 95% of IGF-I$^{-/-}$ mice died at birth. These animals were <60% of the body weight of their wild-type siblings and their lungs were not inflated. Upon dissection and analysis of viscera, it was found that the decrease in weight of the viscera was very small and probably could not account for the total decrease in body weight of the IGF-I$^{-/-}$ animals. In fact, when expressed as percentage body weight the livers and brains of the IGF-I$^{-/-}$ were found to be significantly greater than in wild-type animals (Fig. 2). The only organ which showed a significant reduction from

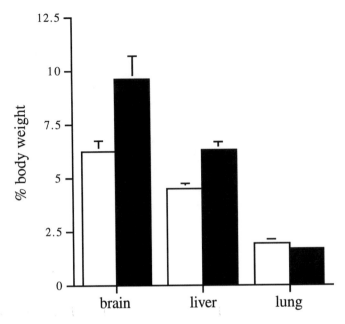

Fig. 2. Organs of neonatal mice from wild type (open bars) and IGF$^{-/-}$ (solid bars) mice expressed as percentage body weight. Means ± 1 SD are shown, there were three mice per group.

wild-type when measured in this fashion was the lung.

Pregnant mice were sacrificed from embryonic day 13.5 to 18.5 and the embryos examined. The homozygous mutant (IGF-I$^{-/-}$) mice were judged to be alive at e18.5 with beating hearts and other vital signs. IGF-I$^{-/-}$ animals were generally smaller at all stages examined, but this was not statistically significant before e15.5. The absolute size of the IGF-I$^{-/-}$ pups and wild-types was variable depending on the genetic background and litter size. Wild-type pups backcrossed for >5 generations onto the C57BL/6J background had a body weight of 1.393 g ± 0.102 and the mean of the IGF-I$^{-/-}$ pups was 0.808 g ± 0.039, whereas on the 129/Sv × C57BL/6J background the mean for wild-types was 1.488 g ± 0.084 and 0.863 g ± 0.072 for the IGF-I$^{-/-}$.

Histopathology of IGF-I$^{-/-}$ mice

The primary alteration noted in the IGF-I$^{-/-}$ neonates and embryos based on histopathologic examination was a generalized muscular dystrophy. This was most easily seen in the diaphragm, heart and tongue which are the muscles most developed at birth and required for pup survival. These muscles appeared less organized in the IGF-I$^{-/-}$ animals [4] and there appeared to be a decrease in the amount of myofibrils. These changes were also seen in all the e17.5 embryos examined. At e13.5 and e15.5

days, muscle changes were detected in some, but not all of the IGF-I$^{-/-}$ animals. In addition, the lungs in the dead IGF-I$^{-/-}$ neonates were not inflated (ataletic). The alveolar septae appeared to be more cellular than those of the wild-type neonates. The lungs of the e17.5 IGF-I$^{-/-}$ embryos were also more cellular with less evidence of alveolar separation and definition than the wild-type controls. There was no difference in the appearance of the lungs at earlier stages. In some animals from all ages, the epidermis appeared hypoplastic with a decrease in the thickness of the cell layers, particularly the strata spinosum. Remaining organ systems showed no detectable abnormalities at any of the stages examined.

In contrast to the IGF-I$^{-/-}$ mice, animals homozygous for the "midi" mutation IGF-I$^{m/m}$ were viable and fertile. These mice were, however, significantly smaller than either wild-type or heterozygous animals (Fig. 1). In addition, the intercross between the full knockout and the midi strain IGF-I$^{m/-}$ is smaller still. Although only a few animals have so far been derived, these are <50% the size of normal at 8 weeks of age.

Conclusion

We have disrupted the mouse IGF-I gene by inserting a copy of the neomycin gene with its own promotor and polyadenylation sites into the start of the IGF-I coding sequence. Expression from two lines with a targeted IGF-I gene was not detectable by reverse transcriptase PCR in homozygote IGF-I$^{-/-}$ mice. In both these lines the phenotype is indistinguishable: that is, reduced muscle mass in the heterozygous mice and decreased size, myodystrophy and substantial perinatal mortality in the homozygous offspring. A third line, expressing low levels of IGF-I, was viable and fertile when homozygous, but the mice were approximately 60% of normal size at 3 months of age.

Based on these results, IGF-I has a profound effect on the size of embryonic and post natal mice. Heterozygosity is associated with a decrease in circulating IGF-I levels and a reduction in mean body weight at birth and throughout life. In all cases the difference between the wild-type and heterozygous body weight is statistically significant. At birth, homozygous IGF-I$^{-/-}$ mice are 58% of the weight of the wild-types and the majority die without breathing. We have found, however, that approximately 5% of the homozygous mutant mice will survive beyond birth for up to 4 months. We do not yet have an explanation for this, though these animals had no detectable IGF-I mRNA or protein and were severely growth retarded. Preliminary results indicated severe effects on both the central and peripheral nervous systems in addition to pronounced dwarfism, muscle underdevelopment and reduced longevity.

Baker et al. [8] and Liu et al. [9] have also inactivated the IGF-I gene in mice. Although the overall growth effect in the homozygous IGF-I$^{-/-}$ mice is comparable, the mice described by Liu et al. do not show the same histopathological changes as the IGF-I$^{-/-}$ animals generated in our laboratory. Whilst the differences in the strains derived by the two groups have yet to be explained, the importance of IGF-I in embryonic and postnatal growth is clearly shown by all of the models.

The availability of mouse strains with genetically defined lesions is an increasingly powerful tool in the study of the role of growth factors and hormones throughout development. Using the well characterized genetics of the mouse and transgenic and embryonal stem cell technology it is possible to produce a veritable titration of endocrine components. The availability of mice with defined defects in IGF-I gene expression permit us to dissect the role of IGF-I not only in development, but also in disease pathogenesis.

Acknowledgements

We thank Arturo Raygoza for technical assistance.

References

1. Mathews LS, Hammer RE, Behringer RR, D'Ercole AJ, Bell GI, Brinster RL, Palmiter RD. Endocrinology 1988;123:2827–2833.
2. Palmiter RD, Brinster RL, Hammer RE, Trumbauer ME, Rosenfeld MG, Birnberg NC, Evans RM. Nature 1982;300:611–615.
3. DeChiara TM, Efstratiadis A, Robertson EJ. Nature 1990;345:78–80.
4. Powell-Braxton L, Hollingshead P, Warburton C, Dowd M, Pitts-Meek S, Dalton D, Gillett N, Stewart TA. Genes Dev 1993;7:2609–2617.
5. Shimatsu A, Rotwein P. J Biol Chem 1987;262:7894–7900.
6. Tybulewicz VLJ, Crawford CE, Jackson PK, Bronson RT, Mulligan RC. Cell 1991;65:1153–1163.
7. Mansour SL, Thomas KR, Capecchi MR. Nature 1988;336:348–352.
8. Baker J, Liu Jeh-Ping, Robertson EJ, Efstratidis A. Cell 1993;75:73–82.
9. Liu Jeh-Ping, Baker J, Perkins AS, Robertson EJ, Efstratiadis A. Cell 1993;75:59–72.

Expression and function of IGFBPs during rodent development

John E. Pintar[1], Joseph Cerro[1], Randal Streck[2], Teresa Wood[3], Leslie Rogler[4], Barrett Green[1] and Anoop Grewal[1]

[1]*Department of Neuroscience and Cell Biology, UMDNJ-Robert Wood Johnson Medical School, Piscataway, New Jersey;* [2]*Department of Neuroscience, Milton Hershey Medical Center, Hershey, Pennsylvania;* [3]*Department of Medicine, Albert Einstein College of Medicine, Bronx, New York; and* [4]*Division of Developmental Toxicology, United States Food and Drug Administration, Little Rock, Arkansas, USA*

Abstract. Genetic analysis in the mouse has shown that ablation of three components of the insulin-like growth factor system — IGF-I, IGF-II and the type 1 IGF receptor — can lead to developmental deficits. We review here the results on the expression patterns of these genes in the context of these genetic studies and also review the fetal expression patterns of the six IGF binding proteins (IGFBPs), which together constitute the third axis of the IGF system. Five of the six IGF binding proteins are expressed in the rat embryo proper as early as e10.5, while at least IGFBP-1, -2, -3 and -5 can be detected in uterine tissue even earlier. Taken together, these results suggest that functional redundancy may explain the absence of a major developmental deficit following genetic ablation of one binding protein, IGFBP-2, that is known to be expressed at high levels in numerous embryonic and fetal cell populations of developmental interest.

Introduction

The insulin-like growth factor (IGF-I and IGF-II) peptides induce cell proliferation and specific differentiative events in vitro. Gene targeting experiments designed to determine whether there is any required role for these peptides in vivo, have proven that both IGFs play essential roles in promoting embryonic growth. Mice genetically lacking IGF-II grow to ~60% of normal body weight, but exhibit no other major structural deficits and continue postnatal growth at normal rates [1,2]. Analogous studies have deleted IGF-I and have shown for the first time that this gene is likewise essential for normal embryonic and early postnatal growth even before the pubertal period when IGF-I is known to mediate growth hormone action [3,4]. Mice homozygous for a null IGF-I mutation additionally have diminished viability, dependent on the strain background, when compared to wild-type mice [3].

The IGF system has two known cellular receptors. The type 1 receptor (IGFR1) is a tyrosine kinase with high homology to the insulin receptor [5,6] and is thought to be the primary transducer of IGF-I and IGF-II activities. A required role for this receptor has also been identified genetically and IGFR1 disruption leads to lethality

Address for correspondence: John E. Pintar. Department of Neuroscience and Cell Biology, UMDNJ-Robert Wood Johnson Medical School, 675 Hoes Lane, Piscataway, NJ 08854, USA.

254

at birth [3]. The structurally distinct type 2 receptor (IGFR2) binds IGF-II strongly, but not IGF-I and is also the mammalian cation-independent mannose–6–phosphate receptor [7]. Mice with a chromosomal deletion of the IGFR2 gene exhibit greater growth than wild-type mice [8], suggesting that the IGFR2 acts principally to inhibit IGF-II activity by internalization. Indeed *Tme* mice, which lack a functional IGFR2 receptor, can be rescued from fetal lethality when crossed to mice lacking IGF-II [9]. The mechanism of IGFR2 action remains unclear, although there is evidence that binding of IGF-II to the IGFR2 can induce calcium influx in reconstituted vesicles through a G-protein-coupled mechanism [10].

Nearly all IGF molecules in the adult serum and tissue fluids form either a binary complex with any one of several IGF binding proteins (IGFBPs) or a ternary complex with IGFBP–3 and an 88 kDa acid-labile subunit [11,12]. To date six members of the IGFBP gene family have been cloned and their respective peptides characterized (reviewed in [13]). In vitro assays have established that the IGFBPs can modulate the binding of IGFs to cell surfaces (and therefore to association with IGF receptors) and can both attenuate and enhance the mitogenic response of several cell lines to IGF treatment (see [14] and other contributions, this volume). The different IGF genes exhibit tissue specificity in their adult expression patterns and also exhibit different responses to hormonal and physiological treatments at both the transcriptional and peptide levels. Taken together, these results suggest that the IGFBPs each play distinct roles in the adult animal.

Results and Discussion

While IGFBPs have received considerable attention in the adult, our studies have been primarily concerned with the expression of IGFBPs during prenatal development. Initially, we have assayed IGFBP mRNA expression during rat and mouse development by in situ hybridization and the embryonic expression patterns of two of the binding proteins, IGFBP–2 and IGFBP–5 have been reported in detail previously [15–20]. More recently, we have begun to examine the expression of other IGFBPs and to extend observations to early postimplantation ages. Using in situ hybridization, we have shown that all six IGFBPs are expressed during early post-implantation and midgestational development, extending our previous studies of older embryos [21]. Each IGFBP has a unique expression pattern, which suggests that each may have a unique role in development. Further, each IGFBP is often coexpressed with other IGFBPs, suggesting that they may also have complicated, combinatorial effects on the behavior of the IGF system. Highlights of the fetal expression patterns at early ages, which will be presented in detail elsewhere, are as follows:
— 1. IGFBP–1 is transcribed solely in the liver during early postimplantation and midgestation development. Further, it is first expressed at appreciable levels at e11.5, which is coincident with the growth that transforms the liver from a relatively small, morphologically indistinct tissue into the largest organ in the body cavity. These observations suggest a direct role in liver development, which is

supported by evidence that IGFBP–1 may mediate major tissue-specific proliferative processes such as postlobectomy liver regeneration [22].

— 2. IGFBP–3 mRNA expression is also apparent by e10.5 in a subset of cells which express IGFBP–5. This subset includes essentially all IGFBP–5-expressing mesenchyme including muscle progenitors, suggesting that while IGFBP–3 and IGFBP–5 may have independent functions in some tissues, they may work in concert or provide redundance in mesenchymal cells. Additional sites of expression include endothelial cells, mesenchyme surrounding the kidney and the dermal fibroblasts surrounding the developing hair follicle (Cerro J et al, in preparation).

— 3. IGFBP–4 and IGF-II mRNAs exhibit expression patterns which are widespread and strikingly similar, particularly in the embryonic and extra-embryonic mesenchyme. Genetic arguments have suggested that an overabundance of IGF-II may be deleterious, and perhaps fatal, to rodent embryos. Since IGFBP–4, which has a higher affinity for IGF-II than for IGF-I, has been shown to be an unusually potent inhibitor of IGF action in several in vitro systems, this coincident expression pattern suggests that the principal role of IGFBP–4 in the embryo is to attenuate the effect of IGF-II. Additionally, in the nervous system, IGFBP–4 mRNA is expressed in the spinal cord in an intriguing pattern that results in an intense band of hybridization across the intermediate zone of the spinal cord. Thus far, this pattern has been seen only in the caudal spinal cord and not the rostral cord, which suggests that IGFBP–4 may be playing an important regulatory role in establishing or maintaining a rostral-caudal axis.

— 4. Finally, IGFBP–6 transcription appears to be nearly ubiquitous in the midgestation embryo, albeit at low levels, but no convincing hybridization above background has been seen at early postimplantation ages. The highest levels of expression are found in a distinct population of cells just beyond the perichondrial layers of developing cartilage. This population is histologically indistinct from the surrounding mesenchyme and appears to project into muscle groups, suggesting that it may represent a connective tissue sheath around muscles.

In previous work, we extensively characterized the temporal and spatial patterns of expression of other IGF system genes and now briefly consider some unexpected results, in light of these expression patterns, that have emerged from genetic experiments. As mentioned above, IGF-II ablation leads to retarded growth of both the fetus and placenta. It remains formally possible that the growth deficit exhibited by IGF-II mutant mice is a consequence of ablated IGF-II expression in extra-embryonic tissues that indirectly affects fetal size; however, the differential onset of the growth deficits in these two fetal regions (e11.5 and e13.5, respectively) [4] argues for separate effects on each tissue. Since size deficits in IGF-II ablated animals begin only at e11 [4], significantly later than IGF-II transcription is initiated [23], this raises the question of whether IGF-II is actually produced at earlier ages. Thus far, although IGF-II has not been directly measured, all other evidence is consistent with IGF-II production. For example, at least at early postimplantation ages, IGF-II E-peptide immunoreactivity can be detected, suggesting that IGF-II mRNA is translated

[23]. Further, we have recently shown that the endoprotease furin exhibits an expression pattern strikingly parallel to IGF-II at early postimplantation ages [24]. Since IGF-II has three potential furin recognition sites, this provides suggestive evidence that an enzyme capable of processing the IGF-II precursor is present and active during the earliest times of IGF-II transcription. This result argues, but does not prove, that the absence of IGF-II effects on growth at ages earlier than e11 do not result from an inability to cleave proteolytically the IGF-II precursor and release active IGF-II.

Much of the previous research on the IGF system supported the idea that IGFs are paracrine and autocrine regulators and the distinctive spatial and temporal expression patterns that characterize not only IGF-II, but also IGF-I and IGFBP expression during embryogenesis are consistent with potentially local IGF effects. For example, the earliest time at which IGF-I expression is detected in the rat is at e9.5 in a distinct population of the cells — the septum transversum — that induces the liver [19]. Thus a potential interaction between the leading edge of invading liver cells that express IGFBP-2 and the septum transversum has been postulated [19]. Thus far, however, no apparent deficits in liver formation have yet been observed in either the IGF-I mutant [3] or the IGFBP-2 knockout. In fact, the genetic evidence to date more generally suggests that the IGF system instead has widespread endocrine effects that belie these specific expression patterns, but there are occasional indications of more specific, localized deficits. For example, type 1 IGF-receptor expression is especially prominent in skeletal muscle at mid and late gestation [25] (Streck, RD and Pintar JE, in preparation) and these cells are clearly hypomorphic in the type 1 IGF receptor knockouts [3]. It is not yet known, however, whether muscle is more affected in its growth than other cell types or whether subgroups of muscle that are especially high in type 1 receptor mRNA (including the pectoral and intercostal groups; Streck RD and Pintar JE, in preparation) show a more severe deficit than muscle subsets with lower levels of type 1 receptor mRNA. Another cell type expressing high levels of type 1 receptor mRNA are the neurons and neuronal precursors of the newly-forming prenatal sympathetic ganglia [25] (Streck RD and Pintar JE, in preparation) which exhibit enhanced mitogenesis in the presence of IGF-I in vitro [26]. The status of sympathetic neuron survival and differentiation in IGF system mutants both in vivo and in culture, should provide insight into the in vivo relevance of these in vitro studies.

As previously reported [19], the IGFBP-2 locus has been successfully targeted by homologous recombination. Germ-line transmission of the altered allele has been achieved, but, somewhat surprisingly, viable and reproductively capable mice homozygous for the mutant IGFBP-2 allele have resulted. The phenotype of this new strain of mice will be reported in detail elsewhere, but several implications of this observation can be discussed. First, as discussed above, all other IGFBPs are expressed throughout the midgestational period in the embryo proper and thus may be able to compensate for the lack of IGFBP-2. In addition, many IGFBPs are expressed early in the decidualizing regions of the uterus (Fig. 1). For example, IGFBP-3 is found lining the endothelial cells of the decidua, while IGFBP-1 lines the uterine lumen and IGFBP-2 is expressed in a cell group separating the dedicua from the rest of the uterus as early as embryonic day 8 in the rat. Finally, IGFBP-5 is, unlike IGFBP-3, highly expressed in the smooth muscle cells of the uterus. Clearly then, in addition to early expression of IGFBPs within the fetus itself, other IGFBPs are potentially available to the developing fetus at even earlier times in locally high levels that could compensate for IGFBP-2 loss in the mutant animals. Compensation for IGFBP-2 absence would not require an increase in other IGFBPs, although in

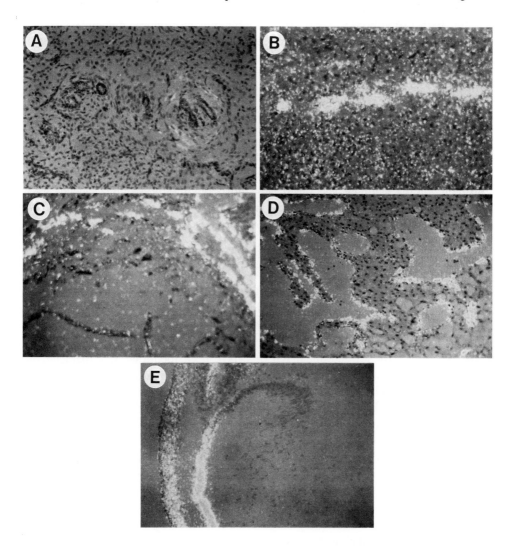

Fig. 1. Expression of different IGFBPs in the uterus of a pregnant rat at embryonic day 8 of gestation. A. IGFBP-1 is found not only in the lining of the initial uterine lumen, but also in the lining of the secondary uterine lumen and glandular epithelium; B. IGFBP-2 is expressed at the border between the expanding decidua and nondecidual uterus; C. and D. IGFBP-3 is found in the endothelial sinusoids of the expanding decidua. E. IGFBP-5 is expressed in both the smooth muscle of the uterus and in uterine cells at the outer extent of the decidual reaction.

MyoD knockouts, myf-5 has been shown to be upregulated [27]. Second, if functional compensation is occurring, multiple knockouts will be required to prove suspected critical roles of some gene products as illustrated by several recent examples. For example, ablation of all γ retinoic acid-receptor isoforms are necessary for a lethal phenotype while mice containing an ablation of only one isoform (RAR-γ-2) are normal [27]. In addition, genetic ablation of the myoD locus, which itself can induce muscle differentiation in fibroblast lines following transfection, has no dramatic effect on skeletal muscle differentiation; neither does ablation of a second transcription factor, myf-5 (reviewed in [28]). Yet a double mutant produces a complete absence of skeletal muscle [29]. These examples of functional compensation between related gene products provide a potential framework for understanding the relatively mild alterations in the IGFBP-2 mice that have thus far been observed. Finally, one final consideration concerns the background strains upon which mutant alleles are examined. The genetic background upon which many mutations are maintained influence genetic penetrance, evidence from the IGF-I null mutation reinforces this point, since the homozygote state is invariably lethal on the 129/Sv background, but can survive to adulthood on an outbred background. The 129/Sv line that has been used to produce many of the ES lines used in targeting experiments is a particularly difficult line to maintain and breed and, most importantly, exhibits several major neuroanatomical features different from most mouse strains. For example, the corpus callosum can be absent or reduced in these mice and this deficiency can vary significantly between individuals [30]. As a result, it is particularly important to carefully compare mutant and wild-type animals on appropriate backgrounds when alterations in nervous system organization or behavior are indicated and to consider that mutations maintained on outbred backgrounds will contain varying genetic contributions from a mouse strain with distinct neuroanatomical features.

From the foregoing, it should be apparent that genetic analysis of IGFBP function in vivo may require disruption of multiple IGFBP genes. To this end, 129/Sv mouse genomic clones for all additional IGFBPs have been identified and characterized. Since the fetal patterns of IGFBP-2 and IGFBP-5 expression occasionally overlapped [20], it is suggested that IGFBP-5 may be especially important in compensating for the absence of IGFBP-2 in IGFBP-2 knockouts. To test directly this possibility, we have successfully targeted IGFBP-5 in embryonic stem cells (Fig. 2) and have, in addition, partially completed the targeting vector for ablation of IGFBP-6 (Fig. 3). Production of mice containing targeted mutations in additional IGFBP loci is thus proceeding and should provide additional insight into the prenatal functions of the IGF system.

DNA was isolated from individual embryonic cells colonies that had been transfected with an IGFBP-5 targeting vector (provided by Peter Rotwein), double selected with G418 and gancyclovir and subjected to PCR using primers from neomycin and upstream regions of the IGFBP-5 gene not included in the targeting vector. Following Southern blotting of the PCR fragments, the blot was hybridized with neomycin labeled by random priming. Several individual colonies show neocontaining bands of the predicted size.

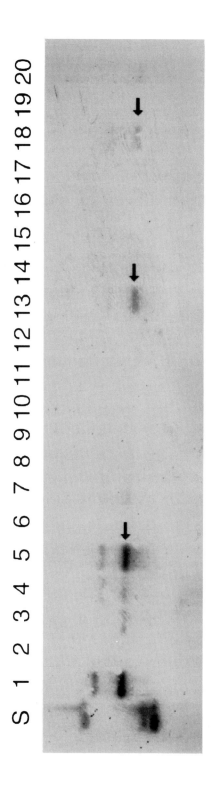

Fig. 2. Targeting of IGFBP-5 in ES cells.

260

A. CLONED REGION OF IGFBP-6 GENE

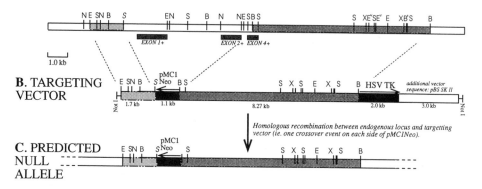

RESULT: *Endogenous sequences which encode for the translation start site, the signal sequence and additional protein-coding sequence are replaced by a neomycin resistance gene with its own promoter.*

Fig. 3. Construction of IGFBP-6 targeting vector. A. Partial restriction map of mouse Sw/129 IGFBP-6 showing restriction fragments containing IGFBP-6 exons; B. Targeting vector constructed by subcloning 5′ and 3′ regions of the IGFBP-6 gene will result in a complete deletion of the transcription start site of exon 1; C. Predicted structure of a targeted IGFBP-6 allele. Abbreviations: B = BamH1; B^s = BssH2 E = EcoR1; E^v = EcoRV; N = Nco1; S = Sac1; X = Xba1.

Acknowledgements

This work was supported by NIH grant NS21970 to JP.

References

1. DeChiara TM, Efstratiadis A, Robertson EJ. Nature 1990;345:78–80.
2. DeChiara TM, Robertson EJ, Efstratiadis A. Cell 1991;64:849–859.
3. Lui J-P, Baker J, Perkins AS, Robertson AJ, Efstratiadis A. Cell 1993;75:59–72.
4. Baker J, Liu J-P, Robertson EJ, Efstratiadis A. Cell 1993;75:73–82.
5. Rubin JB, Shia MA, Pilch PF. Nature 1983;305:438–450.
6. Ullrich, A, Gray A, Tam AW, Yeng-Feng T, Tsubokawa M, Collins C, Henzel W, LeBon T, Kathuria S, Chen E, Jacobs S, Franke U, Ramachandran J, Fulita-Yamaguchi Y. EMBO J 1986;5: 2503–2512.
7. Morgan DO, Edman JC, Standring DN, Fried VA, Smith MC, Roth RA, Rutter WJ. Nature 1987; 329:301–307.
8. Forejt J, Gregorova S. Cell 1992;70:443–450.
9. Filson AJ, Louvi A, Efstratiadis A, Robertson EJ. Development 1993;118:731–736.
10. Okamoto T, Katada T, Murayama Y, Ui M, Ogata E, Nishimoto I. Cell 1990;62:709–718.
11. Barreca A, Minuto F. J Endocrine Invest 1989;12:279–293.
12. Baxter RC, Martin JL, Beniac VA. J Biol Chem 1989;264:11843–11848.

13. Shimasaki S, Ling N. Prog Growth Factor Res 1991;3:43—266.
14. Cohick WS, Clemmons DR. Ann Rev Physiol 1993;55:131—153.
15. Wood TL, Brown AL, Rechler MM, Pintar JE. Mol Endocrinol 1990;4:1257—1263.
16. Pintar JE, Wood TL, Streck RD, Havton L, Rogler L, Hsu MS. Adv Exp Med Biol 1991;293:325—333.
17. Streck RD, Wood TL, Hsu MS, Pintar JE. Dev Biol 1992;151:586—596.
18. Wood TL, Streck RD, Pintar JE. Development 1992;114:59—66.
19. Wood TL, Rogler L, Streck RD, Cerro J, Green B, Grewal A, Pintar JE. Growth Reg 1993;3:3—6.
20. Green B, Jones SB, Streck R, Rotwein P, Pintar JE. Endocrinology 1994;134:954—962.
21. Cerro JA, Grewal A, Wood TL, Pintar JE. Reg Peptides 1993;48:189—198.
22. Mohn KL, Melby AE, Tewari DS, Lax TM, Taub R. Mol Cell Biol 1991;11:1393—1401.
23. Lee JE, Pintar JE, Efstratiadis A. Development 1990;110:151—159.
24. Zengh M, Pintar JE. Developmental expression in rat of proteases furin, PC1, PC2 and carboxy peptidase E. Implications for the maturation of peptide hormone processing. J Neurosci (in press).
25. Bondy C, Werner H, Roberts CT, LeRoith D Mol. Endocrinology 1990;4:1386—1398.
26. DiCicco-Bloom E, Black IB. Proc Natl Acad USA 1988;85:4066—4070.
27. Lohnes D, Kastner P, Dierich A, Mark M, LeMeur M, Chambon P. Cell 1993;73:843—858.
28. Weintraub H. Cell 1993;75:1241—1244.
29. Rudnick MA Schnegelsberg PNJ, Stead RH, Braun T, Arnold HH, Jaenish R. Cell 1993;75:1351—1359.
30. Wahlsten D. Brain Res 1982;239:329—347.

Insulin-like growth factors (IGFs) and IGF binding proteins (IGFBPs) in fetal development: physiology and pathophysiology

Victor K.M. Han, Hitoshi Asano, Douglas G. Matsell, Patric J.D. Delhanty, Jin Hayatsu, Nicole Bassett, Ian D. Phillips, Karen Nygard and Oresta Stepaniuk
MRC Group in Fetal and Neonatal Health and Development, Departments of Pediatrics, Biochemistry and Anatomy, The Lawson Research Institute, The University of Western Ontario, 268 Grosvenor Street, London, Ontario N6A 4V2, Canada

Abstract. Insulin-like growth factors (IGFs) regulate fetal growth and IGF binding proteins (IGFBPs), as modulators of IGF actions, may play a role in this process. To study the role of these peptides in fetal development under normal and pathological conditions, we have cloned ovine specific cDNAs encoding IGF-I and IGF-II and IGFBP-1 to -6. Sequence analyses indicate that the ovine cDNAs to be relatively homologous to those of the human and other species. IGF-II and IGFBP mRNAs, except IGFBP-1, were expressed in many fetal tissues throughout gestation in a developmentally specific manner. In situ hybridization showed IGF-II and IGFBP-5 mRNAs to be localized mainly to mesenchymal cells and IGFBP-2, -3, -4 and -6 mRNAs were localized to both epithelial and mesenchymal cells. IGF-II and IGFBP mRNAs were also expressed in the placental and fetal membranes, indicating that these peptides have an independent paracrine actions in placental development and/or function. Pathological conditions of malnutrition and chronic hypoxemia, known to cause intrauterine growth retardation in fetuses, alter IGFBP, but not IGF-II gene expression. Some of these changes may be due to the effects of nutrition and/or circulating hormones on IGFBP gene expression. Altered expression of mRNAs encoding these peptides were also observed in placentae from pathological pregnancies. The tissue and developmentally specific pattern of IGFBP mRNA expression indicate that the IGFBPs are important paracrine modulators of IGF action during development and are crucial regulators of fetal growth by modulating IGF dependent and independent actions.

Introduction

Polypeptides of the IGF system, namely the IGF peptides (IGF-I and IGF-II), IGF receptors (IGF-I or type 1 IGF receptor and IGF-II/mannose-6 phosphate receptor or type 2 IGF receptor) and six IGF binding proteins (IGFBP-1 to -6) (Fig. 1), are the most well studied paracrine growth factors which play an important role in the regulation of fetal growth and development. For a more complete reference, please refer to our recent review on the involvement of these peptide growth factors in embryonic and fetal development [1]. In this chapter, we will update on some recent developments and new observations made in identifying the mechanisms by which these polypeptides interact to regulate fetal growth.

Address for correspondence: Victor K.M. Han, Rm 3-524 The Lawson Research Institute, 268 Grosvenor Street, London, Ontario N6A 4V2, Canada. Tel.: +1-519-646-6100 Ext 4798. Fax: +1-519-646-6110.

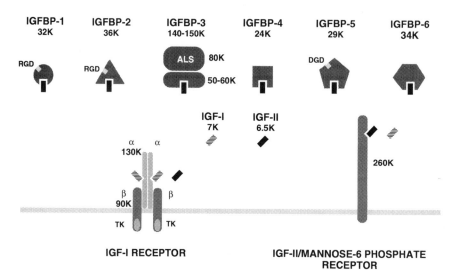

Fig. 1. Peptides of the IGF system.

Gene targeting and disturbance of IGF paracrine actions

IGFs behave as cellular mitogens as well as differentiation factors during development. The most compelling evidence for the importance of these peptides in embryonic and fetal growth, came from recent studies by Liu et al. [2] and Baker et al. [3]. These investigators utilized gene targeting to knock out or disrupt genes encoding IGFs or IGF receptors singly or in combination. Homozygous disruption of IGF-I gene (IGF-I (–/–)) or heterozygous disruption of the paternal allele of the IGF-II gene (IGF-II (p-)) produces growth retarded newborn mice which are 60% of normal birth weight. Depending on the genetic background of the mice, some of the mutants with IGF-I (–/–) genotype die shortly after birth or survive to adult. The latter mice continues to grow with a retarded growth rate compared to the wild-type litter mates and achieve 30% of normal adult weight. Null mutants of IGF-I receptor (IGF-IR), in contrast, die invariably at birth of respiratory failure and exhibit a more severe growth deficiency (45% of normal size) compared to either IGF-I (–/–) or IGF-II (p-) mutants. One of the many interesting concepts that came out of these studies is that there may exist a not yet identified IGF receptor, which is not an IGF-II/mannose-6 phosphate receptor, which mediates additionally the biological actions of IGF-II. This concept was borne of the findings that IGF-I (–/–)/IGF-IR (–/–) double mutants do not differ in phenotype from IGF-IR (–/–) single mutants (45% of normal size), whereas IGF-II (p-)/IGF-IR (–/–) double mutants are growth retarded further (30% of normal size). The investigators also concluded that placental growth is served exclusively by this unknown IGF receptor. However, some questions still remain to be answered as to the mechanisms by which these growth retarded phenotypes occurred. For example, since IGFs mediate the growth and differentiation of many tissues including the endocrine organs, what are the effects on thyroid development? This could explain some of the phenotypic changes observed in the bone; since IGFs interact and regulate the synthesis of other growth factors and IGFBPs, what are the effects on other growth factors and IGFBPs? Alterations in other growth factors like TGF-β and TGF-α could be responsible in part to the phenotypic changes in the bone and skin respectively; could changes in IGFBP-2 synthesis by the developing tissues explain the additional 15% reduction observed by the double mutants of IGF-II (p-)/IGF-IR (–/–)? These are interesting questions that could be easily tested in these genetic models.

Gene expression

Even though in the studies by Baker et al. [3] it was reported that only IGF-IR serves the in vivo mitogenic signalling of IGF-II between embryonic days 11.0 and 12.5 and from 13.5 days onwards, IGF-IR interacts with both IGF-I and IGF-II, these polypeptide transcripts having been identified before these gestational ages. Using reverse transcription-polymerase chain reaction (RT-PCR), Rappolee and Werb [4] have shown that IGF-II and IGF-II receptor transcripts are present from two cell stage onwards and IGF-IR from eight cell stage onwards in the preimplantation mouse embryos (Fig. 2). In contrast, using a similar technique, Watson et al. [5] have demonstrated that in the bovine preimplantation embryos, IGF-I, IGF-II and IGF-IR

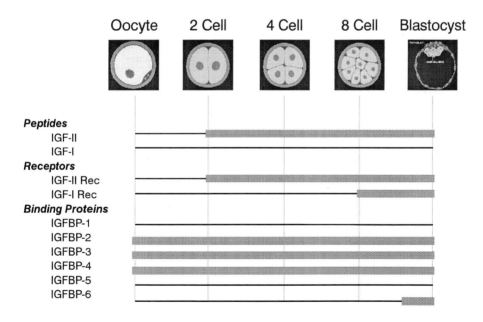

Rappolee & Werb, 1991
Hahnel & Schultz, 1993

Fig. 2. Reimplantation development.

transcripts are expressed continuously throughout from maternal to embryonic stages. Using in situ hybridization, Ohlsson et al. [6], failed to detect any IGF-II transcripts in the human preimplantation embryos. Even though differences in the sensitivity and specificity of the techniques used could explain some of the results, these findings indicate that there are species specific differences in the expression of IGF and IGF receptor genes even in the preimplantation embryos. It is possible that differences between species on the support provided by the secretions of the oviductal cells could account for the differences.

More recently Hahnel and Schultz [7] have shown that not only the IGFs and IGF receptors, but also certain IGFBP transcripts (IGFBP-2, -3, -4 and -6) may be detectable in the preimplantation mouse embryos [8] (Fig. 2), suggesting that the IGF-IGFBP interactions may be initiated early. IGFBP-1 and IGFBP-5 transcripts, however, are not detectable in the early embryos. Using in situ hybridization, we have detected IGFBP-1 mRNA in the liver by 10 days gestation in the mouse embryos and IGFBP-5 mRNA in the mesodermal tissues by 8 days gestation (Fig. 3). In contrast, using northern blot hybridization, IGFBP-1 mRNA is barely detectable in the liver of 50 days gestation ovine fetuses. It increases gradually with gestation, reaches maximum at 123 days gestation and then gradually decreases to term [8]. Liver is the only tissue demonstrated to express IGFBP-1 mRNA, using Northern blotting. In the humans, a similar pattern is also observed. However, if RNAse protection assay is used, low levels of IGFBP-1 mRNA are detectable in other tissues [9]. These findings indicate that, in addition to species specific differences, the methodology used to detect the mRNAs may influence the results.

Studies using gene targeting, have also confirmed the reciprocal parental imprinting of the IGF-II and IGF-IIR (paternal imprinting of the IGF-II gene and maternal imprinting of the IGF-IIR gene), with potential cause of genetic origin for abnormal growth of tissues and organs. This defect is now thought to be the reason for the organ or tissue hypertrophy that is observed in certain overgrowth syndromes of genetic origin e.g., Beckwith-Weideman syndrome. In this syndrome, it is believed to be due to the relaxation of imprinting of the IGF-II gene leading to bi-allelic expression of the IGF-II gene which may possibly lead to overexpresssion of the growth factor at specific organs leading to overgrowth. It is of interest to note that tongue and liver are the organs that are commonly involved in hypertrophy in Beckwith-Weideman syndrome, the same organs which express abundant IGF-II mRNA levels in humans. Perhaps tissue specific overexpression as well as being sensitive target organs to the biologic actions of IGFs, could explain the particular specific organ hypertrophy seen in this syndrome.

In humans, no genetic syndrome or intrauterine growth retarded condition has been linked to either disruption or polymorphism of the IGF or IGF receptor genes. It is therefore more likely that changes in IGF or IGF receptor levels associated with intrauterine growth retardation are due to epigenetic influences that alter the expression of these genes.

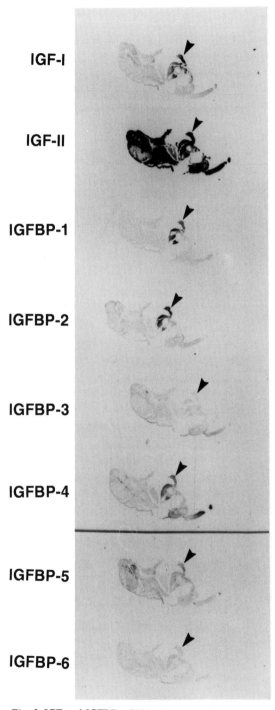

Fig. 3. IGF and IGFBP mRNAs in the newborn mouse.

Species differences

Differences between rodents, sheep and humans in the plasma or serum concentrations of IGF-I and IGF-II during fetal and postnatal life and adults are well described [10]. Even though IGF-II concentrations are higher than IGF-I concentrations in all species, it is only in the rodents that the discrepancy between embryo and mother is pronounced. This is mainly because serum or plasma IGF-II concentrations decrease dramatically in rodents in postnatal life, much more so than any other species. Analysis of IGF-II mRNA levels in the liver of rats indicated the almost nonexistence of IGF-II mRNAs in the adult rat liver, whereas they continue to be detectable in the liver of sheep and humans, albeit at lower levels. The differences in the organization of the IGF-II gene and the promoter structure may be responsible for these differences.

   Similarly, the profiles of IGFBPs in the plasma also differ amongst species (Fig. 4). The profile in the adult mammals appear to be similar with IGFBP-3 being the predominant IGFBP, with lower levels of IGFBP-4. In human and sheep adults IGFBPs with approximately 30 kDa (IGFBP-1, IGFBP-5 or IGFBP-6), are present in lower levels, whereas in the rabbit and rat adults they are present in significantly higher levels. The differences in the fetuses are even more obvious. In the human and sheep IGFBP-3 is the predominant IGFBP, especially in the later gestations [11],

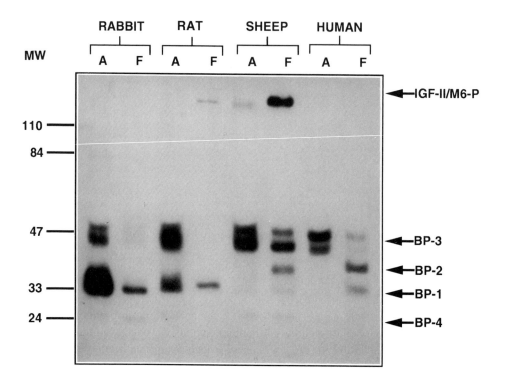

Fig. 4. IGFBPs in plasma of different species.

whereas in the rabbit it is barely detectable even in the later gestation and in the rat it is undetectable. This is also reflected by the level of IGFBP-3 mRNA in the liver of these animals in the fetus and early postnatal ages by both Northern blotting and in situ hybridization. It is of interest to note that the absence of IGFBP-3 in the plasma of rat embryo and fetuses is not due to the lack of IGFBP-3 mRNA expression in other tissues like dorsal mesoderm, dermis and kidney (Fig. 3). These findings suggest that the mRNA that is expressed in these tissues do not contribute to the IGFBP levels in the plasma, and perhaps utilized as a paracrine factor within the tissues. As noted by in situ hybridization studies, these tissues are also sites of abundant expression of IGF-II and therefore potentially targets of paracrine interaction between the two factors. As shown before, IGFBP-3 specific proteases are not responsible for the lack of IGFBP-3 in the plasma.

Physiology

Endocrine vs. paracrine

Traditionally, with classic hormones, endocrinologists have used serum or plasma concentrations to correlate physiology or pathophysiology. However, with IGFs and IGFBPs, which are abundantly expressed in multiple tissues and organs, knowledge of serum or plasma concentrations may not be adequate. Several studies have shown that changes in tissue mRNA levels may not necessarily be accompanied by corresponding changes in serum or plasma concentrations of these peptides. Thus, the concept of physiology in fetuses must extend into paracrinology [12], with measurements of tissue mRNA or peptide levels.

It is however important to note that IGF-I, when used as a pharmacologic agent in either fetuses or growing animals, can be transported into extracellular fluids of target organs to exert biological actions. Since almost all of IGFs in circulation are bound to IGFBPs, the site of biological action of IGFs, obviously, is determined by the IGFBPs. Bar et al. [13] have shown the importance of IGFBPs in the translocation of IGFs across capillaries into the myocardium of adult animals and a similar mechanism may exist in fetuses and in many tissues. The importance of endocrine actions of IGF-I in fetuses is demonstrated by the effects of continuous infusion of the peptide on placental morphometrics and growth of certain fetal organs (Robinson J, personal communication). In these studies, fetal weights are not affected generally and therefore tissue specific responsiveness may play a role.

Tissue specific IGF/IGFBP expression

Since we first described the abundant distribution of IGF mRNAs in the mesenchymal cells of many tissues and organs in the human fetus, studies using in situ hybridization in embryo and fetuses of various species have confirmed similar distribution of IGF mRNAs, with some minor differences. Likewise, IGFBP mRNAs are also expressed in different tissues [11]. Compared to IGFs the cellular distribution of IGFBP mRNAs is more specific and each appears to have a precise spatial and temporal pattern, thus suggesting that these proteins may be involved in regulating the IGF biological function. This pattern is seen in many tissues, but the most convincing evidence is observed in the kidney. This organ also represents the extensive epithelial-mesenchymal interactions that occur in many organs and tissues during development. The ureteric duct of endodermal origin migrates rostrally and interact with the metanephric blastema of the dorsal mesoderm to form the kidney. The ureteric duct in human and mouse fetuses is one of the sites where IGFBP-3 is most abundantly expressed. However, at the point of contact with the metanephric blastema, with the formation of the ampulla, the ureteric duct loses its IGFBP-3 and begins to express IGFBP-2. The aggregated metanephric blastema, which is in contact with the ampulla of the ureteric duct, expresses IGF-II as well as IGFBP-2 and IGFBP-4 [14]. It has long been known that the differentiation processes that occur during nephrogenesis is mediated via the locally synthesized paracrine factors and our findings now suggest that peptides of the IGF system may be involved.

Placenta: important site of IGF-IGFBP interactions

A normally grown and developed placenta is essential for the normal growth and development of the fetus. Placenta not only serves as an important link between the mother and the fetus in the transfer of nutrients and substrates, removal of waste and metabolites, but also an important endocrine organ essential for the maintenance of pregnancy and fetomaternal immunity. Studies using in situ hybridization have indicated that IGF-II is expressed abundantly in the chorionic mesoderm of the villi and intermediate trophoblasts. The latter cells are extremely invasive and serve as the front line cells in interacting with the maternal stromal cells, which subsequently develop into decidual cells. The decidual cells express variable levels of IGFBP mRNAs, the most abundant of which is the IGFBP-1 mRNA. The close proximity of intermediate trophoblast cells of fetal origin and the decidual cells of maternal origin in the basal plate region of the placenta and the fetal membranes, led us to speculate that these cells may be communicating or interacting with each other using these peptides of the IGF system.

Studies in our laboratory using in vitro assays with human first trimester trophoblast cells indicate that the IGF peptides are not mitogens, but promote invasion. Adding IGFBP-1 into the in vitro invasion assay potentiates invasion, the effect which is most obvious in the presence of exogenously added IGF-II [15]. These findings suggest that IGF-II, which is abundantly expressed by the trophoblasts cells, is being utilized as an autocrine promoter of invasion supported by the maternally secreted IGFBP-1. These biological actions may be essential in the normal successful implantation of the conceptus and subsequent formation of a normally functioning placenta.

Pathophysiology

IGFs and IGFBPs are not only involved in the regulation of normal growth and differentiation of the fetus, but also involved in the pathophysiology of intrauterine growth retardation. Studies in both experimental animals and humans present tantalizing evidence for the importance of IGFs and IGFBPs in the pathophysiology of fetal growth retardation (see review [1]). IGF-I concentrations are low and the profiles of IGFBPs may be altered. Previous studies have shown that in the cord blood of IUGR fetuses, IGFBP-3 levels may be decreased and IGFBP-2 and IGFBP-1 levels may be increased. Recent studies by Wang et al. [16], in which they demonstrated that fetal size at birth may be inversely related to fetal plasma IGFBP-1 concentrations, suggest that IGFBP-1 may play a role in the retardation of growth. This IGFBP, which is shown to be an inhibitory binding protein in many in vitro culture conditions, may have an important effect on growth and differentiation of many tissues especially under conditions of decreased IGF-I concentration [17]. However, these concepts are still speculative at the moment because these observations indicate association instead of cause and effect. Since IGFBPs are expressed in multiple fetal tissues and act in paracrine manner, genetic manipulation of the expression of IGFBP genes in transgenic animals either in a positive or a negative manner, may lead us to more conclusive observations.

Regulation of IGF and IGFBP gene expression in the fetus

IGF and IGFBP genes are all expressed in a developmentally specific manner. Under conditions which lead to intrauterine growth retardation, the expression of both IGF and IGFBP genes are altered. More recent studies from many laboratories, indicate that IGFBP levels in the fetal plasma and IGFBP mRNA levels in the tissues are altered in maternal malnutrition, fetal hypoxemia and changes in hormone concentrations.

Maternal undernutrition, and therefore fetal undernutrition, is one mechanism by which growth retardation may be induced in the fetus. Straus et al. [18] have shown that dietary deprivation of maternal rats causes growth retardation in the embryos and concomitant increase in fetal serum IGFBP-1 levels and corresponding increase in hepatic IGFBP-1 mRNA levels. In fetal sheep, we have reported similar changes in the IGFBP-1 levels in the plasma and IGFBP-1 mRNA levels in the liver, when pregnant ewes are subjected to nutritional deprivation [19]. These changes are rapidly corrected when the ewes are refed.

Prolonged fetal hypoxia is another mechanism underlying fetal growth retardation. We have previously shown that when fetal sheep are subjected to prolonged hypoxia by reducing maternal uterine blood flow, growth of specific organs as determined by ^{3}H-thymidine incorporation, is reduced [20]. These fetuses showed an increased expression of IGFBP-1 mRNA and a decreased expression of IGFBP-2 mRNA levels in the liver, with corresponding changes in the levels of IGFBP-1 and IGFBP-2 in the plasma [21]. More recently, we have completed a study in which we addressed the

272

question of whether fetal hypoxemia alone can induce IGFBP-1 gene expression. When fetal sheep are subjected to hypoxemia with varying degrees of acidosis, by putting pregnant ewes in hypoxic conditions, we have shown that IGFBP-1 mRNA levels in the liver and IGFBP-1 levels in the plasma are increased and these levels are inversely correlated with base excess as a measure of circulating and tissue acidosis [22].

Reduction of maternal uterine blood flow causes not only hypoxia, but also changes in circulating fetal hormonal concentrations of catecholamines, glucocorticoids and prostaglandins, as well as disturbance in the transfer of substrates across the placenta, such as amino acids. However, because the IGFBP-1 gene is regulated by intracellular cAMP, we have studied whether these changes observed in the fetus can be explained by the endocrine changes. By infusing epinephrine and norepinephrine to concentrations that one may expect to observe under conditions of reduced uterine blood flow, we have demonstrated that hepatic IGFBP-1 gene expression can be induced, therefore suggesting that the changes in IGFBP-1 levels in fetal hypoxemia and growth retardation conditions may be explained in part by the endocrine changes.

Placenta as a target of altered IGF-II gene expression in IUGR

Pregnancy induced hypertension is an important cause of fetal growth retardation in humans. In this condition, placenta is not only the source of maternal disease, but also a target. Placentae in these pregnancies demonstrate multiple infarcts as a result of narrowing of the maternal spiral arteries and concomitant narrowing of the fetal stem villous arterioles. When IGF-II gene expression is studied by in situ hybridization in these placentae, we have shown that the infarcts are surrounded by fetal intermediate trophoblasts expressing abundant IGF-II mRNA. One of the most interesting findings was that the walls of the stem villous arterioles, which are abnormally thickened, expresses abundant IGF-II mRNA. These findings suggest that IGF-II may also play a role in the placental response to maternal disease and is involved in proliferative reaction of the stem villous arterioles, which contribute to the abnormal placental blood flow observed in these fetuses.

Summary and Conclusions

In recent years, studies in many laboratories, including our own, have suggested that IGFBPs together with IGFs may play an important role in both normal development as well as in the pathophysiology of growth retardation. The temporal and spatial pattern of expression of IGFBPs in many developing tissues suggest that these proteins may be crucial modulators of the actions of IGFs, which are ubiquitously expressed in the mesenchymal elements of the developing tissues. These IGFBPs are expressed in both epithelial and mesenchymal cell types and specific IGFBPs may be utilized to modulate the mitogenic and differentiative actions of IGFs in autocrine and paracrine manner. Altered expression of IGFs and IGFBPs may participate in the pathophysiology of intrauterine growth retardation.

References

1. Han VKM, Hill DJ. In: Schofield P (ed) The Insulin-Like Growth Factors: Structure and Biological Functions. Oxford: Oxford University Press, 1992;178–220.
2. Liu J-P, Baker J, Perkins AS, Robertson EJ, Efstratiadis A. Cell 1993;75:59– 72.
3. Baker J, Liu J-P, Robertson EJ, Efstratiadis A. Cell 1993;75:73–82.
4. Rappolee DA, Werb Z. In: Spencer EM (ed) Modern Concepts of Insulin-Like Growth Factors. Amsterdam: Elsevier Science Publishers, 1991;3–7.
5. Watson AJ, Hogan A, Hahnel A, Wiemer KE, Schultz GA. Mol Reprod Dev 1992;31:87–95.
6. Ohlsson R, Larsson E, Nilsson O, Wahlstrom T, Sundstrom P. Development 1989;106:555–559.
7. Hahnel A, Schlutz GA. Endocrinology 1994;134:1956–1959.
8. Phillips ID, Delhanty PJD, Hill DJ, Han VKM. J Endocrinol 1991;129(suppl):209.
9. Hill DJ, Han VKM, Clemmons DR, Camacho-Hubner C, Wang J. In: Drop SLS, Hintz RL (eds) Insulin-Like Growth Factor Binding Proteins. Amsterdam: Elsevier Science Publishers, 1989;55–61.
10. D'Ercole AJ. In: Spencer EM (ed) Modern Concepts of Insulin-Like Growth Factors. Amsterdam: Elsevier Science Publishers, 1991;9–23.
11. Delhanty PJD, Han VKM. Endocrinology 1993;132:41–52.
12. Hill DJ, Han VKM. J Dev Physiol 1991;15:91–104.
13. Bar RS, Clemmons DR, Boes M, Busby WH, Booth BA, Dake BL, Sandra A. Endocrinology 1991; 127:1078–1086.
14. Matsell DG, Delhanty PJD, Stenpaniuk O, Goodyer C, Han VKM. Kidney Int (submitted).
15. Lysiak JJ, Han VKM, Lala PK. Annual Meeting of the European Placenta Group, Manchester, 1993 (abstract).
16. Wang C-Y, Lim J, English J, Irvine L, Chard T. J Endocrinol 1992;129:459–464.
17. Wang HS, Chard T. J Endocrinology 1992;132:11–19.
18. Straus DS, Takemoto CD. Endocrinology 1990;127:1849–1852.
19. Osborn BH, Fowlkes J, Han VKM, Freemark M. Endocrinology 1992;131:1743–1750.
20. Hooper SB, Bocking AD, White S, Smith A, Challis JRG, Han VKM. Am J Physiol 1991;261: R508–R514.
21. McLellan KC, Hooper SB, Bocking AD, Delhanty PJD, Phillip ID, Hill DJ, Han VKM. Endocrinology 1992;131:1619–1628.
22. Asano H, Richardson B, Han VKM. Ped Res 1993;33:432,75A.

Insulin-like growth factors and muscle cell differentiation

Stephen M. Rosenthal, Don Hsiao, Zhou-Qin Cheng and Lawrence A. Silverman
Department of Pediatrics, University of California, San Francisco, CA 94143-0434, USA

Abstract. Acting through autocrine/paracrine mechanisms, the insulin-like growth factors (IGFs) stimulate the differentiation of skeletal muscle cells. While serum inhibits myogenesis, the IGFs are unique in that they are the only known mitogens that, when free of other serum components, stimulate muscle cell differentiation. The effects of the IGFs are mediated, at least in part, through increased expression of muscle-specific transcription factors and of factors involved in cell-ECM and direct cell-cell interactions. In addition to the IGF-I receptor, which has been previously found to signal IGF-induced myogenesis, recent studies with receptor-selective IGF analogs implicate a role for the IGF-II receptor in this process. Furthermore, IGF binding proteins expressed by skeletal muscle cells inhibit differentiation induced by IGFs.

Introduction

Muscle is an important target tissue for insulin-like growth factor (IGF) action. The expression of IGF peptides, receptors and binding proteins by muscle suggests that a significant component of IGF action in this tissue is mediated through auto-crine/paracrine mechanisms [1–8]. While serum inhibits myogenesis, the IGFs are unique in that they are the only known mitogens that, when free of other serum components, stimulate muscle cell differentiation [9–10]. The following is an overview of the muscle differentiation process and of the potential mechanisms by which the IGFs regulate myogenesis.

Muscle cell differentiation

Muscle cell differentiation is a process whereby mesodermal stem cells become committed to the myogenic lineage as proliferating myoblasts; subsequently these cells cease proliferation and differentiate into fully mature myocytes and multinucleated myotubes. Insight into the mechanisms which regulate muscle cell differentiation has stemmed from the recent discovery of a family of muscle-specific DNA binding proteins homologous to the proto-oncogene c-*myc* [11,12]. When transfected into nonmuscle cells, these peptides all have the ability to convert these cells to muscle cells [11,12].

The discovery of this family of myogenic regulatory factors evolved from an observation reported in 1977 that exposure of mouse C3H-10T-1/2 embryo fibroblast-like cells to 5-azacytidine (5-AZ) led to the development of stable myoblast cell lines [13]. The mechanism proposed for this transformation was 5-AZ-induced inhibition of cellular methyltransferases, resulting in hypomethylation of CpG residues and subsequent activation of specific genes [14]. When DNA from these newly transformed myoblasts was transfected into non-5-AZ-treated fibroblasts, myogenic conversion occurred in approximately 1/15,000 transfected colonies, a frequency thought to be consistent with the probability of transfecting a single locus or a few closely linked loci [15]. Subtraction cDNA hybridization between the transformed myoblasts and the parent fibroblast cell lines ultimately led to the isolation and characterization of a single myogenic regulatory gene, termed MyoD [16]. This gene was found to be expressed in myoblasts and skeletal muscle, but not in smooth or cardiac muscle or in nonmuscle tissues and expression of its cDNA converted fibroblasts to myoblasts [16]. Subsequently, three related mammalian myogenic regulatory genes have been identified and characterized at the molecular level, including myogenin, myf-5 and MRF-4 [17–19]. These peptides dimerize with ubiquitously expressed E2A gene products, bind to the regulatory regions of muscle-specific genes and activate their transcription [12].

The ability of MyoD and related factors to bind DNA and activate muscle-specific transcription, may be modified by peptides whose expression is regulated by the cell cycle. The retinoblastoma gene product (pRB) functions as a ubiquitous growth suppressor when unphosphorylated in the G1 phase of the cell cycle [20–22]. Just prior to the initiation of DNA synthesis (G1/S transition), pRB becomes phosphorylated and functionally inactive [20–22]. The phosphorylated form of pRB promotes proliferation and inhibits myogenesis. When unphosphorylated, pRB is thought to promote differentiation, at least in part, through direct interaction with MyoD or myogenin [22]. The mechanisms which regulate the phosphorylation state of pRB are incompletely understood.

The ability of MyoD and related factors to bind DNA is also influenced by the presence of the c-*myc*-related Id peptide [23]. Proliferating myoblasts express high levels of Id protein which inhibit DNA-binding of MyoD and related factors by competing for their dimerization partners, the E2A gene products [23]. Down-regulation of Id expression is required for muscle cell differentiation and over-expression of Id protein inhibits myogenesis [24].

While all of the MyoD-related factors are expressed exclusively in skeletal muscle and can activate myogenesis, myogenin is the only member of this family which is expressed in all skeletal muscle cell types thus far examined [11,12]. The importance of myogenin in muscle cell differentiation is further supported by the recent observation that mice homozygous for a targeted mutation in the myogenin gene demonstrated a severe reduction in skeletal muscle development [25,26].

The decision of myoblasts to proliferate or enter the differentiation pathway is strongly linked to the cellular environment. This decision is influenced by cell-extracellular matrix (ECM), direct cell-cell interactions, as well as by soluble growth factors. For example, L6E9 skeletal myoblasts plated on laminin or fibronectin differentiate normally, while those grown on fibrillar collagen remain undifferentiated

[27]. The importance of the cellular environment in regulating myogenesis is further supported by recent studies with the cell-surface VLA-4 integrin [28]. Monoclonal antibodies against this integrin, which plays a role in cell-ECM and direct cell-cell interactions, inhibit the differentiation process [28].

The importance of soluble factors in regulating myogenesis is demonstrated by the observation that cells maintained in high serum-supplemented media remain myoblasts and are induced to differentiate when serum is withdrawn [11,12]. Myogenic differentiation triggered by serum depletion is inhibited by basic fibroblast growth factor (FGF) [29] and transforming growth factor-β (TGF-β) [30], though a recent report indicates that TGF-β induces myoblast differentiation in mitogen-rich medium [31].

IGFs and muscle cell differentiation

In contrast to the inhibitory effects of serum on muscle cell differentiation, the IGFs, when free of other serum components, stimulate myogenesis [9,10]. Recent studies implicate an autocrine/paracrine role for IGF-II in muscle cell differentiation. Cloned muscle cells express IGF-II early in the differentiation process, several days before full attainment of the mature muscle cell phenotype [5,6]. In addition, IGF-II antisense oligodeoxynucleotides inhibit this process [32]. Furthermore, FGF, a known inhibitor of myogenesis, markedly inhibits IGF-II gene expression [33].

The mechanisms by which the IGFs stimulate muscle cell differentiation, however, are unknown. Studies from our laboratory have focused on four aspects of IGF-induced myogenesis: 1) exploring the hypothesis that IGF-II, the principal IGF peptide expressed in cultured muscle cells [5,6], stimulates muscle cell differentiation by increasing the expression of myogenin; 2) identifying other genes which play a role in the differentiation process which are regulated by the IGFs; 3) examining which IGF receptor subtypes mediate the effects of IGFs on muscle cell differentiation; and 4) exploring the potential role of IGFBPs in modulating IGF-induced differentiation.

IGFs and myogenin expression

Florini et al. initially reported that IGFs increase myogenin gene expression [34]. In the mouse BC3H-1 muscle cell line, we have demonstrated that treatment with IGFs increases myogenin mRNA in both a time and dose-dependent manner [35]. However, when we examined the relative temporal expression of IGF-II and myogenin, both of which are expressed early in the differentiation process, we found that induction of myogenin mRNA preceded that of IGF-II by 12–24 h [35]. These studies suggest that while IGFs may potentiate myogenin expression, endogenously produced IGF-II may stimulate muscle cell differentiation at a step after the induction of myogenin gene expression has occurred.

Regulation by IGFs of other genes which are important in muscle cell differentiation

An additional mechanism by which IGFs might regulate muscle differentiation is through inhibition of the c-*myc*-related Id peptide [23]. Id is abundant in myoblasts and inhibits differentiation by indirectly inhibiting the ability of myogenin and related peptides to bind to the regulatory regions of muscle-specific genes [23]. At an early step in muscle cell differentiation, Id expression decreases [23]. To explore the potential role of IGFs in the differentiation-associated decrease in Id expression, IGF treatment and differentiation time course studies were carried out. We found that Id mRNA levels were unaffected by IGF treatment and that the decrease in Id expression during differentiation occurred before the induction of IGF-II expression [35].

As muscle cell differentiation is regulated not only by soluble growth factors, but also by cell-ECM and direct cell-cell interactions, we explored the possibility that IGF-II may stimulate myogenesis by regulating the expression of the VLA-4 integrin. VLA-4, a member of a family of cell surface molecules involved in cell-ECM and cell-cell interactions, is expressed in skeletal myocytes and plays an important role in differentiation; antibodies to this integrin inhibit myogenesis [28]. Following treatment of mouse skeletal myoblasts with IGFs, an increase in VLA-4 mRNA was seen in comparison to control cells. In addition, when comparing the relative temporal expression of IGF-II with that of VLA-4 during differentiation, induction of IGF-II mRNA preceded that of VLA-4 [36]. Furthermore, a monoclonal antibody to the VLA-4 integrin inhibited differentiation induced by IGF-II. These data suggest that IGF-II, acting through autocrine/paracrine mechanisms, stimulates muscle cell differentiation, at least in part, by increasing expression of the VLA-4 integrin.

IGF receptor subtypes and muscle cell differentiation

While IGFs stimulate muscle cell differentiation, the role of IGF receptor subtypes in signaling this process has not been firmly established. Previous studies have demonstrated that the tyrosine kinase IGF-I receptor can signal IGF-induced muscle differentiation [37]. To explore a potential role for the IGF-II/cation-independent mannose-6-phosphate receptor [38] in muscle cell differentiation, we treated BC3H-1 cells with native IGF-II or with [Leu^{27}]IGF-II, an analog with normal affinity for the IGF-II receptor, but markedly reduced affinity for the IGF-I receptor [39,40]. The selective affinity of [Leu^{27}]IGF-II for the IGF-II receptor in myoblasts was further demonstrated in cross-linking studies. When ^{125}I-IGF-I was cross-linked to IGF-I receptors, no competition was seen with unlabeled [Leu^{27}]IGF-II despite competition with unlabeled IGF-I or IGF-II. In addition, when ^{125}I-IGF-II was cross-linked to BC3H-1 cells, unlabeled [Leu^{27}]IGF-II competed for binding to IGF-II receptors, but not to IGF-I receptors. When myogenin mRNA was examined in cells treated with IGF-II or the [Leu^{27}]IGF-II analog, IGF-II was more potent in stimulating this marker of differentiation. However, at doses of [Leu^{27}]IGF-II, which did not appear to interact with IGF-I receptors either by binding or cross-linking studies, a 2—3-fold increase in myogenin mRNA occurred in comparison to untreated cells. Similar concentrations of the IGF-II analog also increased the binding of α-bungarotoxin to the nicotinic acetylcholine receptor, a later marker of muscle cell differentiation. While it is conceivable that the effects of [Leu^{27}]IGF-II on myogenesis reflect interaction with the IGF-I receptor at very low affinity, studies with this IGF-II receptor-selective analog provide evidence that the IGF-II receptor may play a role in signaling IGF-II-induced muscle cell differentiation.

As the IGF-I receptor in muscle mediates not only the biological effects of IGF-I, but also plays a role in IGF-II signaling [41,42], we have studied the regulation of IGF-I receptor expression during muscle differentiation. We have demonstrated that specific high affinity IGF-I receptors are present in BC3H-1 mouse myoblasts [6]. To investigate the specificity of ^{125}I-IGF-I binding, competition-inhibition studies were carried out [6]. Specific ^{125}I-IGF-I binding was inhibited by unlabeled IGF-I one-half maximally at 0.14 nM. IGF-II also interacted with the IGF-I receptor, though one-half maximal inhibition of IGF-I binding occurred at 1.3 nM IGF-II. At concentrations of up to 10 nM insulin had little effect in inhibiting IGF-I binding [6].

When myoblasts differentiated into myocytes, we observed a decrease in IGF-I receptor content as determined by Scatchard analysis. IGF-I binding to both myoblasts and myocytes was best fitted by a one-site model. Differentiation was associated with a 60% decrease in IGF-I receptor sites, but no significant change in receptor affinity [6]. BC3H-1 muscle cell differentiation was also associated with decreased IGF-I receptor biosynthesis and mRNA abundance. Metabolic labeling of cells with [^{35}S] methionine followed by immunoprecipitation with an antireceptor, antiserum showed that differentiation was associated with a 50–60% decrease in IGF-I receptor biosynthesis. RNA transfer blots demonstrated a progressive decrease in IGF-I receptor mRNA abundance during differentiation [6].

The observation that an increase in IGF-II peptide gene expression occurred early in the course of differentiation and preceded the decrease in IGF-I receptor gene expression, suggested an autocrine role of IGF-II in IGF-I receptor regulation. This hypothesis was supported by the observation that addition of IGF-II to undifferentiated muscle cells resulted in downregulation of the IGF-I receptor at the levels of binding, mRNA abundance and receptor biosynthesis [6]. In addition we have recently demonstrated that IGF-II induces IGF-I receptor downregulation in muscle cells by stimulating IGF-I receptor protein degradation [43]. In studies with FGF, a known inhibitor of muscle cell differentiation, we observed a marked inhibition of IGF-II peptide expression and an increase in IGF-I receptor expression, further supporting an autocrine/paracrine role for IGF-II in muscle cell IGF-I receptor regulation [33].

To explore which IGF receptor subtypes mediate IGF-I receptor downregulation induced by IGF-II, we studied the effects of the addition of IGF-II and the [Leu^{27}]IGF-II analog to BC3H-1 myoblasts. Concentrations of [Leu^{27}]IGF-II (25–50 ng/ml) were chosen at which this IGF-II receptor-selective analog did not significantly interact with IGF-I receptors, either in binding or in cross-linking studies. Cells were placed in serum-free medium in the presence of vehicle or peptide for 18 h, the time at which maximal IGF-II-induced downregulation of the IGF-I receptor occurs in these myoblasts. Cells were then treated with an acid wash to remove preincubated peptide from the cell surface and binding with [^{125}I]-IGF-I was carried out. IGF-II at 25 and 50 ng/ml caused a 50–60% decrease in IGF-I binding (p < 0.02 vs. untreated cells), while equivalent concentrations of [Leu^{27}]IGF-II had only a minimal effect which was not statistically significant.

As it has been shown that IGF-II pretreatment inhibits not only IGF-I receptor binding, but also IGF-I receptor gene expression [6], we compared the ability of native IGFs and [Leu^{27}]IGF-II to decrease IGF-I receptor mRNA. IGF-I and IGF-II treatment (50 ng/ml) significantly decreased IGF-I receptor mRNA (p < 0.05 vs. control cells). In contrast, [Leu^{27}]IGF-II did not significantly decrease IGF-I receptor mRNA.

While our studies suggest that the IGF-II receptor may play a role in muscle cell differentiation, it does not appear to be involved in signaling IGF-II-induced downregulation of the IGF-I receptor. That IGF-II may stimulate two different responses through distinct receptors or combination of receptors is not unique to differentiating skeletal muscle cells. In the RD human rhabdomyosarcoma cell line, IGF-II stimulates mitogenic effects through the IGF-I receptor and stimulates motility through the IGF-II receptor [44].

The ability of IGF-II to downregulate the IGF-I receptor at the level of gene expression is also not unique to muscle cells. Treatment of T47D human breast cancer cells with progestins results in increased IGF-II secretion and decreased IGF-I receptor biosynthesis and mRNA abundance [45]. Furthermore, treatment of these breast cancer cells with IGF-II induces downregulation of the IGF-I receptor at the level of gene expression [45]. Our studies in muscle cells, however, are the first to demonstrate that downregulation of the IGF-I receptor induced by IGF-II is mediated through the IGF-I receptor.

IGF binding proteins (IGFBPs) and muscle cell differentiation

The role of IGFBPs in myogenesis is not firmly established. Skeletal muscle cells secrete IGFBPs which may enhance or inhibit IGF actions [3,4,7,8]. Studies in which IGF analogs with reduced affinity for IGFBPs were more potent than native IGF-I in stimulating myogenesis provide indirect evidence that these binding proteins inhibit differentiation induced by IGFs [46].

Conclusions

In summary, acting through autocrine/paracrine mechanisms, the IGFs stimulate the differentiation of skeletal muscle cells. The effects of the IGFs are mediated, at least in part, through increased expression of muscle-specific transcription factors and of factors involved in cell-ECM and direct cell-cell interactions. In addition to the tyrosine kinase IGF-I receptor, which has been previously found to signal IGF-induced myogenesis, recent studies with receptor-selective IGF analogs implicate a role for the IGF-II receptor in this process. Furthermore, IGFBPs expressed by skeletal muscle cells inhibit differentiation induced by IGFs.

Acknowledgements

This work was supported by a grant from the NIDDK, NIH (1 R29 DK44181) and aided by Basic Research Grant No. 1-FY92-0700 from the March of Dimes Birth Defects Foundation. Dr. Silverman was a trainee in Pediatric Endocrinology under a program sponsored by the NIDDK, NIH (5 T32 DK07161).

References

1. De Vroede MA, Romanus JA, Standaert ML, Pollet RJ, Nissley SP, Rechler MM. Endocrinology 1984;114:1917–1929.
2. Beguinot F, Kahn CR, Moses AC, Smith RJ. J Biol Chem 1985;260:15892–15898.
3. McCusker RH, Camacho-Hubner C, Clemmons DR. J Biol Chem 1989;264:7795–7800.
4. Tollefsen SE, Lajara R, McCusker RH, Clemmons DR, Rotwein P. J Biol Chem 1989;264:13810–13817.
5. Tollefsen SE, Sadow JL, Rotwein P. Proc Natl Acad Sci USA 1989;86:1543–1547.
6. Rosenthal SM, Brunetti A, Brown EJ, Mamula PW, Goldfine ID. J Clin Invest 1991;87:1212–1219.
7. Ernst CW, McCusker RH, White ME. Endocrinology 1992;130:607–615.
8. Payton JL, Jones SB, Busby WH, Clemmons DR, Rotwein P. J Biol Chem 1993;268:22305–22312.
9. Ewton DZ, Florini JR. Dev Biol 1981;86:31–39.
10. Schmid C, Steiner T, Froesch ER. FEBS Lett 1983;161:117–121.
11. Olson EN. Dev Biol 1992;154:261–272.
12. Edmondson DG, Olson EN. J Biol Chem 1993;268:755–758.
13. Constantinides PG, Jones PA, Gevers W. Nature 1977;267:364–366.
14. Konieczny SF, Emerson CP. Cell 1984;38:791–800.
15. Lassar AB, Paterson BM, Weintraub H. Cell 1986;47:649–656.
16. Davis RL, Weintraub H, Lassar AB. Cell 1987;51:987–1000.
17. Olson EN. Genes Dev 1990;4:1454–1461.
18. Wright WE, Sassoon DA, Lin VK. Cell 1989;5b:607–617.
19. Edmondson DG, Olson EN. Genes Dev 1989;3:628–640.
20. Chen P-L, Scully P, Shew JY, Wang JYJ, Lee W-H. Cell 1989;58:1193–1198.
21. Laiho M, DeCaprio JA, Ludlow JW, Livingston DM, Massague J. Cell 1990;62:175–178.
22. Gu W, Schneider JW, Condorelli G, Kaushal S, Mahdavi V, Nadal-Ginard B. Cell 1993;72:309–324.
23. Benezra R, Davis RL, Lockshon D, Turner DL, Weintraub H. Cell 1990;61:49–59.
24. Jen Y, Weintraub H, Benezra R. Genes Dev 1992;6:1466–1479.
25. Hasty P, Bradley A, Morris JH, Edmondson DG, Venuti JM, Olson EN, Klein WH. Nature 1993;364:501–506.
26. Nabeshima Y, Hanaoka K, Hayasaka M, Esumi E, Li S, Nonaka I, Nabeshima Y-I. Nature 1993;364:532–535.
27. Heino J, Massague J. J Biol Chem 1990;265:10181–10184.
28. Rosen GD, Sanes JR, LaChance R, Cunningham JM, Roman J, Dean DC. Cell 1992;69:1107–1119.
29. Li L, Zhou J, James G, Heller-Harrison R, Czech MP, Olson EN. Cell 1992;71:1181–1194.
30. Massague J, Cheifetz S, Endo T, Nadal-Ginard B. Proc Natl Acad Sci USA 1986;83:8206–8210.
31. Zentella A, Massague J. Proc Natl Acad Sci USA 1992;89:5176–5180.

282

32. Florini J, Magri K, Ewton D, James P, Grindstaff K, Rotwein P. J Biol Chem 1991;266:15917–15923.
33. Rosenthal SM, Brown EJ, Brunetti A, Goldfine ID. Mol Endocrinol 1991;5:678–684.
34. Florini JR, Ewton DZ, Roof SL. Mol Endocrinol 1991;5:718–724.
35. Brown EJ, Hsiao D, Rosenthal SM. Biochem Biophys Res Commun 1992;183:1084–1089.
36. Rosenthal SM, Hsiao D. Pediatr Res 1993;33:S67.
37. Ewton DZ, Falen SL, Florini JR. Endocrinology 1987;120:115–123.
38. Morgan DO, Edman JC, Standring DN, Fried VA, Smith MC, Roth RA, Rutter WJ. Nature 1987; 329:301–307.
39. Beukers MW, Oh Y, Zhang H, Ling N, Rosenfeld R. Endocrinology 1991;128:1201–1203.
40. Sakano K, Enjoh T, Numata F, Fujiwara H, Marumoto Y, Higashihashi N, Sato Y, Perdue JF, Fugita-Yamaguchi Y. J Biol Chem 1991;31:20626–20635.
41. Yu KT, Czech MP. J Biol Chem 1984;259:3090–3095.
42. Kiess W, Haskell JF, Lee L, Greenstin LA, Miller BE, Aarons AL, Rechler MM, Nissley SP. J Biol Chem 1987;262:12745–12751.
43. Rosenthal SM, Brown EJ. Mechanisms of insulin-like growth factor (IGF)-II-induced IGF-I receptor downregulation in BC3H-1 cells. J Endocrinol (in press).
44. Minniti CP, Kohn EC, Grubb JH, Sly WS, Oh Y, Muller HL, Rosenfeld RG, Helman LJ. J Biol Chem 1992;267:9000–9004.
45. Papa V, Hartmann KKP, Rosenthal SM, Maddux BA, Siiteri PK, Goldfine ID. Mol Endocrinol 1991; 5:709–717.
46. Silverman LA, Hsiao D, Rosenthal SM. Pediatr Res 1993;33:S65.

The roles of IGF-I, IGF-II and IGFBPs in myogenesis

Daina Z. Ewton, Karen A. Magri and James R. Florini

Biology Department, Syracuse University, Syracuse, NY 13244, USA

Abstract. IGF-I and IGF-II stimulate both proliferation and differentiation of L6A1 muscle cells. While IGF-I causes a greater proliferative response, IGF-II treatment results in a greater myogenic response. If the proliferative response to IGF-I was reduced, IGF-I activity approached that of IGF-II. The extreme potency of IGF-I analogs with reduced affinity for IGFBPs in stimulating L6A1 differentiation, indicate that the IGFBPs secreted by L6A1 cells are strongly inhibitory to this action of IGF-I. A distinct pattern of expression of IGFBP-4, -5 and -6 mRNA (and secreted protein) in the presence of IGF-I, IGF-II or insulin, suggests that each IGFBP may play a defined role during a specific phase of muscle growth and differentiation.

The IGFs play a unique role in muscle development, stimulating both proliferation and differentiation of cells in culture. In contrast, other mitogens, such as FGF, TGF-β and PDGF, have been shown to be potent inhibitors of muscle differentiation. The usual procedure for stimulating differentiation of muscle cells in culture has been to transfer them from mitogen-rich growth medium to low serum medium. However, we have demonstrated that the addition of IGFs in serum-free medium resulted in not only cell growth, but also extensive differentiation [1].

Additional studies showed that muscle cells express the genes for IGF-II, and to a lesser extent, IGF-I and IGFBPs [2,3]. Thus, myoblast cultures spontaneously differentiating in low-serum medium were actually secreting enough IGF-II to cause autocrine stimulation of their own growth and differentiation [4]. Muscle cell lines which differentiated more rapidly, were found to secrete more autocrine IGF-II and were generally less responsive to exogenous IGFs. Furthermore, an oligomer antisense to IGF-II blocked spontaneous differentiation, which could be overcome by exogenous IGF-II [4]. Recent studies also demonstrated that addition of IGF-I, IGF-II or insulin to L6A1 muscle cultures resulted in decreased steady-state levels of IGF-II mRNA, suggesting that IGFs can regulate their own expression by a negative feedback mechanism [5]. Thus an essential role of the IGFs in controlling growth and differentiation of muscle cells was established.

Early in our studies we concluded that the type 1 IGF receptor mediates IGF and insulin stimulated L6A1 muscle cell differentiation, since the order of potency was IGF-I>IGF-II>insulin, reflecting the relative affinities for the type 1 IGF receptor [6]. Although differentiation was stimulated by lower concentrations of IGF-I, we observed that IGF-II and insulin treatment caused more extensive fusion of myoblasts into myotubes, accompanied by elevated levels of muscle-specific proteins measured

284

under our usual conditions. In addition, the L6A1 cells exhibited a biphasic differentiative response to IGF-I, IGF-II and insulin; differentiation was stimulated at lower concentrations, reached a maximum and then decreased at higher concentrations of the IGFs or insulin. If the actions of IGF-I and IGF-II (and insulin at supraphysiological concentrations) are mediated by the same receptor, why do IGF-I treated cultures differentiate less extensively? Do IGF binding proteins play a role in this puzzling phenomenon? The objectives of this study were to answer these questions about the specific roles of IGF-I and IGF-II and IGFBPs in the regulation L6A1 muscle cell differentiation.

Mitogenic actions of IGF-I delay L6A1 differentiation

At concentrations of IGF-I and IGF-II, which are optimal for the stimulation of L6 differentiation, IGF-I usually caused a greater proliferative response than IGF-II did. Since proliferation and differentiation are mutually exclusive events, this increased mitogenic activity of IGF-I could result in decreased myogenic activity. To investigate this possibility, we compared the effects of IGF-I and IGF-II under culture conditions in which the proliferative response to IGF-I was reduced or eliminated. We found that in L6A1 cultures that had been plated at twice the normal density (conditions in which the cells proliferated less and thus differentiated faster) or if the IGFs were added in the presence of cytosine arabinoside (a DNA synthesis terminator that kills proliferating cells), the activity of IGF-I approached that of IGF-II. Thus, in cultures in which the proliferative signals from IGF-I were reduced, the cells were able to differentiate more effectively [7].

If the proliferative effects of IGF-I delay differentiation by forcing the cells through another cell cycle, the myogenic effects of IGF-I might ultimately be as great as those of IGF-II — only being delayed by the length of the mitogenic response. When we examined the extent of differentiation over an extended period of time, we found that under our normal culture conditions, IGF-I delayed the onset of differentiation by 1 day, when compared to IGF-II; that is, creatine kinase levels in IGF-II treated cells at 3 days were the same as those in IGF-I-treated cells at 4 days [7]. Therefore, IGF-I, acting as a mitogen, caused the cells to proliferate more before differentiation commenced, while IGF-II (which is a less potent mitogen) caused the cells to differentiate sooner.

IGF analogs with reduced affinity for the type 1 receptor

Analogs of IGF-I and IGF-II with reduced affinity for IGF receptors provide a very useful tool for further examining the role of the type 1 receptor in stimulating muscle differentiation. [Leu^{24}]IGF-I, an analog with 32-fold reduced affinity for the type 1 receptor [8], showed a dramatic decrease in activity in stimulating L6A1 differentiation when compared to native IGF-I. Similarly, [Leu^{27}]IGF-II, an analog with 100-fold reduced affinity for the type 1 receptor [9], showed very little activity when compared to native IGF-II [7]. Thus, these analog studies support our earlier conclusions based on relative potencies of IGFs that the type 1 receptor mediated the actions of both IGF-I and IGF-II on L6A1 differentiation.

IGF analogs with reduced affinity for IGFBPs

Since IGFBPs have been shown not only to inhibit, but also to potentiate IGF action [10], IGF analogs with altered affinity for IGFBPs could provide useful information as to the role of IGFBPs in modulating IGF action in L6A1 muscle cells. We found that IGF-I analogs with reduced affinity for IGFBPs, such as LongR^3 IGF-I, were about 10 times more potent than native IGF-I in stimulating L6A1 proliferation, as has been reported in studies with other cell types. Surprisingly, though, they were about 100 times more potent than native IGF-I in stimulating differentiation [7]. This increased potency of these analogs could be seen in all the parameters of differentiation that we measured: fusion of myoblasts into myotubes, increased creatine kinase activity and elevated steady-state levels of myogenin mRNA. In addition, these analogs were also much more potent than native IGF-I in decreasing the steady-state levels of mRNA for IGF-II (Magri et al., manuscript submitted for publication). These results suggested that IGFBPs secreted by L6A1 cells were potent inhibitors of IGF-I action.

In contrast, IGF-II analogs with reduced affinity for IGFBPs were only slightly more potent than native IGF-II in stimulating either proliferation or differentiation (Ewton and Florini, manuscript in preparation). This observation may lead to the initial conclusion that IGFBPs somehow are not as inhibitory to IGF-II action and that the IGFBPs modulate IGF-I and IGF-II actions in different ways. However, these IGF-II analogs also exhibited altered affinities for the type 1 and type 2 receptors which could also account for their lower potency [11].

IGFBPs in L6A1 conditioned media

Several sublines of L6 cells have emerged which differ in their rate of differentiation and in their response to IGFs. We wished to examine the role of IGFBPs in modulating the actions of IGFs by comparing IGFBPs secreted by two such sublines: the more proliferative L6A1 cells, in which the differentiative response to IGFs is delayed, and the more rapidly differentiating L6A1c cells, which exhibit a decreased proliferative response to IGFs. Previous studies by McCusker et al. [12] reported that L6 muscle cells secreted two IGFBPs, ~24 and ~31 kDa, as determined by ligand blotting. Myoblasts secreted a greater percentage of the 24 kDa form, while myotubes secreted a predominance of the 31 kDa form. Ligand blot analysis of conditioned media from the more proliferative L6A1 cells treated for 3 days with IGF-I, IGF-II, insulin or LongR^3 IGF-I, confirmed the presence of ~24 kDa and ~31 kDa IGFBPs (Fig. 1). IGF-I and IGF-II caused the greatest increases in the 31 kDa protein, while insulin and LongR^3 IGF-I had smaller effects. The levels of the 24 kDa protein were increased primarily by IGF-I, while the other factors caused smaller increases. Conditioned media from the more rapidly differentiating L6A1c cultures contained

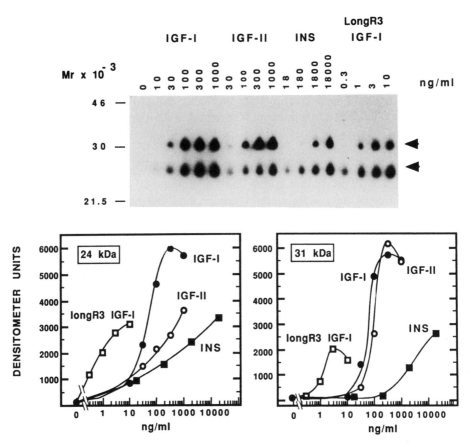

Fig. 1. Ligand blot analysis of IGFBPs in conditioned media of the more proliferative L6A1 cells. L6A1 cells were treated for 3 days with the indicated concentrations of IGF-I, IGF-II, insulin or LongR³ IGF-I (top). The proteins in the conditioned media were separated by SDS-PAGE, blotted onto nitrocellulose, probed with ¹²⁵I-IGF-II and subjected to autoradiography. Densitometric analysis of the ligand blot shown in A (bottom).

the same forms of IGFBPs, but the relative amount of the 31 kDa IGFBP was much greater than the 24 kDa form in IGF-I and IGF-II treated cultures (Ewton and Florini, manuscript in preparation).

We further analyzed the conditioned media by immunoblotting with antibodies to IGFBPs and identified the 31 kDa protein as IGFBP-5, while the 24 kDa band was composed of both IGFBP-4 and IGFBP-6 (Ewton and Florini, manuscript in preparation). The relative levels of the three IGFBPs present in the conditioned media of the more rapidly differentiating L6A1c cells under various conditions are summarized in Fig. 2.

IGFBP-4 and IGFBP-6 could be detected in the media of quiescent cultures in serum-free media and were increased more after incubation with IGF-I than with IGF-

IGFBPs IN CONDITIONED MEDIA

	IGFBP-4	IGFBP-5	IGFBP-6
QUIESCENT CELLS	+	-	+
IGF-I	+ + +	+ + + +	+ + +
IGF-II	+ +	+ + + +	+ +
INSULIN	+	+ +	+

Fig. 2. Relative abundance of IGFBPs in the conditioned media of the more rapidly differentiating L6A1c cells. Conditioned media were collected from cells after 3 days in serum-free medium (quiescent cells), or after the addition IGF-I (100 ng/ml), IGF-II (300 ng/ml) or insulin (1800 ng/ml) and analyzed by ligand and immunoblotting.

II or insulin. No IGFBP-5 could be detected in quiescent cultures, but the levels increased dramatically after IGF-I or IGF-II treatment; the effect of insulin again was less pronounced (Ewton and Florini, manuscript in preparation). Thus muscle cultures that differentiate more rapidly secrete more IGFBP-5, while more proliferative cells secrete more of IGFBP-4. This is in agreement with the report of McCusker et al. [12] that compared IGFBPs secreted by L6 myoblasts and myotubes.

Our initial studies focused on defining which IGFBPs were present in the media under our culture conditions in order to see how they may affect the actions of IGF-I or IGF-II. Therefore we examined IGFBPs that accumulated in the conditioned media over the length of the experiment and did not focus on the regulation of IGFBP secretion by IGFs. If we also took into account the increased proliferation in IGF-treated cultures, we found that while the accumulation of IGFBP-5 was specifically stimulated by IGFs and insulin, the increased levels of IGFBP-4 and IGFBP-6 in the media were largely due to increased number of cells secreting the IGFBPs.

Effect of IGFs and insulin on steady state levels of IGFBP mRNA levels

Northern blot analyses were done to determine whether the effects of the IGFs and insulin on IGFBP protein levels in the conditioned media reflected similar changes in the steady state levels of IGFBP mRNAs. mRNA transcripts for IGFBP-4 (~2.4 kb), IGFBP-5 (~6.0 kb) and IGFBP-6 (~1.3 kb) were readily detectable in IGF-I treated L6A1c cultures (Ewton and Florini, manuscript in preparation). Effects of IGF and insulin treatment on steady state levels of mRNAs are summarized in Fig. 3.

High levels of IGFBP-4 mRNA were present in proliferating myoblasts, but decreased in quiescent cells in serum-free medium or in differentiating cells in serum-

IGFBP-mRNA - STEADY STATE LEVELS

	IGFBP-4	IGFBP-5	IGFBP-6
PROLIFERATING MYOBLASTS	+++	-	++
QUIESCENT CELLS	+	-	+++
IGF-I - day 1	+++	+	++
day 2	+	++	+
IGF-II	+	+++	+
INSULIN	+	+++	+

Fig. 3. Relative abundance of IGFBP mRNAs in L6A1c cells. Total RNA was prepared from myoblasts proliferating in growth medium or from cells maintained for 2 days in serum-free medium (quiescent cells), IGF-I (100 ng/ml), IGF-II (300 ng/ml) or insulin (1800 ng/ml) and was analyzed by Northern blotting.

free medium containing IGF-I, IGF-II or insulin. The one exception to this trend was seen 1 day after the addition of IGF-I where IGFBP-4 mRNA levels remained high (while they were already reduced in IGF-II or insulin-treated cells). If high levels of IGFBP-4 can generally be correlated with a proliferative state, then this observation is consistent with our earlier conclusion that due to the proliferative actions of IGF-I, IGF-I-stimulated differentiation lags 1 day behind that of IGF-II.

IGFBP-5 mRNA, on the other hand, was not detectable in proliferating myoblasts or in quiescent cells, but increased dramatically in cells differentiating in the presence of IGFs or insulin. The effects of IGF-II and insulin, which cause a greater differentiative response, were greater than that of IGF-I.

Proliferating myoblasts exhibited detectable levels of IGFBP-6 mRNA which decreased somewhat with IGF or insulin treatment, but increased substantially in quiescent cells in serum-free medium.

Cell associated IGFBPs in L6A1 muscle cultures

Several reports have described IGFBPs not only released by cells into the medium, but also associated with the cell surface. Cell surface IGFBPs have been shown to potentiate IGF-stimulated mitogenesis in several cell lines [10]. In order to determine whether or not any of the IGFBPs secreted by L6A1c muscle cells into the conditioned media could also be found associated with the cells, we performed ligand blots using whole cell lysates from L6A1c muscle cultures that had been treated with

IGFs or insulin. The results indicated that significant amounts IGFBP-5 were found associated with the cells upon treatment with IGFs or insulin, but barely detectable levels of IGFBP-4 or IGFBP-6 were found (Ewton and Florini, manuscript in preparation). In these studies we did not determine whether or not IGFBP-5 was associated primarily with the cell surface, or is present within the cells.

Discussion

Our studies demonstrate that the growth and differentiation of the rat skeletal muscle cell line L6A1 are under intricate control by the IGF family of growth factors. The complex myoblast IGF system consists of two growth factors (IGF-I and IGF-II), two cell surface receptors (type 1 and type 2) and three IGFBPs (IGFBP-4,-5 and -6). Most effects of IGF-I and IGF-II (and insulin at high concentrations) appear to be mediated by the type 1 receptor, even though L6 myoblasts contain 15 times more type 2 receptors [13]. A role for the type 2 receptor in IGF action on muscle cells has not been established. Since growth factor-induced mitogenic signals appear to be inhibitory to differentiation, the greater potency of IGF-I in stimulating L6A1 cell proliferation appears to result in its lower activity in stimulating differentiation when compared to IGF-II. Muscle cells do not rely on exogenously provided IGFs alone, since they can secrete enough IGF-II to be effective in an autocrine manner [2–4]. The levels of IGF-II mRNA, in turn, are controlled by the IGFs themselves through a negative feedback mechanism [5].

L6A1c muscle cells secrete three IGFBPs, but the effects of IGFs and insulin on the accumulation of the proteins in the media are not directly related to the effects on the steady-state levels of IGFBP mRNAs. IGF-I and IGF-II caused the greatest increases in IGFBP-5 protein levels in the media, while insulin had a smaller effect. In contrast, the steady state levels of IGFBP-5 mRNA were most dramatically stimulated by insulin and IGF-II, with IGF-I having lower activity reflecting the relative activity of these factors in stimulating differentiation. These observations suggest that IGF-I and IGF-II, by binding to secreted IGFBP-5, are also somehow stabilizing the protein to proteolytic degradation or by releasing cell surface associated binding proteins, while the effects of insulin are at the level of mRNA. Similar findings have been reported by others using different cell systems [14–17].

In addition, IGFBP-4, -5 and -6, appear to be expressed by L6A1c muscle cells at specific stages of proliferation or differentiation. IGFBP-4 seems to be associated with a proliferative state, while IGFBP-5 is strongly induced during differentiation; IGFBP-6 may play a role during a quiescent state. The effects of each IGFBP in modulating IGF-I or IGF-II actions may vary since the affinities of the IGFBPs for IGF-I or IGF-II also vary; while IGFBP-4 appears to bind IGF-I and IGF-II with equal affinity, IGFBP-5 and IGFBP-6 have been shown to have much higher affinity for IGF-II [18,19]. Not all skeletal muscle cells may express identical IGFBPs. A recent report by James et al. [20] showed that the mouse C2 muscle cells express only IGFBP-5, while Ernst et al. [21] demonstrated that IGFBP-2 was secreted by the

C2C12 subline.

Our initial data using analogs of IGF-I with reduced affinity for IGFBPs suggest that the IGFBPs produced by L6A1 cells are strongly inhibitory to IGF-I action. However, we do not know which of the IGFBPs is involved. Defining an exact role for each IGFBP in either potentiating or inhibiting the mitogenic or myogenic actions of IGF-I or IGF-II will depend on more extensive studies using purified IGFBPs.

Acknowledgements

We thank Drs. Margaret Cascieri (Merck), Paul Walton, John Ballard (GroPep) and Ron Rosenfeld for the gifts of analogs of IGF-I and IGF-II. We are especially grateful to Drs. Nicholas Ling and Shunichi Shimasaki for providing us with antisera and cDNA probes for IGFBPs, Drs. Mark Benedict for ^{125}I-IGF-II and Eric Olson for the myogenin cDNA probe. We also thank Ciba-Geigy and Eli Lilly for generous supplies of IGF-I and IGF-II, respectively. We gratefully acknowledge the careful technical assistance of Cathleen Jenney and Kathleen Long. Supported by NIH grant HL11551 and USDA grant 9000716.

References

1. Ewton DZ, Florini JR. Dev Biol 1981;86:31—39.
2. Tollefsen SE, Lajara R, McCusker RH, Clemmons DR, Rotwein P. J Biol Chem 1989;264:13810—13817.
3. Tollefsen SE, Sadow JL, Rotwein P. Proc Natl Acad Sci USA 1989;86:1543—1547.
4. Florini J, Magri K, Ewton D, James P, Grindstaff K, Rotwein P. J Biol Chem 1991;266:15917—15923.
5. Magri KA, Ewton DZ, Florini JR. 74th Annual Meeting of the Endocrine Soc, 1992;113 (abstract).
6. Ewton DZ, Falen SL, Florini JR. Endocrinology 1987;120:115—124.
7. Ewton DZ, Magri KA, Florini JR. 75th Annual Meeting of the Endocrine Soc, 1993;1142 (abstract).
8. Cascieri MA, Chicchi GG, Applebaum J, Hayes NS, Green BG, Bayne ML. Biochemistry 1988;27:3229—3233.
9. Beukers MW, Oh Y, Zhang H, Ling N, Rosenfeld RG. Endocrinology 1991;128:1201—1203.
10. Cohick WS, Clemmons DR. Annu Rev Physiol 1993;55:131—153.
11. Francis GL, Aplin SE, Milner SJ, McNeil KA, Wallace JC, Ballard FJ. 75th Annual Meeting of the Endocrine Soc, 1993;492 (abstract).
12. McCusker RH, Camacho-Hubner C, Clemmons DR. J Biol Chem 1989;264:7795—7800.
13. Beguinot F, Kahn CR, Moses AC, Smith RJ. J Biol Chem 1985;260:15892—15898.
14. Conover CA. J Clin Invest 1991;88:1354—1361.
15. Camacho-Hubner C, Busby WH, McCusker RH, Wright G, Clemmons DR. J Biol Chem 1992;267:11949—11956.
16. Martin JL, Ballesteros M, Baxter RC. Endocrinology 1992;131:1703—1709.
17. Neely EK, Rosenfeld RG. Endocrinology 1992;130:985—993.
18. Clemmons DR, Dehoff ML, Busby WH, Bayne ML, Cascieri MA. Endocrinology 1992;131:890—895.
19. Bach LA, Tseng LY-H, Swartz JE, Rechler MM. Endocrinology 1993;133:990—995.
20. James PL, Jones SB, Busby WH, Clemmons DR, Rotwein P. J Biol Chem 1993;268:22305—22312.
21. Ernst CW, McCusker RH, White ME. Endocrinology 1992;130:607—615.

©1994 Elsevier Science B.V. All rights reserved
The insulin-like growth factors and their regulatory proteins
R.C. Baxter, P.D. Gluckman and R.G. Rosenfeld, editors

IGF-I as a paracrine growth factor in developing rat brain

George A. Werther, Vincenzo Russo, Helen Cheesman and Stephanie Edmondson
Centre for Child Growth and Hormone Research, Royal Children's Hospital, Parkville Vic, 3052, Australia

Abstract. We have demonstrated receptors and IGF-I mRNA synthesis in adjacent layers of olfactory bulb (OB) and cerebellum, and our in situ studies with exon-specific riboprobes indicates that only "paracrine" exon 1 IGF-I is expressed. This suggests that paracrine IGF-I systems occur in developing brain. Our serum-free newborn OB organ culture system shows neuronal differentiation in the presence of IGF-I and basic FGF (bFGF). The greater potency of des(1−3) IGF-I suggests IGF binding protein (IGFBP) production. These were identified by ligand and Northern blotting and immunoprecipitation as BP-2 and -3, as well as BP-4 and -5. Their abundance is regulated distinctly by IGF-I and bFGF, involving receptor-dependent and -independent mechanisms. In situ hybridisation on fresh and cultured newborn OBs, shows that IGFBP-2 and BP-4 mRNAs colocalise in glial-rich glomerular layer, similar to IGF-I receptors, while IGFBP-5 localises in the mitral cell (neuron) layer, similar to IGF-I mRNA. IGFBP-3 is only expressed in culture in glial regions, possibly as an injury response. IGFBP-2 is associated with cell membranes, possibly via binding to integrin receptors through its RGD sequence. The distinct localisation of the IGFBPs with sites of IGF-I synthesis or sites of IGF-I action suggests the possibility of unique roles in transport and targeting of IGF-I in its paracrine action in the developing brain.

Introduction

The roles of IGF-I in the brain remain unclear although it has potent effects in vitro on multiple CNS cell types, both glial and neuronal [1,2]. Evidence for widespread likely sites of action comes from findings of ourselves [3] and others [4] demonstrating, by in vitro autoradiography, widespread cell surface receptors in rat brain, with highest density in choroid plexus, olfactory bulb (OB), hippocampus, hypothalamus and cerebellum. The distribution of IGF-I receptors is similar, but distinct from IGF-II/M-6-P and insulin receptors [3,4].

Evidence for paracrine IGF-I systems in brain — source of IGFs in the brain

In contrast to IGF-II [5,6], IGF-I peptide is not detected in cerebrospinal fluid and its messenger RNA is not seen on Northern blotting of whole brain. Solution hybridisation has, however, demonstrated IGF-I mRNA synthesis in OB and cerebellum [7]. By in situ hybridisation we [8], and subsequently others [9,10], demonstrated IGF-I synthesis in specific cell layers in OB (mitral cell layer and granular and glomerular layers), hippocampus and cerebellum. In OB and cerebellum, sites of IGF-I synthesis are adjacent to and overlap IGF-I receptor sites, suggesting paracrine IGF-I systems

[8]. Mechanisms regulating IGF-I expression in these sites remain unknown, but our use of exon-specific riboprobes generated by PCR and subcloning, indicates that only "paracrine" exon 1 IGF-I transcripts (weakly GH-dependent) are expressed in OB (manuscript submitted).

OB organ culture system — a model for intact in vivo brain

In order to further characterise IGF-I action in these likely sites of paracrine action, we developed a serum-free OB organ culture system, utilising 1 day postnatal rat OBs. IGF-I in combination with basic fibroblast growth factor (bFGF) supports differentiated growth in vitro over 6 days, with both neuronal and glial cell markers (respectively neurofilament 150 kDA and glial fibrillary associated protein — GFAP) expressed similarly to freshly obtained day 6 OBs. Protein synthesis and glucose incorporation, both quantified by radio-labelled substrate uptake, were both enhanced additively by IGF-I and bFGF [11]. Des(1—3) IGF-I was more potent than intact IGF-I in support of metabolic and protein synthetic functions and in maintenance of differentiated cell growth (manuscript submitted).

IGF binding proteins (IGFBPs) in the brain — their potential role in paracrine IGF-I actions

The finding that des(1—3) IGF-I is more potent in OB organ culture than intact IGF-I suggests that IGFBPs are synthesized locally. This had been suggested previously in a brain explant organ culture system [12] and is certainly consistent with various findings in brain derived neuronal and glial cultured cell systems [13—15]. Analysis of IGFBPs secreted into conditioned medium from cultured OBs revealed on Western ligand blot four IGFBPs, identified predominantly as BP-2 (32 kDa), and BP-3 (37—42 kDa doublet subject to proteolysis by pregnant serum), as well as minor bands at 29 kDa and 24 kDa, consistent with BP-5 and BP-4. Immunoprecipitation further confirmed the identity of BP-2 (using an antibody from Mat Rechler, NIH) and BP-5 (using an antibody from David Clemmons, Chapel Hill). Messenger RNAs were identified by Northern blotting for BP-2, -4 and -5 (submitted for publication).

Regulation of IGFBPs in the developing OB

The abundance of the IGFBPs is regulated by IGF-I and basic FGF (bFGF), involving receptor-dependent mechanisms, in that IGFBP mRNAs are also regulated. Intriguingly, whereas IGF-I enhances BP-2, BP-4 and BP-5 mRNA, bFGF has opposing effects on BP-4 mRNA, which it enhances and BP-5 mRNA which it reduces, even in the presence of IGF-I. This BP-specific regulation may represent a differentiating effect of bFGF. The regulation of IGFBP abundance by IGF-I involves both receptor-dependent and -independent mechanisms, in that IGF-I analogues with minimal affinity for IGFBPs, such as des(1—3) IGF-I [16] and analogues with minimal receptor affinity, such as [Leu[24]] IGF-I [17], both increase IGFBP abundance in medium [18]. Pons et al. recently demonstrated specific and contrasting regulatory effects of IGF-I and bFGF on expression of IGFBPs by hypothalamic neurons or glial cells in culture [19]. The role of other local growth factors in regulation of IGFBPs in the brain remains unclear.

Localisation of IGFBPs in the developing OB

We examined the anatomical location of IGFBPs and IGF-I mRNA in the developing OB, comparing freshly obtained and cultured newborn OB. Using in situ hybridisation, we established that IGFBP-2 mRNA is expressed in glial cell rich glomerular and external plexiform layers, as recently described in this and other brain regions [20]. We found that IGFBP-4 mRNA, expressed in other brain regions [21], is expressed in similar cell layers, while IGFBP-5 is strongly expressed in neurons of the mitral cell layer together with IGF-I mRNA (manuscript submitted). These findings suggest the possibility that IGFBP-5 is associated with newly-expressed IGF-I and may be involved in its transport to adjacent IGF-I receptor sites, which correspond to sites of BP-2 and BP-4 expression. This further raises the possibility that BP-2 and BP-4 are involved in targeting of the transported IGF-I to its receptor. This might involve attachment of either of these IGFBPs to cell surface, as has been described for BP-3 [22] and BP-5 [23].

Freshly obtained and cultured OBs showed similar distribution of IGFBPs -2, -4 and -5 mRNAs, but only cultured OB showed scattered expression of IGFBP-3 mRNA, associated with greater gliosis, suggesting its involvement in an "injury" response similar to that described in vivo [24].

We examined for possible cellular association of IGFBPs with OB membranes by cross-linking and immunoprecipitation using BP-5 and BP-2 antibodies. Only BP-2 was associated with cell membranes, an interesting finding given its anatomical colocalisation with IGF-I receptors and the potential for a role in targeting of IGF-I to its receptor. The possibility that this cell membrane attachment of BP-2 involved binding to an integrin receptor via its known "RGD" sequence was further investigated. An RGD-containing peptide competed BP-2 away from the cell membrane, consistent with its attachment via RGD sequence. These findings are under further investigation.

Summary and Conclusions

It is now clear that IGF-I plays a central role in the developing postnatal brain, particularly in the OB in the first week of life. A paracrine system, with IGF-I receptors adjacent to sites of IGF-I synthesis, is complemented by a system of

294

IGFBPs associated with sites of IGF-I synthesis and with sites of IGF-I action. An IGFBP (IGFBP-2) associated with sites of IGF-I action, the IGF-I receptor, is also associated with cell surface membranes, probably via its RGD sequence recognised by an integrin receptor. Further understanding on the interaction of IGFBPs in the brain with components of extracellular matrix may point to mechanisms whereby IGFBPs are involved in the paracrine modulation of IGF-I action in the brain and elsewhere.

Acknowledgements

This work was supported by the National Health and Medical Research Council of Australia.

References

1. McMorris FA, Smith TM, DeSalvo S, Furlanetto RW. Proc Natl Acad Sci USA 1986;83:822–826.
2. Recio-Pinto E, Rechler MM, Ishi DN. J Neurosci 1986;6:1211–1219.
3. Werther GA, Hogg A, McKinley M, Oldfield B, Figdor R, Mendelsohn FAO. Neuroendocrinology 1989;1:370–377.
4. Lesniak MA, Hill JM, Kiess W, Rojeski M, Pert CA, Roth J. Endocrinology 1988;123:2089–2099.
5. Hynes MA, Brooks PJ, Van Wyk JJ, Lund PK. Mol Endocrinol 1988;2:47–54.
6. Stylianopoulou F, Herbert J, Soares MB, Efstratiadis A. Proc Natl Acad Sci USA 1988;85:141–145.
7. Rotwein P, Burgess SK, Milbrandt JD, Krause JE. Proc Natl Acad Sci USA 1988;85:265–269.
8. Werther GA, Abate M, Hogg A, Cheesman H, Oldfield B, Hards D, Hudson P, Power B, Freed K, Herington AC. Mol Endocrinol 1990;4:773–778.
9. Bondy C, Werner H, Roberts CT, LeRoith D. Neuroscience 1992;46:909–923.
10. Ayer-Le Lievre C, Stahblom PA, VR Sara. Development 1991;111:105–115.
11. Werther GA, Cheesman H, Russo V. Brain Res 1993;617:339–342.
12. Binoux M, Hossenlopp P, Lassarre, Hardouin N. FEBS Lett 1981;124:178–184.
13. Olson JA Jr, Shiverick KT, Ogilvie S, Buhi WC, Raizada MK. Endocrinology 1991;129:1066–1074.
14. Ocrant I, Fay CT, Parmelee JT. Endocrinology 1990;127:1260–1267.
15. Cheung PT, Smith EP, Shimasaki S, Ling N, Chernausek SD. Endocrinology 1991;129:10–14.
16. Carlsson-Skwirut C, Lake M, Hartmanis M, Hall K, Sara VR. Biochem Biophys Acta 1989;1001: 192–197.
17. Clemmons DR, Cascieri MA, Camacho-Hubner C, McCusker RH, Bayne ML. J Biol Chem 1990; 265:12210–12216.
18. Russo VC, Buchanan C, Werther GA. Ann NY Acad Sci 1993;692:308–310.
19. Pons S, Torres-Aleman I. Endocrinology 1992;131:2271–2278.
20. Lee WH, Michels KM, Bondy CA. Neuroscience 1993;53:251–265.
21. Brar AK, Chernausek SD. J Neurosci Res 1993;35:103–114.
22. Martin JL, Baxter RC. Growth Reg 1992;2:88–89.
23. Jones JI, Gockerman A, Busby WH, Camacho-Hubner C, Clemmons DR. 1993;679–687.
24. Gluckman P, Klempt N, Guan J, Mallard C, Sirimanne E, Dragunow M, Klempt M, Singh K, Williams C, Nikolics K. Biochem Biophys Res Commun 1992;182:593–599.

Insulin-like growth factors in the nervous system: evolution, fetal development, maintenance and tumor formation

Steen Gammeltoft[1], Anne Danielsen[1], Morten Frödin[1], Mette Grønborg[1], Lars B.H. Hansen[1], Ninna R. Holm[1], Katarina Drakenberg[2], Vicki R. Sara[2], Birthe Hultberg[3] and Christer Nilsson[4]

[1]*Department of Clinical Chemistry, Glostrup Hospital, Copenhagen, Denmark;* [2]*Department of Pathology, Karolinska Institute, Stockholm, Sweden;* [3]*Department of Pathology, Bispebjerg Hospital, Copenhagen, Denmark; and* [4]*Department of Molecular Neurobiology, Wallenberg Laboratory, Lund, Sweden*

Abstract. Insulin-like growth factor, IGF-I, and IGF-I receptor are expressed in the brains of the three lower vertebrates: *Cottus scorpius* (sea scorpion), *Raja calvata* (ray) and *Myxine glutinosa* (atlantic hagfish). IGF-I and IGF-II are highly expressed in the fetal mammalian brain and act as mitogens on immature neurons and astrocytes. In adult brain IGF-II is synthesized in the choroid plexus and secreted to the cerebrospinal fluid. Choroid plexus epithelial cells in culture express IGF-II mRNA and secrete immunoreactive protein. Chromaffin cells from fetal, neonatal and adult rat synthesize IGF-II and respond to IGF-II by increased cell proliferation and IGF-II acts synergistically with NGF or bFGF. IGF-II mRNA and immunoreactivity is present in higher amounts in benign meningiomas than in malignant glioblastomas and astrocytomas.

Summary and perspectives

Insulin-like growth factors, IGF-I and IGF-II, are polypeptides structurally similar to insulin which act as mitogens on various cell types via activation of the IGF-I receptor tyrosine kinase. IGF-I and IGF-II receptors are expressed in three representatives of lower vertebrates: the osteichthyes, chondrichtyes and cyclostomi. Competitive binding studies and affinity labelling of brain membranes from *Cottus scorpius* (sea scorpion), *Raja calvata* (ray) and *Myxine glutinosa* (atlantic hagfish) identified a mammalian IGF-I receptor by its binding specificity and the molecular size of its α subunit. There was no evidence for the presence of a mammalian IGF-II/mannose 6-phosphate (Man-6-P) receptor in brains of *Cottus, Raja* and *Myxine*.

During fetal development IGF-I and IGF-II are highly and widely expressed in the nervous system, but their expression declines postnatally. In adult brain IGF-II is synthesized in the choroid plexus and secreted to the cerebrospinal fluid. Furthermore, IGF-II is synthesized in the adrenal medulla. IGF-I and IGF-II act as mitogens on immature neurons and astrocytes from fetal rat brain. Choroid plexus epithelial cells

---

Address for correspondence: Steen Gammeltoft, M.D., Department of Clinical Chemistry, Glostrup Hospital, DK-2600 Glostrup, Denmark.

in culture express IGF-II mRNA and IGFBP-2 mRNA and secrete immunoreactive proteins. Chromaffin cells from fetal, neonatal and adult rats respond to IGF-II by 2- to 10-fold increase in cell proliferation and IGF-II act synergistically with nerve growth factor (NGF) or basic fibroblast growth factor (bFGF). IGF-II mRNA is present in higher amounts in benign meningiomas than in malignant glioblastomas and astrocytomas, whereas the content of immunoreactive IGF-II is similar.

From these data we conclude that IGF-I may have neuroendocrine functions early in vertebrate evolution and that IGF-I and IGF-II may be involved in stimulation of neuronal and glial precursor cell proliferation during fetal development of mammalian brain. In adult mammals IGF-II may act as an autocrine, paracrine or neuroendocrine growth factor in maintenance of choroid plexus epithelium in brain and of chromaffin cells in adrenal medulla. Finally, IGF-II may act as an autocrine growth promotor in intracranial meningiomas.

Introduction

IGF-I and IGF-II, are regulatory peptides showing structural homology to insulin, that regulate cellular proliferation in vertebrates [1,2]. IGFs seem to be well conserved during vertebrate evolution. Amino acid sequences of IGF-I and IGF-II from human and chicken show 84—89% homology. The deduced amino acid sequences of IGF-I cDNA from lower vertebrates like amphibian, osteichthye and cyclostome show 70—84% homology to human IGF-I [3—5].

The cDNA of an insulin-like peptide from amphioxus is equally related to human insulin and IGFs (48%) and may represent a transitional form from which insulin and IGF diverged in early vertebrate evolution [6].

Two types of IGF receptors have been identified in mammals [7,8]. The IGF-I receptor is structurally similar to the insulin receptor and bind IGF-I with higher affinity than IGF-II and insulin only in high concentrations. The IGF-II receptor is identical to the cation-independent Man-6-P receptor and binds IGF-II with much higher affinity than IGF-I and does not crossreact with insulin. The cellular effects of IGF-I and IGF-II seem to be mediated by the IGF-I receptor, whereas the IGF-II/Man-6-P receptor is primarily involved in endocytosis and depredation of IGF-II [9].

IGF-I and IGF-II show mitogenic and insulin-like metabolic effects throughout life [1]. The biological actions of IGF-I and IGF-II have been characterized in vitro where they stimulate DNA and RNA synthesis in variety of cells, but also metabolic effects such stimulation of glucose uptake, glycogen synthesis, amino acid transport and lipid synthesis. Thus IGF-I and IGF-II exert pleiotropic effects like other polypeptide growth factors.

In accordance with the ubiquitous expression of IGF-I and IGF-II during various stages of vertebrate life, they show growth-promoting actions in almost any tissue under various physiological and pathological conditions. Both IGFs are highly and widely expressed during fetal development and growth. Postnatally, the gene expression of IGF-I and IGF-II declines and are restricted to selected tissues. IGF-I is synthesized in several tissues including liver, muscle, kidney, bone, adrenal cortex, ovary and testis, whereas IGF-II is synthesized in brain, heart, kidney, liver, muscle, ovary, testis, skin and adrenal medulla [1,7].

In the nervous system IGF-I and IGF-II are expressed during fetal development of the brain and peripheral nerves. Postnatally, only IGF-II expression is detectable in the choroid plexus and meninges. In the peripheral nervous system IGF-I and IGF-II are expressed in sympathetic ganglia and adrenal medulla. The role IGF-I and IGF-II in the nervous system is poorly understood. In vitro studies of astrocytes and neuronal precursor cells from fetal rat brain in primary culture, show that IGF-I and IGF-II stimulate the proliferation and cell survival [10].

These studies suggest that IGF-I and IGF-II are important proliferation factors during fetal development of the brain. Postnatal functions of IGFs have been studied using cell cultures of sympathetic ganglia and chromaffin cells showing that IGFs stimulate cell proliferation and survival of these cell types. Furthermore IGF-I stimulate epinephrine release from cultured chromaffin cells. In the adult brain the role of IGF-I and IGF-II remains enigmatic.

This review addresses four questions of the role of IGFs in the nervous system. First, the evolution of IGF-I and its receptor in the brain is analyzed by studies of three primitive vertebrates: *C. scorpius*, *R. calvata* and *M. glutinosa*. Their presence in the brain as suggest that IGF-I has neuroendocrine functions early in vertebrate evolution. Secondly, the production and action of IGF-II in the adult choroid plexus has been studied in order to define the role of IGFs in the adult nervous system. Our data suggest that the choroid plexus epithelium is the main site of IGF-II biosynthesis and that IGF-II may have an autocrine function in stimulation of choroid plexus epithelium cell growth. Thirdly, the effect of IGF-II on proliferation of chromaffin cells representing the sympathoadrenal system, was analyzed in order to define a role of IGF-II in the peripheral nervous system. IGF-II stimulates proliferation of chromaffin cells throughout life and acts synergistically with NGF and bFGF. Fourthly, the expression of IGF-II in human intercranial tumors, was analyzed in order to define the role of IGF-II in the human brain tumor growth. IGF-II is expressed in high amounts in meningiomas suggesting a role in autocrine growth regulation.

IGF-I and IGF-I receptor are present in the brain of primitive vertebrates

Using immunohistochemistry, IGF-I-like immunoreactivity has recently been observed in endocrine cells in the intestinal mucosal and in the endocrine pancreas of *C. scorpius, R. clavata* and *M. glutinosa* [11,12]. These species hold pivotal positions in the evolution of the neuroendocrine system. IGF-I immunoreactive perikarya and fibers have been observed in all levels of the *M. glutinosa* brain [11].

IGF-I receptors have been demonstrated in representatives of the osteichthyes, chondrichtyes and cyclostomi [13]. In the three species examined: *Cottus, Raja* and

Myxine the highest binding of ^{125}I-labelled IGF-I or IGF-II was measured in the brain compared with liver and gastrointestinal tract. Competitive binding assay and affinity labelling identified the receptor as the IGF-I receptor described in higher vertebrates based on two criteria: IGF-I and IGF-II are almost equally potent in displacing receptor-bound ^{125}I-IGF-I and ^{125}I-IGF-II and the labelled protein has a molecular size of 100,000—120,000 under reducing conditions.

The peptide specificity is similar to IGF-I receptors human glioma cells [14] and bovine chromaffin cells [15], but different from IGF-I receptors in fetal rat brain neurons, which bind IGF-I with 10 times higher affinity than IGF-II [16]. The molecular size is similar to the α subunit of the neuronal subtype of IGF-I receptor described in mammalian brain, which is smaller than in other tissues [17]. Scatchard analysis of our data showed that IGF-I receptor affinity and concentration in the brains of *Cottus, Raja* and *Myxine* is similar to that described in the rat brain [17].

Remarkably, there was no indication of the presence of the mammalian IGF-II/Man-6-P receptor in the brain of these primitive vertebrates. This is in agreement with previous observations, that although the cation-independent Man-6-P receptor is present in chicken and *Xenopus laevis*, this receptor is unable to bind IGF-II [18]. The data extend the evidence that the IGF-II-binding ability of the Man-6-P receptor is acquired late in evolution and is characteristic of the mammalian species.

In mammals the function of IGF-II binding to the IGF-II/Man-6-P receptor is unclear. The mitogenic effects of IGF-II appear to be mediated through the IGF-I receptor like in other vertebrates, whereas the IGF-II/Man-6-P receptor is involved in endocytosis and degradation of IGF-II [7—9]. Although it remains to be established that IGF-II-like material is also produced in *Cottus, Raja* and *Myxine*, the present results indicate that the biological actions of IGF-II will be mediated via the IGF-I receptor.

IGF-II, IGFBP-2 and IGF-I receptor are expressed in choroid plexus of mammalian brain

Postnatally, IGF-II expression persists in certain tissues and in the central nervous system IGF-II transcripts are mainly located to the choroid plexus and meninges [19—21]. These findings probably explain the relatively high level of IGF-II in the human cerebrospinal fluid compared to serum [22]. In addition, the choroid plexus synthesizes insulin-like growth factor binding protein-2 (IGFBP-2), which preferentially binds IGF-II and is the main IGFBP in both human and rat CSF [23].

IGF-II mRNA is present in primary cultures of highly purified choroid plexus epithelial cells from adult sheep brain and IGF-II is secreted into the medium. Furthermore, IGFBP-2 mRNA is expressed and IGFBP-2 is secreted by the cultured epithelial cells [24]. These data, in combination with unpublished results from in situ hybridization of IGF-II mRNA in adult rat and pig choroid plexus (C. Nilsson et al., in preparation), indicate that, at least in the adult mammal, the epithelium is an important site of IGF-II and IGFBP-2 production in the choroid plexus. Thus, our

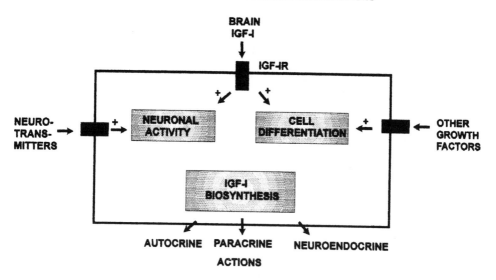

Fig. 1. Model of biosynthesis and actions of IGF-I on brain neurons from primitive vertebrates. A neuronal cell produces and secretes IGF-I that have autocrine, paracrine or neuroendocrine actions in the brain. Brain IGF-I activates the IGF-I receptor and regulates neuronal activity and cell differentiation. Other neurotransmitters and growth factors may act in concert with IGF-I.

data indicate that IGF-II and IGFBP-2 are not produced by separate cell types of the postnatal choroid plexus, as has been suggested in studies of the rat and human fetus [25].

To understand better the role of the IGFs in the choroid plexus the presence of IGF-I receptors and Man-6-P/IGF-II receptors in suspensions of epithelial cells and in Triton X-100-soluble and insoluble fractions of cells have been studied. A large number of IGF-I receptors are present on the cell surface, whereas Man-6-P/IGF-II receptors are detectable only in low amounts on the surface compared with a higher content in the solubilized fraction. Measurements on the insoluble fraction, which is enriched in clathrin-coated pits, showed high binding of IGF-I whereas no binding of IGF-II was seen.

These findings strongly suggest that most Man-6-P/IGF-II receptors in choroid plexus epithelium are found intracellularly. We propose that the Man-6-P/IGF-II receptor is downregulated in choroid plexus epithelial cells, due to the synthesis and secretion of IGF-II into the cerebrospinal fluid. In contrast, the IGF-I receptor, which also binds IGF-II, may resist downregulation in the presence of ligand.

The IGF-I receptor in choroid plexus cells is functional, as shown by the stimulation of tyrosine kinase activity and autophosphorylation of the β subunit by IGF-I, IGF-II and insulin, with decreasing potency [21]. At present, the role of the IGF-I receptor tyrosine kinase in choroid plexus epithelial cells is not known, but one possibility is that it mediates endocrine and autocrine signals of IGF-I and IGF-II in

300

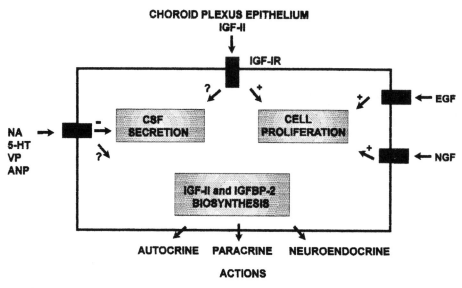

Fig. 2. Model of IGF-II and IGFBP2 biosynthesis and actions in choroid plexus epithelium. IGF-II and IGFBP2 are produced and secreted by choroid plexus epithelial cells and have autocrine, paracrine or neuroendocrine actions in the central nervous system. IGF-II produced in the choroid plexus by epithelials cells acts via the IGF-I receptor and stimulate cell proliferation in concert with other growth factors like EGF and NGF. Various neurotransmitters including nor-adrenaline (NA), 5-hydroxytryptamine (5-HT), vasopressin (VP) and atrial natriuretic peptide (ANP) inhibit cerebrospinal fluid (CSF) secretion. It is not known whether these neurotransmitters regulate IGF-II and IGFBP2 by synthesis. Actions of IGF-II on CSF secretion are unknown.

the continuous replacement of the cells. Preliminary results from our laboratory show that IGF-II stimulates DNA synthesis of cultured epithelial cells from neonatal choroid plexus and that addition of IGF-II antibody to the cell culture blocked DNA synthesis (C. Nilsson, in preparation). These data suggest that IGF-II may be involved in autocrine regulation of choroid plexus epithelial cell growth.

IGF-II stimulate proliferation of chromaffin cells synergistically with NGF or bFGF

Chromaffin-cell division in the rat occurs mainly during fetal and neonatal development, whereas proliferation of adult chromaffin cells is very low [26]. Little is known about the factors that regulate the growth of chromaffin cells. Postnatally, bFGF is present in bovine and rat adrenal medulla [27,28], and bFGF stimulates the proliferation of neonatal rat chromaffin cells [29,30]. It is not known whether NGF is present in the adrenal medulla, but the NGF receptor (p75) has been demonstrated immunocytochemically in chromaffin cells from adult rhesus monkeys and Trk receptors have been found in rat chromaffin cells NGF acts as a mitogen on cultured chromaffin cells from neonatal and adult rats [31].

IGF-II mRNA and immunoreactivity have been demonstrated in adult human and rat adrenal medulla [32]. Human and bovine chromaffin cells express the IGF-I receptor tyrosine kinase [15,33] and IGF-I stimulates catecholamine synthesis and secretion by cultured bovine chromaffin cells in vitro [34]. IGF-I and IGF-II stimulate the proliferation of rat pheochromocytoma PC12 cells [35,36].

IGF-II stimulates the proliferation of chromaffin cells from fetal, neonatal and adult rats in a serum-free culture system. The responsiveness to IGF-I and IGF-II differed significantly with the developmental stage, being highest in neonatal and lowest in adult chromaffin cells. The dose-response relationship of IGFs in neonatal chromaffin cells corresponds to that observed in other cell types and the fact that IGF-I is more potent than IGF-II suggests that the effect is mediated by the IGF-I receptor [37].

In neonatal and adult chromaffin cells, addition of bFGF or NGF stimulated DNA synthesis to approximately the same level as IGF-I or IGF-II. However, the response to bFGF or NGF in combination with either IGF-I or IGF-II was more than additive, indicating that the combined effect of the IGFs and bFGF or NGF is synergistic. The degree of synergism was 2- to 4-fold in neonatal chromaffin cells and 10- to 20-fold in adult chromaffin cells compared with the effect of each growth factor alone. In contrast, the action of bFGF and NGF added together in the absence of IGFs was not synergistic or additive [37]. The apparent postmitotic state of adult chromaffin cells in situ may be induced inhibitory factors in the adrenal gland. Thus, corticosterone and pituitary adenylate cyclase-activating popypsptide 38 inhibit IGF-II- and bFGF-stimulated growth of cultured neonatal and adult chromaffin cells by 75%–95% (M. Frödin, in preparation).

IGF-II acted also as a survival factor on neonatal chromaffin cells and the cell survival was further improved when bFGF or NGF was added together with IGF-II. We propose that IGF-I and IGF-II act in synergy with bFGF and NGF to stimulate proliferation and survival of chromaffin cells during neonatal growth and adult maintenance of the adrenal medulla [37].

These findings may have implications for improving the survival of chromaffin cell implants in diseased human brain. Brain implants of chromaffin cells have been used as dopaminergic donors in patients with Parkinson disease, but the long-term benefit has been hampered by poor survival of the implanted cells [38]. The approach has been abandoned and replaced by transplantation of human fetal ventral mesencephalic cells that seems to give better results [39]. Administration of NGF to brain implants of chromaffin cells in experimental animals has led to improved cell survival [40]. Based on our data a combination of IGF, NGF and bFGF may be more effective than each growth factor alone in improving the survival of the chromaffin cell implants. Thus, implantation of autologous adrenal medullary tissue diseased human brain, should be reconsidered as it may be advantageous over transplantation of heterologous fetal tissue regarding tissue accessibility, immunotolerance and medical ethics.

302

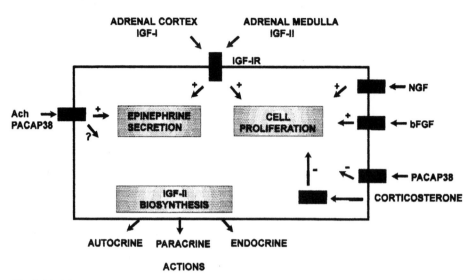

Fig. 3. Model of the IGF-II biosynthesis and actions of IGF-I and IGF-II on the chromaffin cell. IGF-II is produced and secreted and may have autocrine, paracrine or endocrine actions. IGF-I from the adrenal cortex and IGF-II from the adrenal medulla act via the IGF-I (IGF-IR) receptor and stimulate cell proliferation and epinephrine secretion. Chromaffin cell proliferation is stimulated by NGF and bFGF, which act synergistically with IGF-I and IGF-II. Cell proliferation is inhibited by the neuropeptide pituitary adenylate cyclase-activating peptide-38 (PAPAC38) and corticosterone. Acetylcholine (Ach) and PACAP38 stimulate epinephrine secretion. It is not known whether neurotransmitters regulate IGF-II biosynthesis.

IGF-II is expressed in human intracranial meningioma

Aberrant expression of growth factors and their receptors seem to play a role during malignant transformation and tumor development [41]. Studies of human glioblastomas have shown that they express PDGF receptor and EGF receptor [42,43] and that human meningiomas express FGF and EGF receptors [44,45]. IGF-II transcripts and peptides have been isolated from a variety of extracranial tumors [46]. The presence of IGF-II transcripts has been described in two malignant gliomas [47] and IGF-II immunoreactivity has been detected in cyst fluid of three low-grade astrocytomas [48]. IGF-I and Man-6-P/IGF-II receptors have been characterized in meningiomas and glioma cell lines, respectively [14,49].

Recently, we have demonstrated that four human meningiomas express IGF-II transcripts and immunoreactive IGF-II [50]. Other primary intracranial brain tumors like oligoastrocytomas and glioblastomas also contained immunoreactive IGF-II, whereas IGF-II mRNA could not be detected by Northern analysis [50]. It is possible, however, that IGF-II mRNA are present in low amounts and translated to IGF-II peptide in these malignant tumors. It is also possible that plasma is contained in the

303

INSULIN-LIKE GROWTH FACTORS AND MENINGIOMA

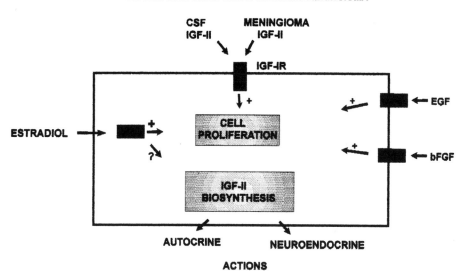

Fig. 4. Model of IGF-II biosynthesis and actions on meningioma cells. IGF-II is synthesized and released by meningioma cells and may have autocrine or neuroendocrine actions. IGF-II produced by choroid plexus epithelial cells and meninges in the cerebrospinal fluid or produced by meningioma cells act via the IGF-I (IGF-IR) receptor and stimulate meningioma cell proliferation. Cell may also be proliferation stimulated by EGF and bFGF. Estradiol may stimulate cell proliferation, possibly via IGF-II biosynthesis and autocrine growth stimulation.

tumors, which could amount to approximately 4% by weight. If the IGF-II concentration in plasma is 500 ng/ml, there might be a significant contamination of tumor extracts amounting to IGF-II levels of 20 ng/g tissue. IGF-II may be involved in regulation of cell growth in meningiomas, because IGF-I receptors, which mediate the effects of IGF-II, are present in primary human meningiomas [49]. BFGF and EGF are also potential growth regulators of meningiomas and may act in concert with IGF-II.

IGF-II is normally produced by the meninges in adult mammals [19,20] and our finding that IGF-II mRNA is present in meningiomas, suggest that the meningioma cell maintains its IGF-II-producing capacity during tumor development. It is notable that the tumors exhibit high levels of a 4.8 kb transcript compared with placenta, because this transcript is the active species in the synthesis of preproIGF-II [9]. This may account for the high levels of IGF-II in the meningioma extracts. Consequently, IGF-II could be regarded as a tumor marker for meningiomas and determination of IGF-II concentrations in the cerebrospinal fluid may be useful in the diagnosis. The transforming potential of IGF-II is unclear, but meningiomas occur predominantly in women, and the tumor has been suggested to be estrogen-sensitive [51–53]. It is possible that IGF-II mediates a tumor-promoting effect of estrogens in meningiomas in analogy with the mechanism operation in mammary carcinoma [54].

In the current study, IGF-II mRNA was not detected in the malignant intracranial astrocytomas and glioblastomas by Northern analysis, indicating that the IGF-II gene may be expressed only at low levels. This stresses the different origin of malignant brain tumors compared with the benign meningiomas. A recent study has reported, however, the expression of IGF-II mRNA in two cases of primary human glioblastoma by Northern analysis [47]. The discrepancy may suggest that glioblastomas are heterogenous or that meningeal or choroidal tissues have contributed to the signal.

References

1. Daughaday WH, Rotwein P. Endocrine Rev 1989;10:68–91.
2. Humbel RE. Biochem 1990;190:445–462.
3. Ballard FJ, Johnson RJ, Owens PC, Francis GL, Upton FM, McMurtry JP, Wallace JC. Gen Comp Endocrinol 1990;79:459–468.
4. Kajimoto Y, Rotwein P. Mol Endocrinol 1990;4:217–226.
5. Nagamatsu S, Chan SJ, Falkmer S, Steiner DF. J Biol Chem 1991;266:2397–2402.
6. Chan Sj, Cao Q-P, Steiner DF. Proc Natl Acad Sci USA 1990;87:9319–9323.
7. Gammeltoft S. In: Martinez J (ed) Processing, Biological Activity and Pharmacology. Chichester: Ellis Horwood, 1989;176–210.
8. Sara VR, Hall K. Physiol Rev 1990;70:591–614.
9. Nielsen FC. Prog Growth Factor Res 1992;4:257–290.
10. Gammeltoft S, Auletta M, Danielsen A, Larsen E, Nielsen FC, Nilsson C, Senen D, Wang E. In: Isaksson O, Westermark B, Betsholtz C (eds) Basic and Clinical Aspects. Amsterdam: Elsevier Science Publishers, 1990;227–241.
11. Reinecke M, Drakenberg K, Falkmer S, Sara VR. Histochemistry 1991;96:191–196.
12. Reinecke M, Drakenberg K, Falkmer S, Sara VR. Reg Peptides 1992;37:155–165.
13. Drakenberg K, Sara VR, Falkmer S, Gammeltoft S, Maake C, Reinecke M. Reg Peptides 1993;43: 73–81.
14. Gammeltoft S, Ballotti R, Kowalski A, Westermark B. C Res 1988;48:1233–1237.
15. Danielsen A, Larsen E, Gammeltoft S. Brain Res 1990;518:95–100.
16. Nielsen FC, Wang E, Gammeltoft S. J Neurochem 1991;58:12–21.
17. Gammeltoft S, Haselbacher GK, Humbel RE, Fehlmann M, Van Obberghen E. EMBO J 1985;4: 3407–3412.
18. Clairmont KB, Czech MP. J Biol Chem 1989;264.
19. Stylianopoulou F, Herbert J, Soares MB, Efstratiadis A. Proc Natl Sci USA 1988;85:141–145.
20. Beck F, Samani NJ, Byrne S, Morgan K, Gebhard R, Brammar WJ. Development 1988;104:29–39.
21. Nilsson C, Blay P, Nielsen FC, Gammeltoft S. J Neurochem 1992,58:923–930.
22. Haselbacher GK, Humbel R. Endocrinology 1982;110:1822–1824.
23. Tseng LYH, Brown AL, Yang YWH, Komanus JA, Orlowski CC, Taylor T, Rechler MM. Mol Endocrinol 1989;3:1559–1568.
24. Hellesen N, Hansen LBH, Nilsson C, Gammeltoft S. Mol Brain Res (in press).
25. Wood TL, Brown AL, Rechler MM, Pintar JE. Mol Endocrinol 1990;4:1257–1263.
26. Tiscler AS, Ruzicka LA, Donahue SR, DeLellis RA. Int J Dev Neurosci 1989;7:439–448.
27. Grothe C, Unsicker K. Histochemistry 1990;94:141–147.
28. Grothe C, Unsicker K. J Histochem Cytochem 1989;37:1877–1883.
29. Claude P, Parada IM, Gordon KA, D'Amore PA, Wagner JA. Neuron 1988;1:783–790.
30. Lillien LE, Claude P. Nature 1985;317:632–634.
31. Tischler AS, Riseberg JC, Hardenbrook MA, Cherington V. J Neurosci 1993;13:1533–1542.
32. Haselbacher GK, Irminger J-C, Zapf J, Ziegler WH, Humbel RE. Proc Natl Acad Sci USA 1987;84: 1104–1106.

33. Dahmer MK, Perlman RL. J Neurochem 1988;51:321–323.
34. Dahmer MK, Hart PM, Perlman RL. J Neurochem 1990;54:931–936.
35. Dahmer MK, Perlman RL. Endocrinology 1988;122:2109–2113.
36. Nielsen FC, Gammeltoft S. Biochem Biophys Res Commun 1988;154:1018–1023.
37. Frödin M, Gammeltoft S. Proc Natl Acad Sci USA (in press).
38. Goetz CG, Olanow CW, Koller WC, Penn RD, Cahill D, Morantz R, Stebbins C, Tanner CM, Klawans HL, Shannon KM. N Engl J Med 1989;320:337–341.
39. Widner H, Tetrud J, Rehncrona S, Snow B, Brundin P, Gustravh B, Björklund A, Lindvall O, Langston JW. N Engl J Med 1992;327:1556–1563.
40. Cunningham LA, Hansen JT, Short MP, Bohn Mc. Brain Res 1991;561:192–202.
41. Heldin C-H, Westermark B. Eur J Biochem 1989;184:487–496.
42. Hermansson M, Nistér M, Betsholtz C, Heldin C-H, Westermark B, Funa K. Proc Natl Acad Sci USA 1988;85:7748–7752.
43. Libermann TA, Razon N, Batal AD, Yarden Y, Schlessinger J, Soreq H. Cancer Res 1984;44:753–760.
44. Takahasi JA, Mori H, Fukumoto M, Igarashi K, Jaye M, Oda Y. Proc Natl Acad Sci USA 1990;87:5710–5714.
45. Shiura RA, Lawrence F, Vogel H, Lee YL, Horoupian DS, Urich H. Cancer 1988;62:2139–2144.
46. Daughaday WH. Endocrinology 1990;127:1–4.
47. Sandberg AC, Engberg C, Lake M, Von Holst H, Sara VR. Neurosci Lett 1988;93:114–119.
48. Glick RP, Unterman TG, Hollis R. J Neurosurg 1991;74:972–978.
49. Kurihara M, Tokunaga Y, Tsutsumi K, Kawwaguchi T, Shigematsu K, Niwa M. J Neurosurg 1989;71:538–544.
50. Hultberg B, Haselbacher G, Nielsen FC, Wulff BS, Gammeltoft S. Cancer 1993;72:3282–3286.
51. Jay JR, MacLaughlin DT, Riley KR, Martuza RL. J Neurosurg 1985;62:757–762.
52. Lesch KP, Gross S. J Neurosurg 1987;67:237–243.
53. Grunberg SM, Daniels AM, Muensch H, Daniels JR, Bernstein L, Kortes V. J Neurosurg 1987;66:405–408.
54. Yee D, Cullen KJ, Sonnmyoung P, Perdue JF, Hampton B, Schwartz A. Cancer Res 1988;48:6691–6696.

Insulin-like growth factor, an autocrine regulator of skeletal cells

Ernesto Canalis

Departments of Research, Medicine and Orthopedic Surgery, Saint Francis Hospital and Medical Center, Hartford, CT 06105-1299 and The University of Connecticut School of Medicine, Farmington, CT 06030, USA

Abstract. Insulin-like growth factors, IGF-I and IGF-II, are growth factors synthesized by skeletal cells and known to increase bone formation. The synthesis of IGF-I and IGF-II is regulated by systemic hormones and locally produced growth factors and their activity is regulated by IGF binding proteins. There is a correlation between the expression of IGF-I and IGF-II and the differentiated function of the osteoblast and bone formation. It is possible that changes in the synthesis or activity of IGF-I and IGF-II are responsible for selective forms of metabolic bone disease. Systemic IGF-I or agents that enhance the synthesis of skeletal IGF-I may have a place in the future treatment of osteopenia.

Initial studies from this laboratory revealed that bone in organ culture secretes growth factor activity [1]. The components of this activity have characterized and it was demonstrated that insulin-like growth factors, IGF-I and IGF-II, are prevalent growth factors secreted by skeletal cells and they have important actions in bone cell function [2–4].

Role of systemic and local IGF in bone remodeling

In the circulation, IGF-I and IGF-II form a complex with IGF binding proteins (IGFBPs) and an acid labile subunit and there is little, if any, free IGF-I or IGF-II available to peripheral tissues. Therefore, the locally secreted IGF-I and IGF-II might play a more important role in the regulation of cell function. Intact calvariae and isolated osteoblasts in culture secrete IGF-I and II and their concentrations in culture medium, are 1–10 nM [3,5]. These levels are 10–30 times lower than those found in serum, but are physiologically relevant since they are similar to the effective concentrations of IGF in bone [2].

The contribution of systemic IGF-I and IGF-II to bone remodeling is uncertain, not only because there may be no free circulating IGF, but also because when IGF-I is administered systemically its effects on bone formation have been inconsistent [6,7]. It is likely that the systemic form of IGF-I, which is derived from the liver and

Address for correspondence: Ernesto Canalis, Department of Research, Saint Francis Hospital and Medical Center, 114 Woodland Street, Hartford, CT 06105-1299, USA.

is growth hormone-dependent, has more relevance to linear growth through cartilage-mediated effects. In contrast, the locally synthesized IGF-I, which for the most part is not growth hormone dependent, may be more important for the maintenance of bone mass.

Actions of IGFs in skeletal tissue

IGF-I and IGF-II have important and similar effects on bone remodeling and it is likely that the IGF-I receptor mediates their anabolic actions in bone (Table 1). IGF-II is about 4—7 times less potent than IGF-I on bone formation [8]. Although IGF-I and IGF-II are modest mitogens, they increase DNA synthesis and the replication of cells of the osteoblastic lineage, presumably preosteoblastic cells, which can differentiate into osteoblasts. A major role of IGFs is the stimulation of the differentiated function of the osteoblast. IGF-I increases osteocalcin synthesis and IGF-I and IGF-II increase type 1 collagen transcripts and synthesis rates [9]. As a result of its effects on the differentiated function of the osteoblast, IGF-I increases bone matrix apposition rates as determined by histomorphometric analysis, therefore it increases bone formation [10].

In addition to their anabolic actions, IGF-I and IGF-II decrease the degradation of collagen in bone cultures and as such they prevent the degradation of bone matrix [8]. This effect is analogous to their actions on cartilage, where IGFs have been shown to decrease the degradation of proteoglycans [11]. The mechanism of the IGF effect on collagen degradation is currently being examined in our laboratory. Initial experiments reveal that IGF-I decreases basal and stimulated interstitial collagenase mRNA expression and this inhibition may be responsible for the decrease in bone collagen degradation. This does not exclude additional possible actions of IGF-I and IGF-II on the expression of tissue inhibitors of metalloproteinases, also known to regulate collagen degradation.

Recently, IGF-I was shown to enhance the recruitment of osteoclasts [12]. Consequently, it could have a role in bone resorption. IGF-II was not found to alter osteoclast recruitment and this observation could reveal subtle differences in the mechanisms of action of IGF-I and IGF-II in bone.

Cultures of osteoblast-enriched cells express receptors for IGF-I and IGF-II [13]. IGF-I binds to a high affinity receptor with a molecular mass of 130 kDa and a dissociation constant of 750 pM and it is believed that this receptor mediates most of the anabolic actions of IGF in bone. IGF-II binds to a high affinity of receptor

---

Table 1. Actions of IGF-I and IGF-II in bone

1. IGFs enhance the differentiated function of the osteoblast and increase collagen synthesis.
2. IGFs have modest mitogenic activity for cells of the osteoblastic lineage.
3. IGFs decrease collagen degradation.
4. IGF-I, but not IGF-II, increases osteoclast recruitment.

with a molecular mass of 240 kDa. This receptor is identical to the mannose-6-phosphate receptor and its function in bone is uncertain. It is possible to regulate the activity of IGF-I and IGF-II by modifying their binding to specific receptors and there is evidence that steroids regulate IGF-I and IGF-II binding to bone cells [14,15]. Cortisol enhances IGF-I binding, but this effect appears to be dependent on cell number and 1,25-dihydroxyvitamin D_3 increases IGF-I binding in selected osteoblast cell lines. From the evidence currently available, it would appear that systemic and local regulators of bone cell function play a more important role in the regulation of IGF-I and IGF-II synthesis and of their binding proteins than on receptor binding.

Regulation of IGF-I synthesis by skeletal cells

Studies from this and other laboratories have shown that IGF-I is synthesized by cells of the osteoblast lineage and that its synthesis is controlled by systemic hormones and local factors (Table 2).

Parathyroid hormone (PTH) appears to be the hormone with the most significant actions on IGF-I synthesis in skeletal cells; it increases IGF-I transcripts and polypeptide levels by 3—4-fold in osteoblast cultures. The level of regulation has not been determined and it is possible that PTH regulates IGF-I synthesis by transcriptional and posttranscriptional mechanisms [16]. The effect of PTH on skeletal IGF-I synthesis seems to be mediated by changes in cyclic AMP. Neither ionomycin nor phorbol esters increase IGF-I synthesis, suggesting that changes in intracellular calcium or protein kinase C activity do not mediate this action of PTH in bone. Growth hormone causes a modest increase in skeletal IGF-I synthesis. This may be because bone cells express a low number of growth hormone receptors or because exon 2 of the IGF-I gene, which contains necessary elements for a growth hormone response, is expressed at low levels in bone cells (Canalis et al., unpublished observations). 17-β-estradiol increases IGF-I transcription in bone cells transfected with estrogen receptors [17].

Table 2. Regulation of IGF-I synthesis in bone cells

Systemic hormones	
Stimulatory:	PTH and related agents
	Growth hormone
	Estradiol
Inhibitory:	Cortisol
	Vitamin D in selected cells
Growth factors	
Stimulatory:	Bone morphogenetic protein
Inhibitory:	Fibroblast growth factor
	Transforming growth factor β
	Platelet-derived growth factor
Other agents	
Stimulatory:	Prostaglandin E_2

Glucocorticoids decrease IGF-I transcript and polypeptide levels in bone cell cultures [18]. Glucocorticoids and IGF-I have opposite effects on bone formation and it is possible that a decrease in IGF-I mediates the inhibitory actions of glucocorticoids on bone formation [19]. Other steroids such as 1,25-dihydroxyvitamin D_3 decrease IGF-I polypeptide levels in selected osteoblast cell lines.

The synthesis of skeletal IGF-I is also modified by factors secreted by bone cells. Prostaglandin E_2, a cyclic AMP inducer, increases IGF-I transcript and polypeptide levels in osteoblast cultures, whereas most mitogens secreted by skeletal cells are inhibitory [20]. Basic fibroblast growth factor, platelet-derived growth factor and transforming growth factor β1 decrease IGF-I transcript and polypeptide levels in osteoblasts [21]. Although the growth factors studied have mitogenic activity, their effect on IGF-I synthesis is independent of their actions on cell cycle and is not modified by DNA synthesis inhibitors. These growth factors tend to inhibit the differentiated function of the osteoblast and this correlates with a decrease in IGF-I synthesis. In contrast, bone morphogenetic protein 2, known to induce the differentiation of mesenchymal cells into cells of the osteoblastic lineage, increases IGF-I synthesis in osteoblast cultures [22,23]. Bone morphogenetic proteins, members of the transforming growth factor β superfamily of polypeptides, have modest mitogenic activity for cells of the osteoblastic lineage, but they increase alkaline phosphatase activity and collagen synthesis, suggesting that they enhance the differentiated function of the osteoblast [24]. It is therefore apparent that growth factors that inhibit the differentiated function of the osteoblast inhibit IGF-I synthesis, whereas factors that increase differentiation augment skeletal IGF-I synthesis. This leads us to believe that the expression of the osteoblastic phenotype and IGF-I expression are correlated.

Regulation of IGF-II synthesis in skeletal cells

Although hormones have been shown to modulate the synthesis of IGF-I in cultured osteoblasts, they do not appear to have effects on IGF-II synthesis (Table 3). Hormones with known actions on bone cell metabolism do not change IGF-II transcripts in osteoblasts after 6 h of treatment and do not change IGF-II polypeptide concentrations in cultured intact calvariae [5,25], suggesting that skeletal IGF-II synthesis is not regulated by systemic hormones. In contrast, locally produced growth factors, including basic fibroblast growth factor, platelet-derived growth factor and transforming growth factor β, inhibit IGF-II mRNA and polypeptide levels (B. Gabbitas and E. Canalis, unpublished observations). This effect is analogous to that observed on IGF-I synthesis, although its onset is slower, and there are small differences in growth factor potency. Similar to the changes observed on IGF-I synthesis, the decrease in IGF-II synthesis is independent of growth factor mitogenic activity and bone morphogenetic protein enhances IGF-II synthesis.

Table 3. Regulation of IGF-II synthesis in bone cells

Systemic hormones	No acute effects
Growth factors	
Stimulatory:	Bone morphogenetic protein
Inhibitory:	Transforming growth factor β
	Basic fibroblast growth factor
	Platelet-derived growth factor

Expression and activity of IGFBPs in bone cells

Skeletal cells synthesize a variety of IGFBPs and their expression and regulation in osteoblasts is cell line specific [26]. Cultures of nontransformed osteoblasts express detectable transcripts for IGFBP-2, 3, 4, 5 and 6, but unstimulated control cultures do not express IGFBP-1. This does not exclude the possibility of IGFBP-1 induction by specific agents. The role of the IGFBPs in bone is somewhat uncertain. For the most part IGFBP-4 has inhibitory activity, whereas IGFBP-5 appears to stimulate cell growth in mouse osteoblast-like cells, suggesting that it has unique anabolic properties [27,28]. Other studies have shown that IGFBP-2 and 3 at high concentrations inhibit bone formation in osteoblast cultures [29,30]. On the other hand, the physiological levels of various IGFBPs in bone are not known and it is possible that the inhibitory effects are due to the use of supraphysiological concentrations. Recently, a number of groups have started to examine the regulation of IGFBPs in skeletal cells. Cyclic AMP inducers, known to stimulate IGF-I synthesis in bone, enhance the synthesis of IGFBP-3, 4 and 5 [31]. In addition, 1,25-dihydroxyvitamin D_3 increases IGFBP-3 and 4 synthesis, suggesting that these changes may play a role in the actions of vitamin D in bone [32]. IGFBPs also are regulated by growth factors. IGF-I and IGF-II increase the levels of skeletal IGFBP-5, however, IGFs increase IGFBP-5 mRNA expression in normal osteoblasts and not in osteosarcoma cell lines [33,34]. It is likely that IGFs have dual regulatory effects on IGFBP-5 involving synthesis as well as polypeptide stabilization, which could be secondary to a decrease in IGFBP proteolytic activity. Fibroblast growth factor increases IGFBP-4 synthesis in osteoblast cell cultures [35]. Studies on the regulation of IGFBPs by growth factors in bone are incomplete and require further investigation.

Relevance of skeletal IGF-I and IGF-II

However, because IGF-I and IGF-II are among the most prevalent growth factors secreted by skeletal cells and have important actions on bone formation, it is reasonable to predict that they play a significant role in bone remodeling and in the maintenance of bone mass. In addition, it is likely that IGF-I and IGF-II are important in the expression of the differentiated function of the osteoblast. It is conceivable that changes in IGF-I and IGF-II synthesis or activity and alterations in IGFBP synthesis

312

or distribution are responsible for selected forms of metabolic bone disease. For instance, it is possible that a decrease in IGF-I synthesis plays a role in the decreased bone formation observed after glucocorticoid exposure. One could speculate that local growth factors that inhibit the differentiated function of the osteoblast as well as IGF-I and IGF-II synthesis, might be overexpressed in some forms of osteoporosis. From a therapeutic point of view, IGF-I could be administered to restore bone mass in the early phases of osteopenia, as long as the bone architecture has been preserved [36]. Unfortunately, the systemic administration of IGF-I causes side effects, which could be circumvented by inducing the synthesis of the locally produced skeletal IGF-I.

Acknowledgements

This work was supported by grants from the National Institutes of Health AR21707, DK42424 and DK45227. The author is thankful to Ms. Cathy Boucher, Bari Gabbitas, Heather Lacy, and Sheila Rydziel for technical support and Ms. Beverly Faulds for secretarial assistance.

References

1. Canalis E, Peck WA, Raisz LG. Science 1980;210:1021–1023.
2. Canalis E. J Clin Invest 1980;66:709–719.
3. Canalis E, McCarthy T, Centrella M. Endocrinology 1988;122:22–27.
4. Canalis E, Pash J, Varghese S. Crit Rev Eukaryot Gene Exp 1993;3:155–166.
5. Canalis E, Centrella M, McCarthy TL. Endocrinology 1991;129:2457–2462.
6. Ibbotson KJ, Orcutt CM, D'Souza SM, Paddock CL, Arthur JA, Jankowsky ML, Boyce RW. J Bone Min Res 1992;7:425–432.
7. Spencer EM, Liu CC, Si ECC, Howard GA. Bone 1991;12:21–26.
8. McCarthy TL, Centrella M, Canalis E. Endocrinology 1989;124:301–309.
9. Canalis E, Lian J. Bone 1988;9:243–246.
10. Hock JM, Centrella M, Canalis E. Endocrinology 1988;122:254–260.
11. Luyten FP, Hascall VC, Nissley PS, Morales TI, Reddi AH. Arch Biochem Biophys 1988;267:416–425
12. Mochizuki H, Hakeda Y, Wakatsuki N, Usui N, Akashi S, Sato T, Tanaka K, Kumegawa M. Endocrinology 1992;131:1075–1080.
13. Centrella M, McCarthy TL, Canalis E. Endocrinology 1990;126:39–44.
14. Bennett A, Chen T, Feldman D, Hintz RL, Rosenfeld RG. Endocrinology 1984;115:1577–1583.
15. Kurose H, Yamaoka K, Okada S, Nakajima S, Seino Y. Endocrinology 1990;126:2088–2094.
16. McCarthy TL, Centrella M, Canalis E. J Biol Chem 1990;265:15353–15356.
17. Ernst M, Rodan GA. Mol Endocrinol 1991;5:1081–1089.
18. McCarthy TL, Centrella M, Canalis E. Endocrinology 1990;126:1569–1575.
19. Canalis E. Endocrinology 1983;112:931–939.
20. McCarthy TL, Centrella M, Raisz LG, Canalis E. Endocrinology 1991;128:2895–2900.
21. Canalis E, Pash J, Gabbitas B, Rydziel S, Varghese S. Endocrinology 1993;133:33–38
22. Wozney JM, Rosen V, Celeste AJ, Mitsock LM, Whitters MJ, Kriz RW, Hewick RM, Wang EA. Science 1988;242:1528–1534.
23. Sampath TK, Rashka KE, Doctor JS, Tucker RF, Hoffmann FM. Proc Natl Acad Sci 1993;90:6004–6008.

24. Chen TL, Bates RL, Dudley A, Hammonds RG, Amento EP. J Bone Min Res 1991;6:1387−1393.
25. McCarthy TL, Centrella M, Canalis E. Endocrinology 1992;130:1303−1308.
26. Hassager C, Fitzpatrick LA, Spencer EM, Riggs BL, Conover CA. J Clin Endocrinol Metab 1992;75:228−233.
27. Mohan S, Bautista CM, Wergedal J, Baylink DJ. Proc Natl Acad Sci USA 1989;86:8338−8342.
28. Andress DL, Birnbaum RS. J Biol Chem 1992;267:22467−22472.
29. Feyen JH, Evans DB, Binkert C, Heinrich GF, Geisse S, Kocher HP. J Biol Chem 1991;266:19469−19474.
30. Raisz LG, Fall PM, Gabbitas BY, McCarthy TL, Kream BE, Canalis E. Endocrinology 1993;133:1504−1510.
31. LaTour D, Mohan S, Linkhart TA, Baylink DJ, Strong DD. Mol Endocrinol 1990;4:1806−1814.
32. Moriwake T, Tanaka H, Kanzaki S, Higuchi J, Seino Y. Endocrinology 1992;130:1071−1073.
33. Conover CA, Kiefer MC. J Clin Endocrinol Metab 1993;76:1153−1159.
34. Conover CA, Bale LK, Clarkson JT, Torring O. Endocrinology 1993;132:2525−2530.
35. Chen TL, Chang, LY, Digregorio DA, Perlman AJ, Huang Y-F. Endocrinology 1993;1382−1389.
36. Ebeling PR, Jones JD, O'Fallon WM, Janes CH, Riggs BL. J Clin Endocrinol Metab 1993;77:1384−1387.

©1994 Elsevier Science B.V. All rights reserved
The insulin-like growth factors and their regulatory proteins
R.C. Baxter, P.D. Gluckman and R.G. Rosenfeld, editors

A role for IGF-I during myeloid cell growth and differentiation

Keith W. Kelley and Sean Arkins

Laboratory of Immunophysiology, Department of Animal Sciences, University of Illinois, 207 Plant and Animal Biotechnology Laboratory, 1201 West Gregory, Urbana, IL 61801, USA

Introduction

Since the classical demonstration by Smith [1] that removal of the pituitary gland affects integrity of a primary lymphoid organ, the thymus gland, concerted efforts have focused on understanding the role of pituitary hormones in regulating the growth, development and integrity of immune tissues. These efforts have disclosed that pituitary hormones, in particular growth hormone (GH) and prolactin (PRL), influence many aspects of development, differentiation and function of cells of the immune system (reviewed in [2–4]). The somatomedin hypothesis, as elaborated by Salmon and Daughaday [5], proposed that the effects of GH were indirect, being mediated by a secondary molecule, which they termed a somatomedin. In the intervening years, development of an understanding of the IGF family has been accompanied by a parallel increase in the perception that many of the effects of GH on lymphoid and myeloid cells might be mediated by IGFs. In addition to the classical endocrine response mode, cells and tissues of the immune system now evidence paracrine and autocrine IGF synthesis and response modes. In support of the latter postulate are the findings that lymphoid and myeloid cells produce the IGF triad of peptides, receptors and binding proteins. This article summarizes recent developments in the IGF-I-immune system axis, highlighting the role of the macrophage as a source of autocrine and paracrine IGF-I and proposing a role for macrophage-derived IGF-I as an important growth factor during myeloid differentiation.

IGF-I modulates effector functions of myeloid cells

A fundamental tenet of the endocrine-immune axis is that ablation of an endocrine organ should affect host resistance to disease. This phenomenon has been demonstrated in the case of hypopituitary dwarf animals in which the development and function of a number of immune compartments is compromised. Accordingly, the administration of growth hormone to hypopituitary dwarf mice reverses defects in both intrathymic development and hematopoiesis [6,7]. Additionally, we have shown that the implantation of growth hormone secreting cells can reverse the thymic involution and the reduction in macrophage and neutrophil superoxide anion secretion in aged rodents [8—10]. Existing data thus strongly implicate a role for pituitary GH in the maintenance of reticuloendothelial tissues and regulation of immune responses [3]. Despite many indirect experiments, some dating back to the early part of this century, supporting the postulate that somatotropin and somatomedins influence disease resistance, firm experimental support was not available until we recently investigated the effects of hypophysectomy on bacterial disease resistance using a rat model. These results showed that hypophysectomized rats had reduced resistance to the lethal effects of *Salmonella typhimurium* and that resistance could be significantly enhanced by the administration of GH [11]. The protective effects of GH are, at least partially, mediated through the macrophage since peritoneal macrophages from hypophysecto- mized rats had a significant impairment in their ability to kill *S. typhimurium* in vitro and this bactericidal capacity was significantly augmented, 75—95%, by GH.

We have explored one aspect of this GH-mediated enhancement of macrophage bactericidal activity by defining the effects of GH in vivo and in vitro on the ability of myeloid cells to produce reactive oxygen intermediates (ROI) upon stimulation with soluble or particulate stimuli [10—14]. ROI are key mediators of the inflammato- ry, microbicidal and tumoricidal activities of macrophages and neutrophils. These experiments showed that the enhanced resistance of GH-treated rats to an experimen- tal infection with *S. typhimurium* is correlated with the ability of macrophages from these animals to generate toxic oxygen metabolites. This ability of macrophages to respond to priming by GH with an enhanced release of ROI is conserved across species and is also shared by another cell type of the myeloid lineage, the neutrophil [14—16]. In the latter cell type both GH and IGF-I effectively prime for enhanced ROI release (Fig. 1). Macrophages can also be primed for enhanced ROI release by IGF-I and another member of the myeloid lineage, the basophil, responds to exogenous IGF-I with increased histamine release [17]. In our model of neutrophil priming, GH-mediated priming for enhanced ROI release appears to be direct and not mediated through the intermediate synthesis and release of IGF-I, since an antibody to the IGF-I receptor does not affect GH-mediated priming, but effectively abrogates IGF-I priming [14]. This does not appear to be the case for the macrophage, however, since GH-mediated enhancement of low density lipoprotein (LDL) uptake and degradation by these cells can be abrogated by an antibody to IGF-I [18], suggesting that this function is mediated through the induction of IGF-I synthesis.

IGF-I and hematopoiesis

Because of the limited life span of mature blood cells, pluripotent stem cells within the bone marrow must continuously replicate and give rise to committed progenitors. These committed progenitors are guided in their growth, differentiation and commit- ment to a specific lineage by a set of glycoprotein growth factors, called the colony stimulating factors (CSF) [19,20]. The identities and relative concentrations of CSFs that progenitor cells encounter during development, determine the lineage to which a cell differentiates [21,22]. Committed progenitors thus become restricted in their

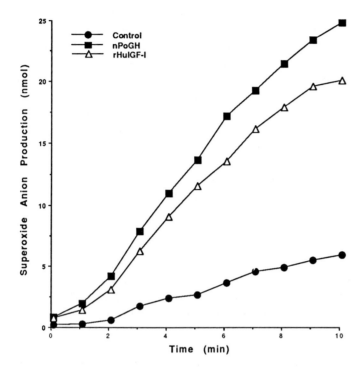

Fig. 1. Porcine neutrophils are primed for enhanced superoxide anion (O_2^-) release by treatment with porcine GH, (PoGH, 500 ng/ml), or IGF-I (rHuIGF-I, 500 ng/ml). Isolated neutrophils were treated for 4 h in vitro and stimulated with 100 ng/ml of phorbol myristate acetate. Superoxide anion production was measured over a time course by the reduction of ferricytochrome *c*. Data are from [14].

development along one of eight major lineages, eventually maturing into mature blood cells. In addition to the CSFs, a number of growth factors (e.g., platelet-derived growth factor [23] and fibroblast growth factor [24]) have been shown to enhance proliferation or to have a permissive action in the growth of early progenitors. There is an accumulating body of data that IGF-I plays a role in maintaining the survival and promoting the differentiation of a variety of cell types within the hematopoietic microenvironment [25].

Erythropoiesis

It has long been recognized that GH stimulates erythropoiesis in vitro [26]. More recently, similar effects have also been reported in vivo, e.g., GH reverses the normocytic-normochromic anemia in hypophysectomized animals [4] and increases the hematocrit values of azidothymidine-treated mice [7]. Some of the earliest evidence of a role for IGF-I in modulation of hematopoietic events, came from studies demonstrating an effect of relatively impure somatomedin preparations on hematopoietic cells. Colony formation of erythroid cells from embryonic mouse liver and adult bone marrow was stimulated by physiological IGF-I concentrations [27]. These findings have now been corroborated in a number of laboratories with recombinant IGF-I. Neonatal rats treated with IGF-I in vivo show a significant increase in bone marrow erythropoietic cell precursors [28] and IGF-I-stimulated erythropoiesis in hypophysectomized rats appears to be mediated both directly and indirectly, through the stimulation of increased erythropoietin (Epo) [29]. These growth promoting effects are also seen in vitro in the absence of either serum or Epo [30]. Comparable effects have also been reported for IGF-II by Dainiak and Kreczko [31] and Sanders et al. [32], although these also appear to be mediated through the type 1 receptor [33]. A detailed methodological understanding of the effects of IGF-I on erythroid development is still lacking, but a recent study suggests that this peptide synergizes with Epo to prevent apoptosis and, in the presence of low Epo concentrations, enhances the maturation of erythroid cells [34].

Lymphopoiesis

While the effects of IGF-I on development of nonerythroid lineages has received less attention, accumulating evidence, nonetheless, suggests that this growth factor also influences both lymphoid and myeloid developmental compartments. The involution of primary and secondary lymphoid tissues induced by hypophysectomy or diabetes can be reversed by exogenous IGF-I [35,36]. In addition, exogenous IGF-I administration to adult pituitary intact mice induces significant increases in spleen and thymus growth [37]. Augmented size of these organs is also associated with significant increase in the number of T and B cells and some increase in mitogen responsiveness. The site of IGF-I action in these studies is largely unknown. It is conceivable, however, that IGF-I may act in one, or more, motifs. The proliferation of T cell progenitors, normal T cells, T lymphoblasts and B cells is augmented by IGF-I [38-44], so it is possible that IGF-I acts within the spleen or thymus to promote local proliferation of lymphocytes. Alternatively, IGF-I can act as a chemoattractant, at least for T cells [39], and might enhance the thymic immigration of T cell precursors. The latter postulate is supported by the finding that thymocytes of IGF-I-treated mice show an increased expression of the PNA receptor, a marker of immature thmocytes [37], and by the demonstration that thymic macrophages in young children express IGF-II [45]. In the case of B cells, IGF-I, in addition to promoting proliferation [44,46], may play a role in the actual commitment to differentiation of lymphoid precursors, as evidenced by the synergy between IGF-I and IL-7 in promoting cytoplasmic μ-heavy chain expression in pro-B cells [47]. Since IGF-I administration can also enhance antibody formation in pituitary intact adults [37], the area of B cell growth and differentiation will undoubtedly receive more attention in the future. A comparable role for IGF-I in T cell differentiation has not been demonstrated although it is noteworthy that pre-T cell lineages respond to IGF-I, but not to any of the cytokines that were known in 1990 [38].

Myelopoiesis

While it is only relatively recently that GH and IGF-I have been implicated as directly modulating the development and differentiation of myeloid cell lineages within the bone marrow, indirect evidence has existed for some time that pituitary insufficiency is associated with defects in the myeloid compartments of the immune system. Our laboratory reported some time ago that synthesis and release of tumor-necrosis factor-α (TNF-α) and O_2^- were reduced in aged rats and that both of these parameters could be reversed by the implantation of pituitary glands beneath the kidney capsule [9]. Macrophages from hypophysectomized rats similarly show a reduced release of TNF-α upon in vitro stimulation with lipopolysaccharide, which was reversed by in vivo GH treatment [48]. In addition, we have also demonstrated that the implantation of GH-secreting cells into aged rats reverses the defective bacterial killing of gram-negative bacteria by bone-marrow derived neutrophils [10].

While these effects could be interpreted as the actions of GH and IGF-I on mature effector cells, an alternative hypothesis is that these hormones influence myeloid development directly. The latter explanation is supported by the demonstration that GH increases IL-3 and granulocyte-macrophage-CSF (GM-CSF) progenitors in both normal BALB/c mice and in mice with severe combined immune deficiency (SCID) [7] and by the demonstration that GM-CSF and members of the IGF family of peptides synergize to enhance proliferation of human myeloid leukemia cells [49]. The concept of synergy between IGFs and CSFs is also entirely in accord with the finding that GH and IGF-I synergize with GM-CSF to enhance granulocyte development in vitro. In the latter instance, enhancement by GH requires the presence of bone marrow adherent cells, presumably as a source of IGF-I since the effects of GH can be abrogated by an antibody directed against the IGF-I receptor [50]. A role for IGF-I in macrophage differentiation has also been suggested by the results of Scheven and Hamilton [51] and more recently by Rodriguez-Tarduchy et al. [52], who found that the addition of IGF-I prevents apoptosis in IL-3-derived bone-marrow lineages upon withdrawal of this cytokine.

IGF-I synthesis by leukocytes

We have recently undertaken a characterization of IGF-I mRNAs in different cell lineages within the murine immune system [53]. Our rationale was that while there was much anecdotal evidence indicating that leukocytes could produce IGF-I, there existed no definitive data on the relative levels of production by various cell lineages or on the effects of activation or differentiation of these cells on IGF-I expression. Using a ribonuclease expression cassette, which incorporated a β-actin cDNA sequence as an internal control [54], we have quantitated relative IGF-I mRNA in a number of tissues. The results (Fig. 2) showed that cells from spleen and thymus, as well as T and B cell lines, express extremely low levels of IGF-I mRNA. Freshly-isolated bone marrow cells (day 0), resident peritoneal macrophages and premyeloid

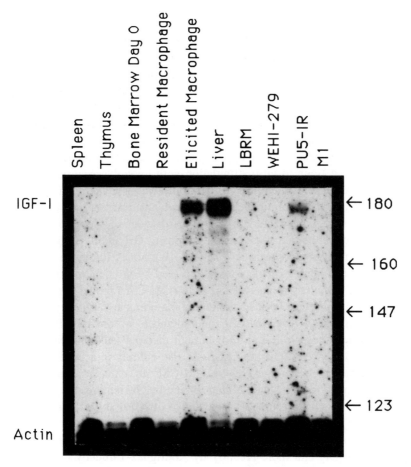

Fig. 2. Relative expression of IGF-I mRNA in murine tissues and cell lines. All lanes contained 12.5 µg total RNA and were simultaneously hybridized with IGF-I and β-actin antisense transcripts from an expression cassette [54]. Lane 1, splenocytes; lane 2 thymocytes; lane 3, freshly isolated bone marrow; lane 4, resident peritoneal macrophages; lane 5, thioglycollate elicited peritoneal macrophages; lane 6, liver; lane 7, LBRM T cells; lane 8, WEHI-279 B cells; lane 9 PU5-1R macrophages; lane 10, M1 premyeloid cells. Data are from [53].

cells (M1) also express negligible transcripts. In contrast, both peritoneal macrophages elicited by an inflammatory stimulus and a macrophage cell line (PU5-1R) express abundant IGF-I mRNA.

These data suggested that cells of the macrophage lineage are the primary source of autocrine-paracrine IGF-I mRNA and that the induction of IGF-I transcripts is associated with activation or differentiation events in macrophages. Accordingly, we then examined the effects of differentiation status on expression of IGF-I mRNA by myeloid cells. We measured IGF-I mRNA expression in bone marrow populations undergoing differentiation to a macrophage phenotype under the influence of the macrophage-specific CSF, macrophage colony stimulating factor (M-CSF or CSF-1). The results (Fig. 3) show that IGF-I mRNA levels, which are virtually absent from freshly isolated bone marrow (lane 1), are induced at very high levels as these cells differentiate into mature macrophages. We have since measured absolute transcript levels in CSF-1 macrophages using a competitive quantitative polymerase chain reaction technique [55]. These data demonstrated that CSF-1 induces an increase from $2 \times 10^6 \times 110 \times 10^6$ IGF-I molecules per μg total cellular RNA as bone-marrow-derived progenitors differentiate into macrophages in vitro. This level of expression

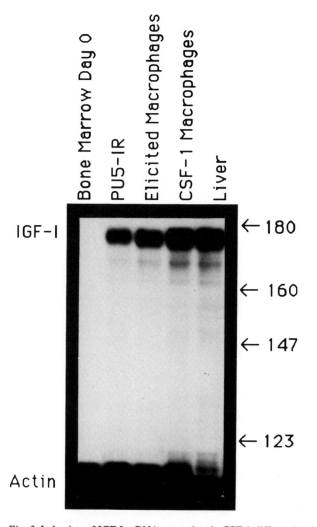

Fig. 3. Induction of IGF-I mRNA transcripts in CSF-1-differentiated murine bone marrow macrophages. Each lane contained 12.5 μg total cellular RNA and was simultaneously hybridized to IGF-I and β-actin antisense transcripts produced from a riboprobe cassette, as described by [54]. Lane 1, freshly isolated bone-marrow cells; lane 2, PU5-1R macro-phages; lane 3, thioglycollate-elicited peritoneal macrophages; lane 4, day 6 CSF-1 differentiated macrophages; lane 5, liver. A labeled pBR322 digest was run in an adjacent lane as a size marker. Data are from [53].

is comparable to that of the liver where we detected 104×10^6 IGF-I molecules per µg total cellular RNA.

These data provide further evidence that IGF-I may influence immune events through a paracrine circuit. The cell type which actually produces IGF-I at local immune foci had received very little attention, until recently. The emerging picture is that a number of leukocyte subsets are actually capable of producing IGF-I. Merimee et al. [44] found that transformed, but not nontransformed, B cells released IGF-I into the culture medium in response to stimulation with GH. Geffner et al. [42] have also provided convincing data that the enhancement of T-lymphoblast cell lines by GH was actually mediated by local synthesis of IGF-I and could be abrogated by antibodies directed against either IGF-I or the IGF-I receptor. This group also found low, but measurable levels, of IGF-I in the medium conditioned by these cells. Our data do not implicate a role for nontransformed T or B cells as a major source of paracrine IGF-I. The levels of IGF-I mRNA produced by splenocytes and thymocytes were consistently 20–40-fold lower than those detected in differentiated macrophage preparations (Fig. 2 and 4). Other workers [56,57] have reported IGF-I production by splenocytes, but this may arise from macrophages within this heterogeneous population. At least in the adult rodent, IGF-I appears to be the main form of IGF produced by leukocytes (Fig. 4). This may not be the case in young children in which IGF-II seems to predominate in thymic epithelial tissues [45].

The IGF binding proteins (IGFBPs) are important soluble factors which can

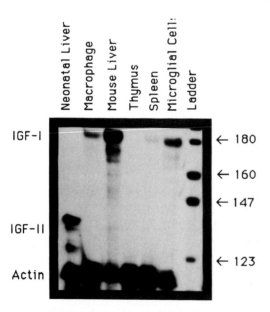

Fig. 4. Relative expression of IGF-I mRNA in leukocytes. Total cellular RNA was simultaneously hybridized with antisense transcripts to IGF-I exon 4 and β-actin derived from an expression cassette [54] and a 135 nucleotide IGF-II antisense transcript. Lane 1, neonatal mouse liver; lane 2, elicited pertoneal macrophages; lane 3, adult mouse liver; lane 4, thymocytes; lane 5, splenocytes; lane 6, CSF-1 differentiated microglial cells; lane 7, molecular size marker. Thirty micrograms of total RNA from spleen and thymus were used in the hybridization; all other samples contained 12.5 µg. Data are from [53].

inhibit, enhance or prolong the metabolic and mitogenic effects of IGF-I. Six different IGFBPs have been isolated and cloned from both rats and humans and these show preferential distribution to various tissue and body fluids [58]. Presently, there is only limited information about IGFBP expression in leukocytes. Neely et al. [59] reported that six out of 12 human leukemic lymphoblast cell lines produced IGFBP-2 or IGFBP-4. Both Nyman and Pekonen [60] and Domene et al. [57] have demonstrated the presence of IGF-I mRNA transcripts for IGFBP-2, -3 and -4 in normal human and rat lymphocytes, but neither have definitely established that all of these IGFBPs were translated into protein and secreted. Preliminary experiments from our laboratory indicate that mature macrophages are the primary source of an IGFBP which we have tentatively identified as IGFBP-4 (Li et al., unpublished). Indeed, the relative abundant production of this binding protein by mature myeloid cells suggests that this might constitute a very effective mechanism for controlling IGF-I levels within the hematopoietic environment [61,62]. The potential regulation of IGFBP levels by IGFBP protease-mediated proteolytic cleavage in this environment has not been explored. There are many other instances in which IGFBP proteolytic cleavage can affect IGF tissue targeting (e.g., Cohen et al. [63]) and since activated macrophages produce particularly high levels of proteases [64] this mechanism warrants attention.

Role of macrophage-derived IGF-I

Of all growth factors, IGF-I is perhaps the most likely candidate for involvement in autocrine/paracrine regulation of immune cell functions. This peptide has been shown to be produced by a wide variety of tissues, is involved in growth and metabolic processes and regulates cellular differentiation and proliferation, all of which are key features of immune homeostasis. In fact, immunologists have been inadvertently employing IGF-I for years by using insulin at supraphysiological concentrations in serum-free media, thus ensuring occupancy and stimulation of the IGF-I receptor. As yet, we can only speculate on the role of the apparently abundant IGF-I production by macrophages. Two independent lines of investigation suggest that this peptide may be involved as: 1) a participant in the peripheral inflammatory and repair processes; and 2) an autocrine or paracrine growth factor in supporting myelopoiesis.

In the periphery, macrophage-derived IGF-I has been alternatively cast as villian and hero in inflammatory and repair processes. In 1988 Rom and colleagues [65] first characterized a growth factor for fibroblasts from alveolar macrophages of humans with asbestosis. This alveolar macrophage-derived growth factor (AMDGF) stimulated IGF-I receptors to phosphorylate a tyrosine-containing artificial substrate, stimulated fibroblast proliferation in a serum-free complementation assay and the latter activity could be inhibited in a dose-responsive manner with an anti-IGF-I monoclonal antibody. An antisense IGF-I RNA transcript hybridized to alveolar macrophage mRNA, but not to monocyte mRNA, suggesting that the ability to produce IGF-I mRNA might be a reflection of differentiation status. More recently, this group [66] examined the regulation of IGF-I mRNA expression in a human macrophage-like cell line, U937, and suggested that mononuclear phagocytes may be unique in having a preformed, stored, releasable pool of IGF-I. The clinical significance of AMDGF was apparent when it was demonstrated that in vitro exposure of macrophages to agents such as chrysotile asbestos, which can cause pulmonary fibrosis in vivo, resulted in the release of IGF-I into the medium [65]. These findings have been recently corroborated in a murine system by Noble et al. [67] using bone-marrow-derived macrophages, although these authors found asbestos to be a less potent stimulant of IGF-I synthesis than hyaluronic acid. The latter, which is an extracellular matrix component, appears to drive IGF-I gene expression by interacting with its ligand on macrophages, CD44, in a TNF-α-dependent fashion. It is conceivable that monocytes arriving at a wound site may be induced to transcribe and translate IGF-I [68] by interacting with matrix components produced during the early stages of the inflammatory response. This model is also in keeping with the report that advanced glycosylation end (AGE) product-modified proteins, which accumulate on proteins as a function of age, trigger the synthesis and release of IL-1β, TNF-α and IGF-I in human monocytes [69]. Since the accumulation of AGE-modified proteins is a normal component of tissue turnover, these results could be interpreted as casting macro-phage-derived IGF-I in the role of a growth factor which facilitates normal tissue remodeling, rather than being involved exclusively in the pathogenesis of fibrosis and granulomatous diseases. The latter explanation is also in keeping with the presence of IGF-I mRNA transcripts in wound macrophages [68] and with the, now, well established role of IGF-I in wound healing [70].

The ontogeny of IGF-I expression in developing macrophages, that we have described, suggests that this peptide may have an autocrine or paracrine role in the expansion or the differentiation of myeloid progenitors within the bone marrow environment. A paracrine role for IGF-I within the bone marrow is indeed indicated by the finding that IGF-I synergizes with IL-7 to promote pro-B cell rearrangement [47] and that a bone marrow stromal cell line produces both IGF-I and an IGF-I binding protein [61]. Both GH and IGF-I, thus, seem to be somewhat comparable to the colony stimulating factors (e.g., G-CSF and GM-CSF) in that these hormones can influence both the differentiation and the effector functions of phagocytic cells. We propose that IGF-I shares at least three properties with the CSFs: programmed cell death, DNA synthesis and effector functions.

Programmed cell death

Both the CSFs and IGF-I are able to maintain the viability of myeloid progenitors in vitro. Gene directed cellular death, or apoptosis, is increasingly recognized as part of the repertoire of responses of differentiating cells [71] and IGF-I is now known to prevent apoptosis in IL-3 dependent cell lines [52] and in erythroid progenitors [34].

DNA synthesis

Both IGF-I and the CSFs can stimulate proliferation of progenitor cell populations

[51,72,73] and myeloid leukemic cells [49,74]. The interaction of IGF-I with the IGF-I receptor may indeed be obligatory in the proliferation of hematopoietic cells since expression of the IGF-I receptor is required for entry of the promyelocytic cell line, HL-60, into S phase [73] and is also an early event in the anti-CD3-mediated activation of T cells [41]. In addition, antisense oligonucleotides directed against the IGF-I receptor sequence inhibit DNA synthesis in HL-60 cells and the differentiation of HL-60 cells to a macrophage phenotype is associated with a decrease in IGF-I receptor mRNA levels [73]. A recent report indicates that IGF-II can synergize with IL-3 to enhance myelopoiesis of CD34+ human progenitors [75].

Effector functions

A number of the colony stimulating factors can, in addition to promoting differentiation, influence the activities of mature myeloid cells in the periphery. For example, GM-CSF is chemotactic and stimulates O_2^- secretion from neutrophils, promotes neutrophil phagocytosis and stimulates the release of IL-1 and TNF-α from macrophages (reviewed in [21]). Similarly, IGF-I is chemotactic, at least for T cells [39], primes neutrophils and macrophages for enhanced release of O_2^- [12,76] and primes basophils for enhanced release of histamine [17]. In addition, the uptake and degradation of LDL's by macrophages is stimulated by IGF-I [18]. In neuronal cells, IGF-I has been shown to shift from promoting proliferation to supporting differentiation [77]. This motif is also a possible modus operandi for IGF-I in bone marrow, although evidence in support of this idea does not yet exist.

Conclusions

Among murine leukocytes, macrophages are the major cells which express transcripts for IGF-I. Elicited macrophages and macrophage cell lines consistently express 20–40-fold higher levels of IGF-I transcripts than those found in T or B cells or in the thymus or spleen. A potential role for IGF-I in macrophage differentiation is suggested by the finding that CSF-1 induces IGF-I transcripts by 50–100-fold as bone marrow progenitors differentiate into macrophages in vitro. Preliminary data indicate that a 25 kDa IGFBP, presumably IGFBP-4, is also synthesized by this macrophage population. These data show that IGF-I mRNA is induced by CSF-1 as bone marrow progenitors differentiate in vitro. We suggest that the IGFs share several properties with colony stimulating factors and are involved in regulating hematopoiesis.

Acknowledgements

This work was supported in part by grants to Keith W. Kelley from the National Institutes of Health (AG06246) and the US Department of Agriculture (92-37206-7777).

326

References

1. Smith PE. Anat Rec 1930;47:119—129.
2. Kelley KW. Biochem Pharmacol 1989;38:705—713.
3. Kelley KW, Arkins S, Li YM. Brain Behavior Immun 1992;6:317—326.
4. Berczi I, Nagy, E. In: Ader R, Cohen N, Felton D (eds) Psychoneuroimmunology II. San Diego; Academic Press, 1991:339—376.
5. Salmon WD, Daughaday WH. J Lab Clin Med 1957;49:825—836.
6. Murphy WJ, Durum SK, Anver MR, Longo DL. J Immunol 1992;148:3799—3805.
7. Murphy WJ, Tsarfaty G, Longo DL. Blood 1992;80:1443—1447.
8. Kelley KW, Brief S, Westly HJ, Novakofski J, Bechtel PJ, Simon J, Walker EB. Proc Natl Acad Sci USA 1992;83:5663—5667.
9. Davila DR, Edwards CK, Arkins S, Simon J, Kelley, KW. FASEB J 1990;4:2906—2911.
10. Fu Y-K, Arkins S, Li YM, Dantzer R, Kelley, KW. Infect Immun 1994;62:1—8.
11. Edwards CK, Yunger LM, Lorence RM, Dantzer R, Kelley KW. Proc Natl Acad Sci USA 1991;88: 2274—2277.
12. Edwards CK, Ghiasuddin SM, Schepper JM, Yunger LM, Kelley KW. Science 1988;239:769—771.
13. Edwards CK, Ghiasuddin SM, Yunger, LM, Lorence RM, Arkins S, Dantzer R, Kelley KW. Infect Immun 1992;60:2514—2521.
14. Fu Y-K, Arkins S, Wang BS, Kelley KW. J Immunol 1991;146:1602—1608.
15. Wiedermann CJ, Niedermuhlbichler M, Beimpold H, Braunsteiner H. J Infect Dis 1991;164:1017—1020.
16. Wiedermann CJ, Niedermuhlbichler M, Geissler D, Beimpold H, Braunsteiner H. Br J Haematol 1991;60:513—516.
17. Hirai K, Miyamasu M, Yamaguchi M, Nakajima K, Ohtoshi T, Koshino T, Takaishi T, Morita Y, Ito K. J Immunol 1993;150:1503—1508.
18. Hochberg Z, Hertz P, Maor G, Oiknine J, Aviram M. Endocrinology 1992;131:430—435.
19. Metcalf D. The Hemopoietic Colony Stimulating Factors. Amsterdam; Elsevier, 1984.
20. Metcalf D. Nature 1989;339:27—30.
21. Nicola NA. Annu Rev Biochem 1989;58:45—77.
22. Gliniak BC, Rohrschneider LR. Cell 1990;63:1073—1083.
23. Michalevics R, Francis GE, Price G, Hoffbrand AV. Leuk Res 1985;9:399—405.
24. Gabbianelli M, Sargiacomo M, Pelosi E, Testa U, Isacchi G, Peschle C. Science 1990;249:1561—1564.
25. Dainiak N. Exp Hematol 1993;21:1405—1407.
26. Golde DW, Bersch N, Li CH. Science 1977;196:1112—1113.
27. Kurtz A, Jelkman W, Bauer C. FEBS Lett 1982;49:105—108.
28. Philipps AF, Persson B, Hall K, Lake M, Skottner A, Sanengen T, Sara VR. Pediatr Res 1988;23: 298—305
29. Kurtz A, Zapf J, Eckardt K-U, Clemons G, Froesch ER, Bauer C. Proc Natl Acad Sci USA 1988;85: 7825—7829.
30. Werther GA, Haynes K, Johnson GR. Growth Factors 1990;3:171—179.
31. Dainiak N, Kreczko S. J Clin Invest 1985;76:1237—1242.
32. Sanders M, Sorba S, Dainiak N. Exp Hematol 1993;21:25—33.
33. Merchav S, Silvian—Drachsler I, Tatarsky I, Lake M, Skottner A. J Clin Endocrinol Metab 1992;73: 447—452.
34. Boyer SH, Bishop TR, Rogers OC, Noyes AN, Frelin LP, Hobbs S. Blood 1992;80:2503—2512.
35. Guler HP, Zapf J, Scheiwiller E, Froesch, ER. Proc Natl Acad Sci USA 1988;85:4889—4893.
36. Binz K, Joller P, Froesch P, Binz H, Zapf J, Froesch ER. Proc Natl Acad Sci USA 1990;87:3690—3694.
37. Clark R, Strasser J, McCabe S, Robbins K, Jardieu P. J Clin Invest 1993;92:540—548.
38. Gjerset RA, Yeatgin J, Volkman SK, Vila V, Arya J, Haas M. J Immunol 1990;145:3497—3501.

39. Tapson VF, Boni-Schnetzler M, Pilch PF, Center DM, Berman JS. J Clin Invest 1988;82:950–957.
40. Kooijman R, Willems M, Rijkers GT, Brinkman A, van Buul-Offers SC, Heijnen CJ, Zegers JM. J Neuroimmunol 1992;38:95–104.
41. Johnson EW, Jones LA, Kozak RW. J Immunol 1992;148:63–71.
42. Geffner ME, Bersch N, Lippe BM, Rosenfeld RG, Hintz RL, Golde DW. J Clin Endocrinol Metab 1990;71:464–469.
43. Geffner ME, Bersch N, Golde DW. Brain Behavior Immun 1992;6:377–386.
44. Merimee TJ, Grant MB, Broder CM, Cavalli-Sforza LL. J Clin Endocrinol Metab 1989;69:978–984.
45. Geenen V, Achour I, Robert F, Vandersmissen E, Sodoyez JC, Defresne MP, Boniver J, Lefebvre PJ, Franchimont P. Thymus 1993;21:115–127.
46. Freund GG, Kulas DT, Mooney RA. J Immunol 1993;151:1811–1820.
47. Landreth KS, Narayanan R, Dorshkind K. Blood 1992;80:1207–1212.
48. Edwards CK, Lorence RM, Dunham DM, Arkins S, Yunger LM, Greager JA, Walter RJ, Dantzer R, Kelley KW. Endocrinology 1991;128:989–996.
49. Oksenberg D, Dieckmann BS, Greenberg PL. Cancer Res 1990;50:6471–6477.
50. Merchav S, Tatarsky I, Hochberg Z. J Clin Invest 1988;81:791–797.
51. Scheven BAA, Hamilton NJ. Biochem Biophys Res Commun 1991;174:647–653.
52. Rodriguez-Tarduchy G, Collins MKL, Garcia I, Lopez–Rivas A. J Immunol 1992;149:535–540.
53. Arkins S, Rebeiz N, Biragyn A, Reese DL, Kelley KW. Endocrinology 1993;133:2334–2343.
54. Biragyn A, Arkins S, Kelley KW. J Immunol Meth 1994;168:235–244.
55. Liu Q, Arkins S, Biragyn A, Minshall C, Dantzer R, Parnet P, Kelley KW. Neuroimmunomodulation 1994;1:33–41.
56. Baxter JR, Blalock JE, Weigent DA. Endocrinology 1991;129:1727–1734.
57. Domene HM, Meidan R, Yakar S, Zila S-O, Cassorla F, Roberts CT Jr, LeRoith D. Endocrinology 1994 (in press).
58. Shimisaki S, Ling N. Prog Growth Factor Res 1991;3:243–266.
59. Neely EK, Smith SS, Rosenfeld RG. Acta Endocrinologica (Copenh) 1991;124:707–714.
60. Nyman T, Pekone F. Acta Endocrinologica 1993;128:168–172.
61. Abboud SL, Bethel CR, Aron DC. J Clin Invest 1991;88:470–475.
62. Cohen P, Lamson G, Okajima T, Rosenfeld RG. Mol Endocrinol 1993;7:380–386.
63. Cohen P, Graves JCB, Peehl DM, Kamarei M, Giudice LC, Rosenfeld RG. J Clin Endocrinol Metab 1992;75:1046–1053.
64. Pluznik DH, Fridman F, Reich R. Exp Hematol 1992;20:57–63.
65. Rom WN, Basset P, Fells GA, Nukiwa T, Trapnell BC, Crystal RG. J Clin Invest 1988;82:1685–1693.
66. Nagaoka I, Trapnell BC, Crystal, RG. J Clin Invest 1990;85:448–455.
67. Noble PW, Lake FR, Henson PM, Riches DWH. J Clin Invest 1993;91:2368–2377.
68. Rappolee DA, Mark D, Banda MJ, Werb Z. Science 1988;241:708–712.
69. Kirstein M, Aston C, Hintz R, Vlassara H. J Clin Invest 1992;90:439–446.
70. Lynch SE, Colvin RB, Ankoniades HN. J Clin Invest 1989;84:640–646.
71. Williams GT, Smith CA, Spooncer E, Dexter TM, Taylor DR. Nature 1990;343:76–79.
72. Fairbairn LJ, Cowling GJ, Reipert BM, Dexter TM. Cell 1993;74:823–832.
73. Reiss K, Porcu P, Sell C, Pietrzkowski Z, Baserga R. Oncogene 1992;7:2243–2248.
74. Pepe MG, Ginztion NH, Lee PDK, Hintz RL, Greenberg PL. J Cell Physiol 1987;133:219–227.
75. Schwartz GN, Hudgins WR, Perdue JF. Exp Hematol 1993;21:1447–1454.
76. Edwards CK, Arkins S, Yunger LM, Blum A, Dantzer R, Kelley KW. Cell Mol Neurobiol 1992;12:499–509.
77. Pahlman S, Meyerson G, Lindgren E, Schalling M, Johansson I. Proc Natl Acad Sci USA 1991;88:9994–9998.

In vitro interactions between IGFs and haemopoietic growth factors: effects on blasts from patients with acute myeloid leukemia

S. Merchav[1,2], A. Carter[1,3], I. Silvian-Drachsler[1], L. Naiderman[1], M. Hirsh[2] and A. Skottner[4]

Haemopoiesis Unit, [1]The Bruce Rappaport Faculty of Medicine and [2]Family Institute for Research in the Medical Sciences, Technion and [3]Department of Hematology, Rambam Medical Center, Haifa Israel; and [4]Pharmacia Kabi Peptide Hormones, Stockholm, Sweden

Abstract. In vitro studies of the mitogenic effects of insulin-like growth factors (IGFs) on freshly isolated human acute myeloid leukemia (AML) blasts demonstrate that IGF-I and IGF-II induce a proliferative response in these cells mainly by interacting with (autocrine or paracrine) haemopoietic growth factors (HGFs). AML blasts also resemble normal human myeloid progenitors in sensitivity to IGFs, as well as in similar dose-dependent magnitude of response to either IGF-I or IGF-II.

These findings demonstrate that while IGFs may play a role in the proliferative expansion of leukemic blasts, malignant transformation of human myeloid progenitors is not reflected in abnormal biological response to these growth peptides.

Introduction

Previous studies performed by us have shown that insulin-like growth factors, IGF-I and IGF-II, enhance the in vitro growth and maturation of human marrow myeloid progenitors in cultures stimulated with haemopoietic growth factors (HGFs), such as Interleukin-3 (IL-3), granulocyte-macrophage colony-stimulating factor (GM-CSF) and granulocyte CSF (G-CSF) [1,2]. Both IGFs were found to exert a synergistic effect upon HGF-induced progenitor cell growth, since neither peptide could stimulate the formation of colonies when added alone.

While IGFs appear to play a role in the normal process of myelopoiesis, it is presently unknown if these peptides are also involved in acute myeloid leukemia (AML). Membrane receptors for IGF-I and IGF-II have been detected on human myeloid leukemic cell lines [3,4], the latter found to proliferate following stimulation with these peptides. Nevertheless, the mitogenic effect of IGFs on freshly isolated leukemic blasts and their possible interactions with HGFs in inducing the proliferative expansion of such cells, have not yet been evaluated.

Direct stimulation of leukemic blast cell growth by HGFs [5–7] is not the only mechanism involved in the proliferative expansion of such cells. Additional cytokines, such as IL-1 and tumor necrosis factor (TNF), have been shown to exert their mitogenic effects on AML blasts via induction of autocrine GM-CSF production by the cells [8,9]. Spontaneous production of IL-1 by AML blasts also exerts a mitogenic effect via HGF production by the cells [10,11].

In the present investigation, we evaluated the capacity of IGF-I and IGF-II to stimulate the in vitro growth of freshly isolated AML blasts. Direct IGF stimulation of AML proliferation, mitogenesis via induction of autocrine GM-CSF and synergistic interactions with haemopoietic growth factors, are described and discussed.

Methods

Isolation of highly enriched leukemic blasts

Peripheral blood or marrow aspirates from 11 freshly diagnosed AML patients were obtained with informed consent, according to specifications of the Helsinki committee. The French-American-British classification [12] of AML in these patients is shown in Table 1.

Samples were drawn under sterile conditions in heparinized syringes, diluted 3-fold in Hanks' Balanced Salts Solution and subjected to Ficoll-Hypaque gradient centrifugation. Buoyant mononuclear cells consisting of >85% blasts were subjected to adherent cell depletion by plastic adherence, followed by T-cell depletion with AET-treated sheep erythrocytes. Only cell suspensions containing >95% blasts as determined by morphology and cytochemistry, were employed for the studies described below.

Blast cell proliferation

Highly enriched AML blasts were incubated at 37°C in a fully humidified incubator of 7.5% CO_2 in air. Cells were grown at 1×10^6/ml in 96-well dishes, under serum-free culture conditions, as previously described [1]. Cultures (triplicates) were pulsed with 0.25 µCi ^{3}H-thymidine following 4 days of incubation for a period of 4 h and radioactivity determined in a β-scintillation counter.

Table 1. Characteristics of AML patients investigated

Patient	Age	Sex	FAB classification
1	20	F	M1
2	17	M	M2
3	64	M	M5
4	66	F	M5
5	45	F	M1
6	48	M	M5
7	42	F	M4
8	51	M	M4
9	31	M	M2
10	44	F	M4
11	40	M	M4

Growth factors

The factors employed in this study were: purified recombinant human (rh) IGF-I (1U/60 ng protein) or IGF-II (Pharmacia-Kabi, Stockholm, Sweden), 5 ng/ml rhIL-3 (5×10^7 U/mg protein; Genetics Institute, Cambridge, MA.), 2.5 ng/ml rhGM-CSF or 2.5 ng/ml rhG-CSF (1×10^8 U/mg protein; AmGEN, Thousand Oaks, CA). In some experiments polyclonal αGM-CSF antibodies were used (1:500 dilution; Genetics Institute).

Results

Stimulation of AML blasts with recombinant human IGF-I or IGF-II, induced a proliferative response in only three of the 11 samples evaluated (pts #1–#3; Table 1). As shown in Fig. 1, a significant ($p < 0.05$) response in these samples was already induced by 0.6 ng/ml of each peptide, with maximal proliferation detected at 3 ng/ml. The response of each patient AML sample to either IGF-I or II was found to be within the same order of magnitude.

In order to evaluate whether the observed mitogenic effects of both IGFs on the above AML blasts were mediated via induction of autocrine GM-CSF by the leukemic cells [8,9], the proliferative response to both peptides was examined in the presence of anti-GM-CSF antibodies. As shown in Fig. 2, αGM-CSF inhibited the proliferative response of AML blasts to IGF-I and IGF-II, but did not influence the incorporation of ^{3}H-thymidine in control cultures of unstimulated cells. The mitogenic effects of both peptides in blast cell cultures of pt #2 were completely abrogated by α-GM-CSF, while some, albeit minor, residual proliferation was still detected in blast cell cultures of pts #1 and #3.

The above findings detected with αGM-CSF indicated that stimulation of AML

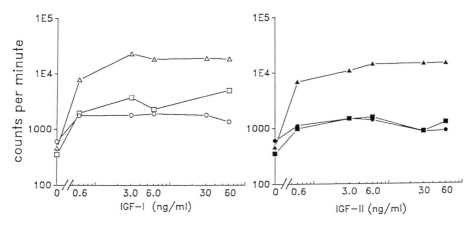

Fig. 1. Effect of IGFs on AML blast cell proliferation. AML blast cells from pt. #1 (triangles), #2 (circles) and #3 (squares). IGF-I (left) or IGF-II (right).

332

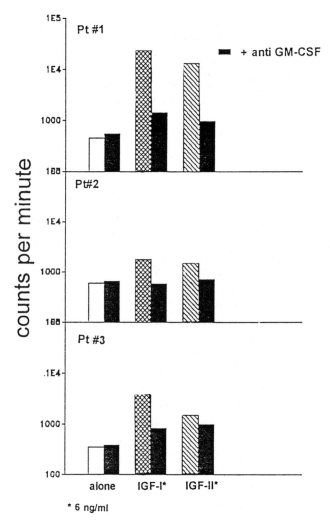

Fig. 2. Abrogation of IGF-induced AML proliferation by anti-GM-CSF antibodies.

blasts from these patients with IGFs results in the presence of both these peptides as well as GM-CSF, in the immediate surroundings of the cells. Some insight as to the type of interactions between IGFs and GM-CSF, which induce a mitogenic response in these AML blasts, was obtained by comparing the expected added effects of each individual type of growth factor to that detected in the presence of both. As shown in Table 2, the proliferative response of AML blasts from pt #1 to IGF-I or IGF-II was much higher than the calculated added individual effects of GM-CSF and either peptide, the latter determined in the presence of αGM-CSF. These findings indicate that IGFs and GM-CSF exert a synergistic effect upon the proliferative activity of pt #1 AML blasts.

Table 2. Interactions between IGFs and GM-CSF

Additive	Pt#1			Pt#3		
	—	IGF-I	IGF-II	—	IGF-I	IGF-II
None	460	18,305	14,120	354	2,275	1,543
αGM-CSF	544	1,440	964	385	819	989
GM-CSF	6,494	18,418	14,416	746	1,576	1,835

Results are expressed as counts per min. IGF-I and IGF-II were added at 6 ng/ml.

While the response of AML blasts from sample #3 was generally low, the same type of analysis as above indicated an additive, rather than synergistic, effect of both IGFs and GM-CSF on the cells. In both cases, the detection of a similar mitogenic effect in blast cell cultures stimulated by IGFs alone and in cultures stimulated with combined exogenous IGFs + GM-CSF, demonstrates that the amount of autocrine GM-CSF produced in response to IGFs is sufficient to maximally stimulate the cells.

Only 3/11 AML samples evaluated exhibited a proliferative response to direct stimulation with IGFs (Fig. 1). In order to circumvent the possible inability of the remaining 8 AML samples to produce autocrine HGFs [8–11], the mitogenic effects of both peptides on the latter (pts #4–#11) were evaluated in the presence of HGFs, specifically IL-3, GM-CSF and G-CSF. Table 3 demonstrates the proliferative response of two AML blast cell samples (#4 and #5) to IGF-I and IGF-II, detected in the presence of HGFs. While each peptide failed to exert a mitogenic effect when added alone, they both interacted synergistically with IL-3 and GM-CSF (pt #4) or with IL-3 alone (pt #5).

We did not detect any proliferative response to IGF stimulation, alone or in the presence of HGFs, in the remaining 6/11 AML samples evaluated. This could not be attributed to the absence of IGF membrane receptors, found to be expressed when evaluated on three of the nonresponding AML blast cell samples (samples #6–#8; data not shown).

Evidence that membrane receptor expression is not necessarily indicative of IGF-mediated response is also provided by our studies of the effect of IGF-I on mature myeloid cells, i.e., circulating neutrophils, whose functional activity is primed by a variety of cytokines, including GM-CSF [13]. These cells have been shown to express

Table 3. Synergistic interactions between IGFs and HGFs

Additive	Pt#4				Pt#5			
	—	IL-3	GM-CSF	G-CSF	—	IL-3	GM-CSF	G-CSF
—	166	805	416	257	1,204	38,397	806	1,101
IGF-I	209	3,493	1,250	318	1,033	52,747	1,226	1,302
IGF-II	275	1,888	1,062	459	1,273	48,608	870	1,072

IGF-I and IGF-II were added at 30 ng/ml.

IGF binding sites [3], identified as type 1 membrane receptors by the use of αIR-3 monoclonal antibodies (Table 4).

Irrespective of the expression of IGF-I membrane receptors on circulating human neutrophils (955 ± 55 receptors/cell; kDa 1.27 ± 0.3 nM), IGF-I failed to exert any stimulatory priming effect on neutrophil functions such as degranulation (lysozyme secretion) [14] or respiratory burst (NBT reduction) [15], whether alone or in the presence of GM-CSF (Fig. 3).

Discussion

We have investigated the role of IGFs in acute myeloid leukemia by evaluating the capacity of IGF-I and IGF-II to stimulate the proliferation of freshly isolated AML blasts. Of the 11 patient samples evaluated, only three exhibited a significant proliferative response to both peptides, when added alone. The effective concentrations inducing AML growth in these samples were similar to those we previously found to enhance colony formation by normal granulocytic progenitors [2], suggesting that the malignant behaviour of human myeloid progenitors is not associated with alterations in IGF responsiveness. The similar dose-dependent magnitude of response of AML blasts to both IGF-I and IGF-II not only resembles that of normal myeloid progenitors [2], but has also been described for a human myeloid leukemic cell line, AML-193 [4]. Although not directly evaluated, we may assume, in view of the above studies, that the mitogenic effect of IGF-II on freshly isolated AML blasts is also exerted via the type 1 membrane receptor.

The growth-promoting effects of IGFs on normal haemopoietic progenitors is strictly dependent upon the presence of HGFs [1,2,16]. It is not surprising, therefore, that blast cell proliferation induced directly by IGF-I and IGF-II involved the induction of autocrine GM-CSF production by the cells. Two additional AML samples exhibited a mitogenic response to both IGFs in cultures containing exogenous HGFs. Taken together, these findings suggest that the mechanism of myeloid progenitor cell response to IGFs does not alter as a result of malignant transformation and that these peptides may modulate, rather than play a primary role in, the proliferative expansion of these cells.

In two samples (#2 and #3) responding to IGFs, some mitogenic activity was still detected in the presence of anti-GM-CSF antibodies. One possible explanation for

Table 4. Inhibition of IGF-I binding to human neutrophils by αIR-3

Binding	−αIR-3 (counts per minute)	+αIR-3 (counts per minute)
Total	131 ± 21	60 ± 13
Nonspecific	43 ± 5	45 ± 5
specific	88 ± 20	15 ± 8

^{125}I-IGF-I was added at 1.5 pM (41 Ci/mM). α IR-3 was added at 100 nM (15 μg/ml). Results represent the mean ± SEM of three independent experiments.

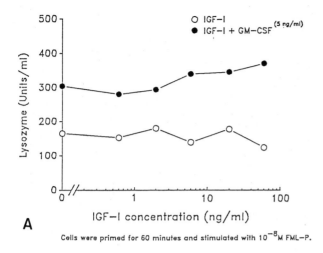

A

Cells were primed for 60 minutes and stimulated with 10^{-8}M FML–P.

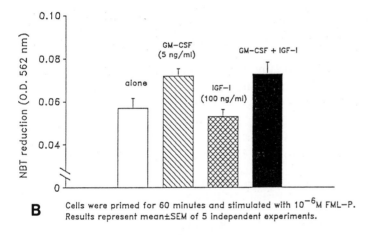

B

Cells were primed for 60 minutes and stimulated with 10^{-6}M FML–P.
Results represent mean±SEM of 5 independent experiments.

Fig. 3. Effect of IGF-I on neutrophil functional activity. Left, degranulation (lysozyme secretion). Right, respiratory burst (NBT reduction).

these findings is that IGFs may also induce a direct, albeit minor, mitogenic effect on human AML blasts. A direct proliferative response to IGFs was also detected in cultures of human promyelocytic HL60 and AML-193 leukemic cell lines [3,4]. Alternatively, IGFs may induce the production of additional growth factors by the leukemic blasts (i.e., IL-6) [10,11], whose activity is not neutralized with anti-GM-CSF antibodies.

We did not detect any proliferative response to IGF stimulation, alone or in the presence of HGFs, in 6/11 AML samples evaluated. This could not be attributed to a complete lack of proliferative activity of these cells, since a response to at least one of the HGFs tested was observed in five of the samples. IGF membrane receptors

336

were also detected in three nonresponding samples. The heterogeneity in biological response to IGFs is not an unusual finding in the type of cells investigated in this study. A lack of correlation between mitogenic stimulation and membrane receptor expression has also been demonstrated in studies of the effects of HGFs on freshly isolated AML blasts [17,18].

While IGFs appear to act synergistically with HGFs in stimulating mitogenic processes of both normal and malignant myeloid cells, we have failed to detect any interactions between these growth factors in stimulating metabolic processes (functional activation) of nonproliferating, circulating neutrophils. In view of the widespread metabolic effects of IGFs [19], it is difficult to envisage that the signalling pathways induced by the latter are restricted to myeloid cell cycling alone. Further studies of the role of these peptides in neutrophil function, i.e., adhesion, chemotaxis, migration etc. [13], are currently under way.

Acknowledgements

We thank Drs S. Clark (Genetics Institute) and L. Souza (AmGEN) for their kind supply of recombinant HGFs. We are also greatly indebted to Prof. J.J. Van Wyk for supplying us with αIR-3.

This work was supported in part by grants from by Pharmacia-Kabi Peptide Hormones, the Israel Cancer Association, the Rappaport Institute and the A. Tufeld Cancer Research Fund.

References

1. Merchav S, Tatarsky I, Hochberg Z. J Clin Invest 1988;81:791.
2. Merchav S, Lake M, Skottner A. J Cell Physiol 1993;157:178.
3. Pepe MG, Ginzton NH, Lee PDK, Hintz RL, Greenberg PL. J Cell Physiol 1987;133:219.
4. Oksenberg D, Diekmann BS, Greenberg PL. Cancer Res 1990;50:6471.
5. Delwel R, Dorssers L, Touw I, Wagemaker G, Lowenberg G. Blood 1987;70:333.
6. Miyauchi J, Keller CA, Yang YC, Wong GG, Clark SC, Minden MD, Minkin S, McCulloch EA. Blood 1987;70:333.
7. Kelleher C, Miyauchi J, Wong GG, Clark SC et al. Blood 1987;69:1498.
8. Delwel R, Buitenen C, Kaushansky K, Schipper P et al. Exp Hematol 1989;17:520.
9. Carter A, Silvian-Drachsler I, Tatarsky I. Am J Hematol 1992;40:245.
10. Oster W, Cicco NA, Klein H, Hirano T, Kishimoto T, Lindemann A, Mertelsmann RH, Hermann F. J Clin Invest 1989;84:451.
11. Beauchemin V, Villeneuve L, Rodriguez-Cimadevilla JC, Rajotte D, Kenney JS, Clark SC, Hoang T. J Cell Physiol 1991;148:353.
12. French American British (FAB) Cooperative Group. Ann Int Med 1995;103:620.
13. Steinbeck MJ, Roth JA. Rev Infect Dis 1989;11:549.
14. Lopez AF, Williamson DJ, Gamble JR, Begley GC, Harian JM, Klebanoff SJ, Waltersdorph A, Wong GG, Clark SC, Vadas MA. J Clin Invest 1986;78:1220.
15. Pick E. Meth Enzymol 1986;132:407.
16. Merchav S, Silvian-Drachsler I, Tatarsky I, Lake M, Skottner A. J Clin Endocrinol Metab 1992;74:447.

17. Budel LM, Touw IP, Delwel R, Clark SC, Lowenberg B. Blood 1989;74:565.
18. Budel LM, Touw IP, Delwel R, Clark SC, Lowenberg B. Blood 1989;74:2668.
19. Van Wyk JJ. In: Li CH (ed) Hormonal Proteins and Peptides, vol XII. New York; Academic Press, 1984;82-120.

Reproduction

Regulation of intrafollicular IGFBPs: possible relevance to ovarian follicular selection

Eli Y. Adashi

University of Maryland School of Medicine, Department of Obstetrics and Gynecology, Division of Reproductive Endocrinology, Baltimore, MD 21201, USA

Abstract. A growing body of information relevant to the rat model has documented the existence of a complete (ovarian) intrafollicular insulin-like growth factor (IGF)-I system, replete with a ligand (IGF-I), a receptor (type 1), and IGF binding proteins (IGFBP-4 and -5). According to current views, the primary, if not sole, role of bioavailable (unbound) intrafollicular IGF-I may be the amplification of FSH action in granulosa cells. It is this FSH-amplifying property of IGF-I which underlies our proposed hypothesis that the intrafollicular IGF-I system may be a determinant of follicular fate. More specifically, it is hypothesized that the net (i.e., bioavailable) intrafollicular IGF-I activity (as defined by the IGF-I/IGFBP ratio) may effect selection by way of amplification, thereby distinguishing follicles destined to ovulate from those destined to succumb to atresia. According to this view, favorably endowed (i.e., IGF-I-replete/IGFBP-deplete) follicles are afforded a selective advantage (i.e., increased FSH sensitivity) in that optimal (amplified) FSH action is assured by the ready bioavailability of unbound IGF-I. Support for this hypothesis can be derived from the observation that healthy follicular granulosa cells are IGF-I-replete, but IGFBP-4 and -5-deplete, the reverse pattern being displayed by atretic counterparts. Moreover, the FSH-dependent maturation of follicles in vivo and of granulosa cells in vitro, is associated with inhibition of the expression of granulosa cell-derived IGFBP-4 and -5.

The hypothesis

According to current views, the primary if not sole role of intrafollicular insulin-like growth factor, IGF-I, may be the amplification of FSH action at the level of the granulosa cell, a facilitatory function in keeping with the often exponential nature of follicular development. The present proposal seeks to evaluate the hypothesis that the (ovarian) intrafollicular IGF-I system may be a determinant of follicular fate. More specifically, it is hypothesized that the net intrafollicular IGF-I activity (as defined by the IGF-I/IGF binding protein (IGFBP) ratio) may produce selection by way of amplification, thereby distinguishing follicles destined to ovulate from those destined to succumb to atresia. According to this view, favorably endowed (i.e., IGF-I-replete/IGFBP-deplete) follicles are afforded an advantage (i.e., increased FSH

Address for correspondence: Eli Y. Adashi, M.D., University of Maryland School of Medicine, Department of Obstetrics and Gynecology, Division of Reproductive Endocrinology, 405 W. Redwood Street, 3rd Floor, Baltimore, MD 21201, USA. Tel.: +1-410-706-4050. Fax: +1-410-328-8389.

sensitivity) in that optimal (amplified) FSH action is assured by the ready bioavailability of unbound IGF-I.

Evidence supporting the hypothesis

1. Healthy and atretic follicles display disparate patterns of expression of key components of the intrafollicular IGF-I system. Indeed, healthy follicular granulosa cells are IGF-I-replete, but IGFBP-4/IGFBP-5-deplete, the reverse pattern being displayed by atretic counterparts [1—4];
2. The gonadotropin-dependent maturation of follicles in vivo is associated with inhibition of the expression of granulosa cell IGFBP-4 [5] and IGFBP-5 transcripts [6];
3. The FSH-dependent differentiation of granulosa cells under both in vitro [7—9] and in vivo [9] circumstances is associated with the inhibition of the constitutive accumulation of IGFBP-4 and IGFBP-5 and;
4. Granulosa cell-derived IGFBPs regulate the bioavailability of endogenously-derived IGF-I by way of sequestration [10], a feature responsible for their well-documented antigonadotropic property [5,6].

Background

The rat intrafollicular IGF-I system

General
Although the central role(s) of gonadotropins in folliculogenesis is well accepted, the variable fate of follicles afforded comparable gonadotropic support, suggests the existence of additional intraovarian modulatory systems [11]. According to this view it is the highly regionalized and appropriately timed expression of select local regulatory loops which may account for the otherwise inexplicable process of follicular selection [11]. Amongst potential intraovarian regulators, IGF-I has been the subject of particularly intense investigation [12]. These studies disclosed the existence of an intraovarian autocrine control mechanism [13] wherein IGF-I may serve as the central signal, and the granulosa cell (schematically illustrated in Fig. 1)

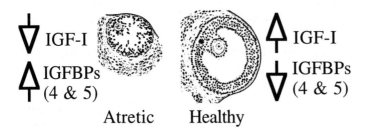

Fig. 1.

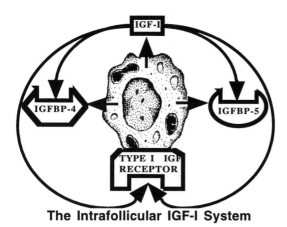

The Intrafollicular IGF-I System

Fig. 2.

its site of production [1,14—16], reception [17—22], sequestration [2—5,7—9,23,24] and action [22—35]. Stated differently, there exists a complete intrafollicular IGF-I system [36], replete with a ligand (IGF-I), a receptor (type 1) and IGFBP-4 and -5 (Fig. 2). Although several species have been the subject of such investigation [37,38], this summary limits itself to the rat model in the interest of brevity. Although the rat ovary is also a site of IGF-II production [39], reception [18,22,40,41] and action [18,22], the progressive postnatal decline in ovarian IGF-II content [40] and the resistance of type 2 IGF receptors to hormonal regulation strongly argue against a meaningful role for this principle in adult rat ovarian physiology.

Projected role of the intrafollicular IGF-I system: selection by way of amplification
According to current views, the primary, if not the sole, role of intrafollicular IGF-I may be the amplification of FSH action at the level of the granulosa cell, a facilitatory function in keeping with the often exponential nature of follicular development. This possibility is supported by a growing body of information documenting IGF-I-mediated amplification of FSH action [22—34] as well as by the demonstration of compromised FSH action under IGF-I-deplete circumstances [10,23,24,42—46]. It is this amplifying property of IGF-I coupled with its selective expression in healthy (but not atretic) follicles [1], which may underlie its projected ability to initiate and/or maintain the process of follicular selection.

Intrafollicular IGF-I: the ligand
Ovarian IGF-I gene expression has been readily detected at birth, preceding the formation of morphologically distinct follicular units [16]. Thereafter, ovarian IGF-I gene expression progressively increases to a peak between days 15 and 25 [40]. Of all adult organs tested, the ovary displays the third highest level of IGF-I gene expression, the liver and uterus being the most active in this regard [47]. These observations support the notion that locally, rather than circulatory-derived IGF-I,

may play a role in ovarian physiology. Cellular localization studies have clearly established the granulosa cell as the sole somatic ovarian cell concerned with IGF-I gene expression [1,15,16] and translation [14]. Most importantly healthy follicles proved IGF-I-replete, whereas atretic follicles proved IGF-I-deplete [1]. These observations suggest that IGF-I may play a positive role in the context of follicular selection and that IGF-I gene expression may be positively correlated with follicular health.

Although the hormonal regulation of whole ovarian IGF-I gene (or protein) expression under (unperturbed or pharmacologically-manipulated) in vivo circumstances has been explored [15,48,49], the utility of this information is uncertain given the highly-regionalized pattern of ovarian IGF-I expression [1,16]. In this connection special mention must be made of in situ hybridization studies wherein ovarian IGF-I gene expression proved resistant to both hypophysectomy and PMSG replacement [16]. Comparable in vitro studies revealed IGF-I gene expression to be short-lived in primary cultures of whole ovarian dispersates or in isolated granulosa cells [50]. Specifically, note was made of irreversible and relatively rapid (within 24 h) decrements in IGF-I (but not type 1 IGF receptor) gene expression, the preservation of which required the concurrent provision of pharmacological concentrations of both insulin and dexamethasone [50].

That granulosa cell-derived IGF-I may be a functional autocrine regulator has been repeatedly documented [22–30]. Although the precise cellular mechanism(s) through which IGF-I amplifies FSH action remain a matter of study, preliminary observations suggest interactions at site(s) both proximal and distal to cAMP generation [32–34].

Intrafollicular type 1 IGF receptors
Ovarian type 1 IGF receptor gene expression has been readily detected at birth at a point preceding the formation of morphologically distinct follicular units [16]. Thereafter, type 1 IGF receptor mRNA levels and [^{125}I]IGF-I binding have been shown to increase 10-fold to a maximum between postnatal days 20–25 [40]. Cellular localization studies established that the granulosa cell is endowed with high affinity low capacity type 1 IGF receptors, the functional characteristics of which conform to those observed in other cell types also studied [16–22].

In vivo as well as in vitro studies revealed the ability of FSH to upregulate granulosa cell type 1 IGF receptors [16,17,19–21], an effect due to enhancement of binding capacity rather than affinity for which a transcriptional component has been demonstrated [16]. Given the pivotal role of FSH in follicular development, this finding strongly suggests that the acquisition of IGF-I responsiveness may be part of granulosa cell ontogeny and that FSH may condition the granulosa cell to respond optimally to IGF-I. Heterologous receptor upregulation was not limited to FSH, similar increments having been observed for luteotropic, β_2-adrenergic and somatogenic (but not lactogenic) granulosa cell agonists [19,20]. Activation of GnRH receptors proved inhibitory to FSH-supported granulosa cell type 1 IGF receptors [21]. Despite such remarkable hormonal responsiveness, type 1 IGF receptors (unlike IGF-I) transcripts appear evenly distributed within the follicle and between follicles irrespective of maturational stage or health status. Consequently, a role for type 1 IGF-I receptors as a determinant of follicular fate appears unlikely at this time.

Intraovarian IGFBPs

General

IGFBPs constitute a heterogenous group of at least six distinct (variably glycosylated) 20–30 kDa gene products [48] capable of binding IGFs (but not insulin) with affinities in the 10^{-10}–10^{-9} M range (Table 1). Current views favor the notion that IGFBPs may not only transport IGFs but may also regulate their bioavailability and perhaps presentation to cognate cell surface receptors [51]. In this connection, both stimulation [52–59] and inhibition [58,59] of IGF binding and action have been reported. Thus, the synthesis and secretion of IGFBPs may play a major role in the regulation of IGF hormonal action at the target cell level regardless of the extracellular concentrations of the IGFs under study. Although structurally distinct, IGFBPs may appear functionally homogeneous given their common ability to sequester IGFs. However, more detailed evaluation, as applied to the ovary (see below), strongly argues that intraovarian IGFBP-2–6 are heterogeneous in terms of their cellular localization, hormonal responsiveness, relative affinity for IGFs and hence antigonadotropic potential.

Identity and cellular localization of rat ovarian IGFBPs
Molecular probing, in situ hybridization, western ligand blotting, deglycosylation analysis and immunoprecipitation studies documented the rat ovary as a highly-compartmentalized (hormonally-dependent) site of IGFBP-2–6, but not IGFBP-1 [2], expression (Table 2).

IGFBP-4 and IGFBP-5 proved granulosa cell-selective [2,5,6], the latter constituting the major species [7–9,24] comprised of a nonglylcosylated doublet (a pronounced 28 kDa moiety and a less prominent 29 kDa protein). IGFBP-4 in turn is primarily represented by a nonglycosylated 24 kDa species along with a minor glycosylated 27 kDa moiety [5,7–9,24]. Although IGFBP-2, IGFBP-3 and IGFBP-6 are theca-interstitial cell-exclusive [2,10,24,54], the mixed cellular nature of the theca-

Table 1. Known rat IGFBPs

IGFBP (#)	Residue (#)	MW (kDa)[a]	Glycosylation (status)	RGD (status)
1	247	26.8	Possible O-Linkage (×1)	+
2	270	29.6	Negative	+
3	265	28.8	Possible N-Linkage (×4)	−
4	233	25.7	Possible N-Linkage (×1)	−
5	252	28.4	Negative	−
6	201	21.5	Negative	−

[a]Predicted size of nonglycosylated mature protein.

346

Table 2. Rat ovarian IGFBPs: identification and cellular localization

IGFBP	mRNA (#)	Ovarian compartment	MW (kDa)[a]	Immunoreactivity (status)	Glycosylation (status)	Reference
2	+	Theca-Interstitial	28	+	–	[2,12]
3	+	Theca-Interstitial	46	ND	+	[2,13]
4	+	Granulosa	24 & 27	+	+	[2,3,57]
5	+	Granulosa	28 & 29	+	–	[4,57]
6	+	Theca-Interstitial	ND	ND	ND	[58]

ND = Not done; [a]Observed size(s) of glycosylated or nonglycosylated protein.

interstitial cell preparations employed precludes more definite conclusions as to the nature of the cell type involved.

Granulosa cell-derived IGFBPs are selectively expressed in atretic, but not healthy antral follicles

Given in situ hybridization studies, IGFBP-4 and IGFBP-5 were noted to be differentially expressed in atretic and healthy antral follicles. Specifically, healthy antral follicles proved IGFBP-deplete, whereas atretic follicles proved IGFBP-replete [2-6]. Given the established IGF-I-sequestering activity of these IGFBPs [5,6,10,42–46], it is tempting to speculate that their high level of expression in atretic follicles may be causally related to the attendant growth failure and ultimate demise (assuming that a net decrease in intrafollicular bioavailable IGF-I may be detrimental to follicular health). Importantly, such unfavorable intrafollicular IGFBP economy may be further compounded by the low level of IGF-I gene expression characteristic of the atretic state [1]. Thus, the combined impact of an IGFBP-replete and an IGF-I-deplete intrafollicular environment may be associated with the initiation and/or maintenance of the atretic process. Whether or not altered intrafollicular IGF-I activity is relevant to the programmed cell death underlying the atretic process [59] remains unknown at this time.

IGFBPs are antigonadotropins by virtue of their IGF-I-sequestering property

Of the known IGFBPs, all except IGFBP-6 have been noted to display antigonado-tropic activity. Specifically, a note was made of the ability of exogenously-added IGFBP-1–5 to attenuate FSH-supported steroidogenesis by cultured rat granulosa cells [5,6,10,42–44,46,54]. Moreover, the intrabursal administration of IGFBP-3 was noted to attenuate hCG-triggered ovulation in PMSG-primed immature rats [44]. Although the precise cellular mechanism(s) underlying the apparent antigonadotropic activity of IGFBPs remains a matter of study, sequestration of endogenous IGF-I is almost undoubtedly at play [10,42,43,45,46] According to this view, the resultant IGF-I-deplete state precludes IGF-I-mediated amplification of gonadotropin action thereby resulting in a net antigonadotropic effect. Although such a mechanism may well underlie the antigonadotropic activity of all the relevant IGFBPs, the equation of antigonadotropism with IGF-I sequestration was particularly rigorously documented for IGFBP-1 [41,45] even though the latter is not expressed in the rat ovary.

FSH inhibits the accumulation of granulosa cell-derived IGFBPs
The ability of FSH to modulate the elaboration of granulosa cell-derived IGFBPs, was documented under both in vivo [7] and in vitro [7–9] circumstances. Specifically, treatment of cultured granulosa cells with FSH (≥10 ng/ml) has been shown to inhibit the elaboration of IGFBP-5 [7,8], an effect requiring the activation of the A-kinase transduction pathway [9]. Qualitatively comparable results (albeit at a lower response sensitivity level) were obtained for the elaboration of IGFBP-4 [7–9]. The disparate response sensitivities of distinct IGFBP species suggest a potent mechanism through which FSH may determine the relative distribution pattern of granulosa cell-derived IGFBPs and the consequent overall IGFBP responsiveness of this cell type. The inhibitory FSH action is all the more noteworthy in light of the generally stimulatory effect exerted by FSH at the level of the granulosa cell. Conceivably then, this apparently inhibitory action of FSH may in effect constitute a net stimulatory gain since granulosa cell-derived IGFBPs are inhibitory to IGF (and thus inevitably to gonadotropin) hormonal action [6].

Acknowledgements

Financial assistance used for this research is from NIH Research Grants HD-19998 and HD-30288. The author also wishes to thank Ms. Cornelia T. Szmajda for her excellent assistance in the preparation of this manuscript.

References

1. Oliver JE, Aitman TJ, Powell JF, Wilson CA, Clayton RN. Endocrinology 1989;124:267–2679.
2. Nakatani A, Shimasaki S, Erickson GF, Ling N. Endocrinology 1991;129:1521–1529.
3. Erickson GF, Nakatani A, Ling N, Shimasaki S. Endocrinology 1992;130:625–636.
4. Erickson G, Nakatani A, Ling N, Shimasaki S. Endocrinology 1992;130:1867–1878.
5. Putowski LT, Choi DS, Mordacq J et al. In vivo hormonal regulation of insulin-like growth factor binding protein-5 mRNA in the immature rat ovary. Mol Cell Endocrinol 1994 (submitted).
6. Putowski LT, Choi DS, Scherzer et al. Rat ovarian insulin-like growth factor binding protein-4: a hormonally-dependent granulosa-derived antigonadotropin. Endocrinology 1994 (submitted).
7. Adashi EY, Resnick CE, Hernandez ER, Hurwitz A, Rosenfeld RG. Endocrinology 1990;126:1305–1307.
8. Adashi EY, Resnick CE, Hurwitz A, Ricciarelli E, Hernandez ER, Rosenfeld RG. Endocrinology 1991;128:754–760.
9. Adashi EY, Resnick CE, Tedeschi C, Rosenfeld RG. Endocrinology 1993;132:1463–1468.
10. Ui M, Shimonaka M, Shimasaki S, Ling N. Endocrinology 1989;125:912–916.
11. Adashi EY, Rohan RM. Trends Endocrinol Metab 1992;3:243–248.
12. Adashi EY. Reprod Fertil Dev 1992;4:497–504.
13. Adashi EY, Resnick CE, Hurwitz A, Ricciarelli E, Hernandez ER, Roberts CT Jr., LeRoith D,

348

Rosenfeld RG. Growth Reg 1992;2:10–16.
14. Hansson H-A, Nilsson A, Isgaard J, Billig H, Isaksson O. Skottner A, Andersson IK, Rozell B. Histochemistry 1988;89:403–410.
15. Hernandez ER, Roberts CH, LeRoith D, Adashi EY. Endocrinology 1989;125:572–574.
16. Zhou J, Chin E, Bondy C. Endocrinology 1991;129:3281–3288.
17. Adashi EY, Resnick CE, Svoboda ME, Van Wyk JJ. J Biol Chem 1986;261:3923–3926.
18. Davoren JB, Kasson BG, Li CH, Hsueh AJW. Endocrinology 1986;119:2155–2162.
19. Adashi EY, Resnick CE, Hernandez ER, Svoboda ME, Van Wyk JJ. Endocrinology 1988;122:194–201.
20. Adashi EY, Resnick CE, Svoboda ME, Van Wyk JJ. Endocrinology 1988;122:1383–1390.
21. Adashi EY, Resnick CE, Vera A, Hernandez ER. Endocrinology 1991;128:3130–3138.
22. Adashi EY, Resnick CE, Rosenfeld RG. Endocrinology 1989;126:216–222.
23. Adashi EY, Resnick CE, Svoboda ME, Van Wyk JJ. Endocrinology 1984;115:1227–1229.
24. Adashi EY, Resnick CE, Svoboda ME, Van Wyk JJ. Endocrinology 1985;116:2135–2142.
23. Adashi EY, Resnick CE, Ricciarelli E, Hurwitz A, Hernandez ER, Rosenfeld RG, Carllson-Skwirut C, Francis GL. J Clin Invest 1992;90:1593–1599.
24. Adashi EY, Resnick CE, Hernandez ER, Hurwitz A, Rosenfeld RG. Mol Cell Endocrinol 1990;74:175–185.
25. Davoren JB, Hsueh AJW, Li CH. Am J Physiol 1985;249:E26–E33.
26. Adashi EY, Resnick CE, Brodie AMH, Svoboda ME, Van Wyk JJ. Endocrinology 1985;117:2323–2320.
27. Hutchinson LA, Findlay JK, Herington AC. Mol Cell Endorinol 1988;55:61–69.
28. Adashi EY, Resnick CE, Svoboda ME, Van Wyk JJ. Endocrinology 1985;116:2369–2375.
29. Adashi EY, Resnick CE, Svoboda ME, Van Wyk JJ, Hascall VC, Yanagishita M. Endocrinology 1986;118:456–459.
30. Bicsak TA, Tucker EM, Cappel S, Vaughan J, Rivier J, Vale W, Hsueh AJW. Endocrinology 1986;119:2711–2719.
31. Zhien ZZ, Carson RS, Herington AC, Lee VWK, Burger HG. Endocrinology 1987;120:1633–1638.
32. Adashi EY, Resnick CE, Svoboda ME, Van Wyk JJ. Endocrinology 1986;118:149–156.
33. Adashi EY, Resnick CE, Svoboda ME, Van Wyk JJ. Biol Reprod 1986;34:81–88.
34. Adashi EY, Resnick CE, May JV, Knecht M, Svoboda ME, Van Wyk JJ. Endocrinology 1988;122:1583–1592.
35. Adashi EY, Resnick CE, Rosenfeld RG. Mol Cell Endocrinol 1994;99:279–284.
36. Adashi EY, Resnick CE, Hurwitz A, Ricciarelli E, Hernandez ER, Roberts CT Jr., LeRoith D, Rosenfeld RG. Human Reprod 1991;6:1213–1219.
37. Hammond JM, Mondschein JS, Samaras SE, Canning SF. J Steroid Biochem Mol Biol 1991;40:411–416.
38. Giudice LC. Endocrine Rev 1992;13:641–669.
39. Hernandez ER, Roberts CT Jr., Hurwitz A, LeRoith D, Adashi EY. Endocrinology 1990;127:3249–3251.
40. Levy MJ, Hernandez ER, Adashi EY, Stillman RJ, Roberts CT Jr., LeRoith D. Endocrinology 1992;131:1202–1206.
41. Hernandez ER, Hurwitz A, Botero L, Ricciarelli E, Hernandez ER, Roberts CT Jr., LeRoith D, Adashi EY. Mol Endocrinol 1991;5:1799–1805.
42. Shimasaki S, Shimonaka M, Ui M, Inouye S, Shibata F, Ling N. J Biol Chem 1990;265:2198–2202.
43. Bicsak TS, Shimonaka M, Malkowski M, Ling N. Endocrinology 1990;126:2184–2189.
44. Bicsak TS, Long N, DePaolo LV. Biol Reprod 1991;44:599–603.
45. Adashi EY, Resnick CE, Ricciarelli E, Hurwitz A, Kokia E. Botero LF, Tedeschi C, Hernandez ER, Koistinen R, Rutanen EM, Seppala M. In: Genazzani AR, Petraglia F (eds) Hormones in Gynecological Endocrinology. Carnforth: Parthenon, 1992;255–261.
46. Adashi EY, Resnick CE, Rosenfeld RG, Powell DR, Koistinen R, Rutanen EM, Seppala M. In: Leroith DR, Raizada MK (eds) Current Directions in Insulin-Like Growth Factor Research. New

York: Plenum Publishing Corporation, 1994 Adv Exp Med Biol 343:377–385.

47. Murphy LJ, Bell Gl, Friesen HG. Endocrinology 1987;120:1279–1282.
48. Davoren JB, Hsueh AJW. Endocrinology 1986;118:888–890.
49. Carlsson B, Carlsson L, Billig H. Mol Cell Endocrinol 1989;64:271–275.
50. Botero LF, Kokia E, Ricciarelli E, Roberts CT Jr., LeRoith D, Adashi EY, Hernandez ER. Endocrinology 1993;132:2703–2708.
51. Clemmons DR. J Dev Physiol 1991;15:105–110.
52. Clemmons DR, Elgin RG, Han VKM, Casella SJ, D'Ercole AJ, Van Wyk JJ. J Clin Invest 1986;77: 1548–1556.
53. DeVroede MA, Tseng LY-H, Katsoyannis PG, Nissley SP, Rechler MM. J Clin Invest 1986;77:602–613.
54. Elgin RG, Busby WJ Jr., Clemmons DR. Proc Natl Acad Sci USA 1987;84:3254–3258.
55. Frauman AG, Tsuzaki S, Moses AC. Endocrinology 1989;124:2289–2296.
56. Knauer DJ, Smith GL. Proc Natl Acad Sci USA 1980;77:7252–7256.
57. Ling NC, Liu X-J, Malkowski M, Erickson G, Shimasaki S. IX Ovarian Workshop, Ovarian Cell Interactions: Genes to Physiology. Chapel Hill, NC, 1992.
58. Rohan RM, Ricciarelli E, Kiefer MC, Resnick CE, Adashi EY. Endocrinology 132:2507–2512.
59. Hurwitz A, Adashi EY. Mol Cell Endocrinol 1992;84:C19–C23.
60. Ricciarelli E, Hernandez ER, Hurwitz A, Kokia E, Rosenfeld RG, Schwander J, Adashi EY. Endocrinology 1991;129:2266–2268.
61. Ricciarelli E, Hernandez ER, Kokia E, Rohan RM, Tedeschi C, Botero L, Rosenfeld RG, Albiston AL, Herington AC, Adashi EY. Endocrinology 1992;130:3092–3094.
62. Drop SLS. J Clin Endocrinol Metab 1992;74:1215–1216.

©1994 Elsevier Science B.V. All rights reserved
The insulin-like growth factors and their regulatory proteins
R.C. Baxter, P.D. Gluckman and R.G. Rosenfeld, editors

Insulin-like growth factors (IGFs), IGF binding proteins (IGFBPs) and IGFBP protease in human uterine endometrium: their potential relevance to endometrial cyclic function and maternal-embryonic interactions

L.C. Giudice[1], J.C. Irwin[1], B.A. Dsupin[1], L. de las Fuentes[1], I.H. Jin[2], T.H. Vu[2] and A.R. Hoffman[2]

Departments of [1]Gynecology & Obstetrics and [2]Medicine, Stanford University Medical Center, Stanford, CA 94305 and Medical Service, Veteran Administration Medical Center, Palo Alto, CA 94304, USA

Introduction

The lining of the uterus, the endometrium, is the anatomic prerequisite for blastocyst implantation. It is composed of several cell types, including glandular and surface epithelium, stroma, vascular endothelium and smooth muscle, fibroblasts and cells of the immune system (reviewed in [1]). During the proliferative (estradiol (E_2)-dominant) phase, endometrial cellular components proliferate [2] and endometrial thickness increases about 10-fold, peaking at ovulation. After ovulation, in the secretory phase and under the influence of progesterone, cellular differentiation and proliferation occur. Endometrial epithelium secretes high levels of glycoproteins and carbohydrates into the glandular lumen and stromal cells decidualize. In addition, spiral arteries proliferate preparing for contact with the fetal placenta, if implantation occurs [2]. Inappropriate development of cellular constituents of the endometrium can lead to infertility and repetitive miscarriages. In the absence of implantation, the functionalist layer of the endometrium is shed and the cellular and structural changes begin anew with a new menstrual cycle. In the presence of implantation the endometrium assumes new functions: nourishing the developing embryo, protecting it from maternal rejection and preventing its overzealous invasion into the maternal myometrium.

During the menstrual cycle, most cellular components of endometrium respond to changing levels of circulating steroid hormones [2] that act primarily or secondarily through a group of endogenously produced growth factors [3]. Interest in the insulin-like growth factors (IGFs) in human endometrium was prompted by two landmark studies. The first was the report of marked E_2-dependence of IGF-I mRNA in rat endometrium [4] and the second was the finding that a major secretory product of human endometrial stromal cells was identical to IGF binding protein-1 (IGFBP-1)

Address for correspondence: L.C. Giudice, M.D., Ph.D, Department of Gynecology and Obstetrics, Stanford University Medical Center, Room HH333, Stanford, CA 94305-5317, USA.

352

[5]. During the past 5 years, our laboratory has extensively investigated the IGF axis in human endometrium across the menstrual cycle and in endometrial decidua during the first trimester of pregnancy [6—8]. In addition, we have used long term cultures of human endometrial stromal cells [9] as a model in which to investigate the effects of the IGFs on stromal proliferation and differentiation [10—13]. In the current monograph, IGF, IGFBP and IGF receptor gene expression in this tissue, as well as stromal cell response to IGF peptides and the secretion of a novel IGFBP-4 protease by endometrial stromal cells, are reviewed.

IGF, IGFBP and IGF receptor gene expression

IGF-I and IGF-II mRNA expression in human endometrium was investigated [8] by a solution hybridization ribonuclease protection assay, using ^{32}P-labeled riboprobes for IGF-I, IGF-II and β-actin and the results are shown in Fig. 1. IGF-I gene expression was primarily in proliferative and early secretory endometrium and there was abundant IGF-II gene expression in mid-late secretory endometrium and early pregnancy decidua. Northern analysis, using IGF-I and IGF-II cDNA probes, confirmed these findings and revealed multiple IGF-I mRNAs (2—7.6 kb) expressed primarily in proliferative and early secretory endometrium and IGF-II mRNAs (1.4—6.0 kb) expressed primarily in secretory endometrium and early pregnancy decidua [8]. The preferential expression of IGF-I mRNA in the proliferative (E$_2$-dominant) phase supports the hypothesis that IGF-I is a mediator of E$_2$'s action (i.e., an "estromedin") in human endometrium. The expression of endometrial IGF-II mRNA in the mid-late secretory phase and in early pregnancy supports a role for IGF-II in differentiative functions of the endometrium, perhaps in tissue remodeling

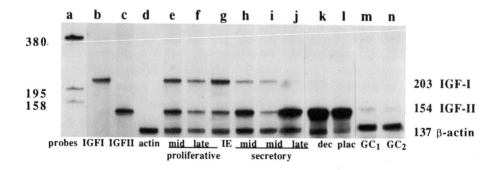

Fig. 1. IGF-I and IGF-II gene expression assessed by solution hybridization-ribonuclease protection assay. Lane a, riboprobes for IGF-I, IGF-II and β-actin, as shown. Lanes b—d, protected fragments using individual riboprobes (IGF-I, IGF-II and β-actin, respectively) and 2.5 μg midproliferative endometrium total RNA. Protected fragments using all three riboprobes simultaneously with 2.5 μg total RNA from: mid and late proliferative endometrium (lanes e and f, respectively), interval endometrium (midcycle) (lane g), midsecretory endometrium (lanes h and i); late secretory endometrium (lane j), early pregnancy decidua (lane k, dec); midgestation placenta (lane l, plac), luteinizing human granulosa cells (GC) from two patients undergoing in vitro fertilization (lanes m and n). With permission from [8].

in early pregnancy or in endometrial tissue shedding in the absence of implantation or as one of several modulators of maternal-embryonic/fetal interactions (see below).

IGFBP-1 is a major secretory product of decidualized endometrium, with mRNA expression first detected by Northern blotting and by in situ hybridization histochemistry in the late secretory phase, exclusively in stromal cells [8,14]. We have recently investigated IGFBP-1—6 gene expression in endometrium using Northern blotting, the results are shown in Fig. 2. IGFBP-1 was abundantly expressed in mid and late secretory endometrium (panel labeled "IGFBP-1", lanes g, i and j). It was not, however, expressed in an endometrial sample from a patient with luteal phase deficiency (lane h), probably reflecting an inadequate response to progesterone for stromal decidualization and therefore IGFBP-1 production. In uterine endometrial decidua samples obtained from subjects with ectopic pregnancies, variable amounts of IGFBP-1 mRNA expression have been observed (e.g., lane k), whereas in other samples IGFBP-1 mRNA expression is abundant [12]. This may reflect decreased progesterone support with some ectopic gestations. IGFBP-2, -3 and -6 mRNAs are differentially expressed in secretory compared to proliferative endometrium (Fig. 2), whereas IGFBP-4 mRNA expression is not cycle-dependent and IGFBP-5 is preferentially expressed during the proliferative phase. The sample from a patient with luteal phase deficiency is very similar to that of proliferative endometrium, again reflecting inadequate response to high levels of circulating progesterone.

With regard to IGF receptors in human endometrium, conflicting results have been reported. In one study, total IGF binding increased in the secretory phase [15], which may be due to increased type 1 and/or type 2 receptors and/or to high levels of IGFBP-1 during the secretory phase. In another study [16], noncycle-dependence was noted for the type 1 IGF receptor. We have recently found an increase in both type 1 and type 2 IGF receptor mRNA by a solution hybridization ribonuclease protection assay [8], although whether IGF receptor protein is cycle-dependent remains uncertain and awaits further studies using IGF analogues that have low affinities for the IGFBPs and preferential affinity for the type 1 or type 2 receptor.

IGF action on endometrial stromal cells

Long term cultures of human endometrial stromal cells [9], provide a model in vitro system to examine steroid and peptide growth factor effects on these cells that undergo proliferation and differentiation (decidualization) in the secretory phase in response to progesterone in vivo [2]. In vitro, epidermal growth factor (EGF) and progesterone (P) promote stromal decidualization, characterized by a specific cellular phenotype and heralded by the production of prolactin and IGFBP-1 (Fig. 3, lane a (28 kDa band)) [9,17—19]. In addition to IGFBP-1, we have found that decidualized endometrial stromal cells also secrete IGFBP-3, -2 and -4 (Fig. 3) [6,10,11]. Relaxin, a structural homologue of the IGF peptides, stimulates IGFBP-1 secretion from these cells [18], whereas insulin inhibits IGFBP-1 mRNA expression and protein synthesis [11,12,20] at concentrations that are compatible with it acting via the insulin receptor

354

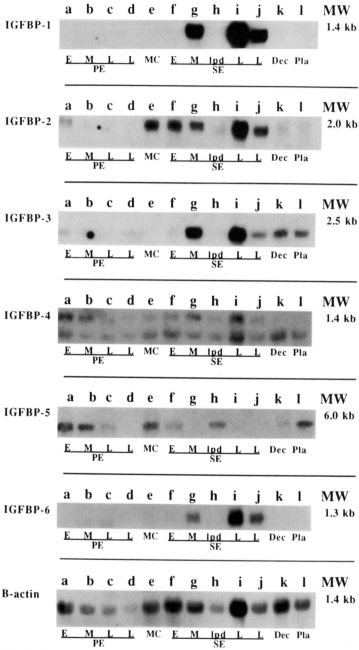

Fig. 2. Northern analysis of endometrial, decidual and placental total RNA (20 µg/well) probed with human IGFBP-1–6 and β-actin cDNA probes. Samples from early (E), mid (M) and late (L) stages of proliferative phase endometrium (PE) and secretory phase endometrium (SE) are shown at the bottom of each panel. Samples from midcycle (MC), from a patient with luteal phase deficiency (lpd), from ectopic gestation uterine decidua (Dec) and term placenta (Pla) are also shown. The same filter was used after stripping and reprobing. Complementary DNA probes used are shown on the left and mRNA transcript sizes are on the right (in kilobases (kb)).

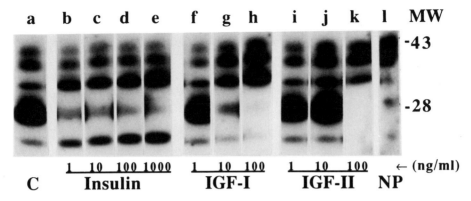

a   b   c   d   e   f   g   h   i   j   k   l   MW

-43

-28

1 10 100 1000   1 10 100   1 10 100   ← (ng/ml)
C   Insulin   IGF-I   IGF-II   NP

Fig. 3. Autoradiograph of a Western ligand blot of conditioned media from endometrial stromal cells cultured for 10 days with EGF (20 ng/ml) and progesterone (1 μM), with no further additions (lane a), or in the presence of insulin (lanes b—e), IGF-I (lanes f—h) or IGF-II (lanes i—k), at various concentrations (ng/ml) as indicated; lane l, nonpregnant female serum (NP). Molecular weight markers are indicated on the right margin, expressed in kDa.

(Fig. 3, lanes b—e). The inhibiting effect of insulin on IGFBP-1 has also been observed with term decidua cells [21]. Increasing concentrations of IGF-I and IGF-II also inhibit IGFBP-1 production by decidualized endometrial stromal cells (Fig. 3, lanes f—k) [11]. However, when IGFBP-1 in conditioned media from decidualized endometrial stromal cells is quantitated by immunoassay, the effects of low doses of the IGF peptides is biphasic (Fig. 4, upper panel). Low levels of IGF peptides increase IGFBP-1 secretion by these cells, whereas higher levels decrease IGFBP-1. Most striking is the observation that in the presence of low levels of IGFs, IGFBP-1 increases and stromal proliferation is inhibited (Fig. 4, lower panel), whereas in the presence of higher levels of IGFs, IGFBP-1 is in inhibited and concomitant stromal cellular proliferation occurs. These data support an inhibitory role for IGFBP-1 on IGF action on these cells and demonstrate that the IGF-induced changes of IGFBP-1 levels in stromal cultures are associated with changes in the biological responses of stromal cells to IGFs. A recent study from our laboratory has shown that IGF analogues with low affinity for IGFBPs are approximately 10-fold more potent than IGF-I in stimulating stromal cell growth (JC Irwin, LC Giudice, unpublished data). These data can be reconciled by the hypothesis that IGFBPs in media conditioned by these cells are saturated with IGF peptides and at low concentrations IGFs complex with unsaturated cell surface-associated IGFBP-1, thereby promoting its release from the cell membrane, by nonreceptor mediated mechanisms, as has been found for other IGFBPs [22—24]. This can then permit access to the type 1 IGF receptor at higher IGF concentrations to inhibit further production of IGFBP-1 and to stimulate endometrial cellular mitosis.

In addition to IGF effects on IGFBP-1 secretion by decidualized endometrial stromal cells, there was also a marked effect on IGFBP-4 with increasing concentrations of IGF peptides that was not observed at any concentration of insulin (Fig. 3).

356

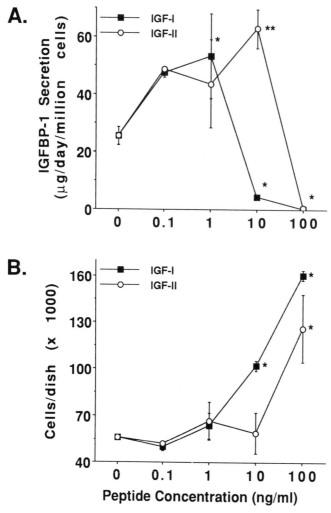

Fig. 4. Dose-dependent regulation of IGFBP-1 secretion (panel A) and cell proliferation (panel B) in decidualized endometrial stromal cultures by IGF-I and IGF-II. Stromal cells were induced to decidualize in culture with EGF (20 ng/ml) and progesterone (1 µM) for 12 days, with the indicated concentrations of IGF-I (■) or IGF-II (O). IGFBP-1 was assayed in 2-day conditioned medium, and the values represent the mean ± SEM (bars) of duplicate or triplicate cultures, assayed in duplicate. $p < 0.05$ (*), $p < 0.01$ (**) compared to no peptide. After 14 days of treatment cells were trypsinized and counted and the values represent the mean ± SEM (bars) of duplicate or triplicate cultures. $p < 0.01$ (*) compared to no peptide.

IGF-I analogues that have markedly decreased affinities for IGFBPs, but bind to the type 1 IGF receptor have no appreciable affect on IGFBP-4 (JC Irwin, LC Giudice, unpublished results). These observations suggest that with decidualized endometrial stromal cells, the decrease in IGFBP-4 in response to IGFs is probably not a receptor-mediated event and may be a consequence of specific IGF:IGFBP interactions. We

357

have hypothesized that IGF:IGFBP-4 interactions result in partial proteolysis of IGFBP-4, rendering it less readily detectable by Western ligand blotting. This hypothesis was tested in a cell-free system, using media from endometrial stromal cells cultured in the absence of IGF peptides. These media were incubated with no added peptide or with IGF-II for varying amounts of time and then were analyzed by Western ligand blotting (Fig. 5). IGFBP-4 was stable throughout the incubation when control medium was used which contained no exogenously added peptide (lanes a–e), but it was undetectable by 3 h of incubation when IGF-II was exogenously added (lanes f–j). Using ^{125}I-IGF-II cross-linked to recombinant human IGFBP-4 as substrate, we have found proteolysis of IGFBP-4 when incubations were with control medium with and without exogenously added IGF-II (JC Irwin, LC Giudice, unpublished data). These experiments have lead to the conclusion that endometrial stromal cells secrete an IGFBP-4 protease into conditioned medium and that the interaction of IGF peptide with IGFBP-4 results in a conformational change, rendering IGFBP-4 a substrate for this enzyme. The presence of an IGF-dependent IGFBP-4 protease has also been described with fibroblast and term decidual culture systems [25–27]. It is likely that common mechanisms have evolved to control IGF:IGFBP-4 interactions in a variety of systems and may include other post-translational modifications in addition to proteolysis.

Summary and Conclusions

We have found that IGF-I and IGFBP-5 mRNAs are differentially expressed in proliferative phase endometrium, whereas IGF-II, IGFBP-1, -2, -3 and -6, and the IGF receptor mRNAs are differentially expressed in secretory phase endometrium. Preliminary evidence shows that IGF mRNAs are expressed exclusively in

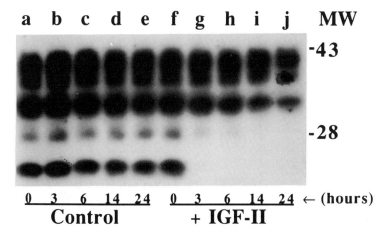

Fig. 5. Autoradiograph of a Western ligand blot of endometrial stomal cell conditioned media incubated in a cell-free system without added IGF-II peptide (Control, lanes a–e) or with IGF-II (100 ng/mL) (+IGF-II, lanes f–j) for 0,3, 6, 14 and 24 h at 37°C.

endometrial stromal cells, whereas IGF receptor mRNAs are expressed in both stroma and epithelium [28]. It is likely (Fig. 6) that stromally-derived IGF-I stimulates proliferation of glandular epithelium by paracrine mechanisms and stromal cells by autocrine mechanisms, resulting in the hallmark of cellular proliferation so characteristic of proliferative phase of the menstrual cycle, before ovulation. IGF-II in late secretory endometrium and in early pregnancy may modulate decidual function. We speculate that locally produced IGF-II may control the secretory activity of decidualized stromal cells throughout the endometrium and may regulate, along with other modulators, the amount of IGFBP-1 in the environment of the invading trophoblast. IGFBP-1, in turn, may modulate the amount of bioavailable IGFs in the microenvironment of the invading trophoblast and may participate with, e.g., EGF, in the differentiation of cytotrophoblasts to syncytiotrophoblasts [29].

While IGFBPs have traditionally been thought of as modulators of IGF action and serve to prolong their half-lives in the circulation, IGF-independent actions of IGFBP's cannot be ignored. For example, IGFBP-3 binds to specific cell receptors and may affect cellular mitosis [30] and IGFBP-1 binds by its RGD sequence [31] to $\alpha_5\beta_1$ integrin, a specific cellular receptor for the extracellular matrix protein, fibronectin and alters cellular motility [32]. It has been shown that the anchoring villus of the invading fetal placenta expresses primarily $\alpha_5\beta_1$ integrin [33]. We propose that this invasive cytotrophoblast phenotype (also called the "intermediate trophoblast" [34]) invading into the maternal decidua is "confronted" by high concentrations of IGFBP-1 which interacts via its RGD sequence with $\alpha_5\beta_1$ integrin on the invading intermediate trophoblast cell membrane (Fig. 7). We further propose that the interactions between IGFBP-1 and the intermediate trophoblast serve to alter invasiveness of this highly invasive trophoblastic phenotype. It is of interest that

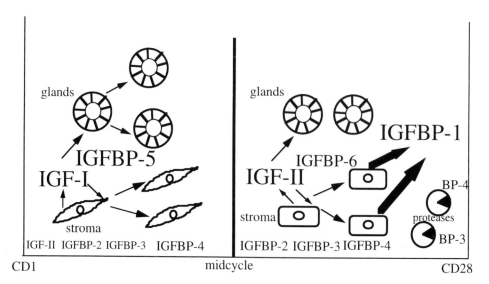

Fig. 6. Model of IGF action and IGFBP expression in human endometrium during the menstrual cycle (see text).

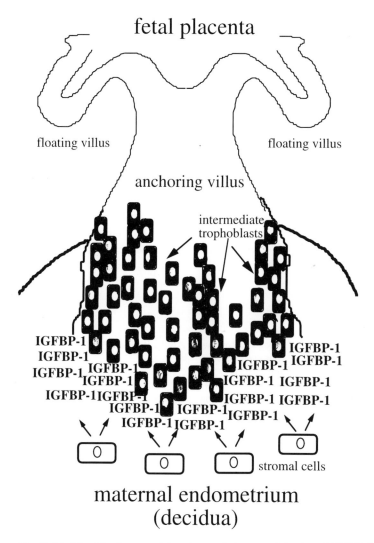

fetal placenta

floating villus   floating villus

anchoring villus

intermediate
trophoblasts

IGFBP-1
IGFBP-1
IGFBP-1 IGFBP-1
IGFBP-1
IGFBP-1 IGFBP-1
IGFBP-1
IGFBP-1 IGFBP-1
IGFBP-1

IGFBP-1 IGFBP-1
IGFBP-1 IGFBP-1
IGFBP-1 IGFBP-1
IGFBP-1 IGFBP-1
IGFBP-1 IGFBP-1
IGFBP-1

stromal cells

maternal endometrium
(decidua)

Fig. 7. Model of fetal-maternal interface and the potential roles of IGFBP-1 in limiting intermediate trophoblast invasiveness and in modulating the amount of IGF-I and IGF-II available to maternal and fetal compartments.

during intermediate trophoblast invasion into the maternal decidua, proteolysis of extracellular matrix components occurs [35] and that IGFBP-1 is the only IGFBP for which no BP-protease has (yet) been described. It is possible that IGFBP-1 is relatively resistant to proteolysis and would survive well in the microenvironment of the invading, protease-secreting intermediate trophoblast. Thus, the presence of abundant IGFBP-1 in maternal decidua suggests that it may have a dual role, as a modulator of IGF action and as a modulator of decidua/ trophoblast interactions. The presence of other IGFBPs may serve to modulate further IGF availability to IGFBP-1 and to IGF receptors.

Acknowledgements

The authors gratefully acknowledge the following colleagues for generously providing cDNA probes: IGF-I, Drs. D Le Roith and C Roberts, National Institutes of Health, Bethesda, MD; IGF-II, Dr G Bell, University of Chicago, Chicago, IL; β-actin, Dr L Kedes, University of Southern California, Los Angeles, CA; IGFBP-1, Dr D Powell, Baylor College of Medicine, Houston, TX; IGFBP-2, Dr. J. Schwander, University of Basel, Basel; IGFBP-3, Dr. W. Wood, Genentech, South San Francisco, CA; and IGFBP4-6, Drs. S. Shimasaki and N Ling, The Whittier Institute, La Jolla, CA. The authors also gratefully acknowledge Diagnostic Systems Laboratories, Webster, TX for the IGFBP-1 immunoassay kits. This work was supported by NIH HD25220 (LCG) and NIH DK36054 (ARH) and the Research Service of the Department of Veterans Affairs.

References

1. Giudice LC, Ferenczy A. In: Adashi EY, Rock JA, Rosenwaks Z (eds) Reproductive Endocrinology, Surgery and Technology. New York: Raven Press, 1994.
2. Noyes RW, Hertig AT, Rock J. Fertil Steril 1950;1:3–25.
3. Giudice LC. Fertil Steril 1994;61;1–17.
4. Murphy LJ, Murphy LC, Freisen HG. Mol Endocrinol 1987;1:445–450.
5. Koistinen R, Kalkinnen N, Huhtala M-L, Seppala M, Bohn H, Rutanen E-M. Endocrinology 1986; 118:1375–1378.
6. Giudice LC, Lamson G, Rosenfeld RG, Irwin JC. Ann NY Acad Sci 1994;646:295–307.
7. Giudice LC, Milkowski DA, Lamson G, Rosenfeld RG, Irwin JC. J Clin Endocrinol Metab 1991;72; 779–787.
8. Giudice LC, Dsupin BA, Vu TH, Lin IL, Hoffman AR. J Clin Endocrinol Metab 1993;76:1115–1122.
9. Irwin JC, Kirk D, King RJB, Quigley MM, Gwatkin RBL. Fertil Steril 1989;52:761–768.
10. Giudice LC, Milkowski DM, Fielder PJ, Irwin J. Human Reprod 1991;6:632–640.
11. Giudice LC, Dsupin BA, Irwin JC. J Clin Endocrinol Metab 1992;75:1235–1241.
12. Irwin JC, Dsupin BA, De la Fuentes L, Giudice LC. Reg Peptides 1993;48:165–177.
13. Irwin JC, De la Fuentes L, Giudice LC. Growth factors and decidualization in vitro. Ann NY Acad Sci (in press).
14. Julkunen M, Koistinen R, Suikkari A-M, Seppala M, Janne OA. Mol Endocrinol 1990;4:700–707.
15. Rutanen E-M, Pekonen F, Makinen T. J Clin Endocrinol Metab 1988;66:173–180.
16. Strowitzki T, von Eye HC, Kellerer M, Haring HU. Fertil Steril 1993;59:315–322.
17. Irwin JC, Utian WH, Eckert RL. Endocrinology 1991;129:2385–2392.
18. Bell SC, Jackson JA, Ashmore J, Zhu HH, Tseng L. J Clin Endocrinol Metab 1991;72:1014–1024.
19. Rosenberg M, Mazella J, Tseng L. Ann NY Acad Sci 1991;622:138–144.
20. Tseng L, Gao J-G, Chen R, Zhu HH, Mazella J, Powell DR. Biol Reprod 1992;47:441–450.
21. Thrailkill KM, Clemmons DR, Busby WH Jr., Handwerger S. J Clin Invest 1990;86:878–883.
22. Neely EK, Rosenfeld RG. J Clin Endocrinol Metab 1992;130:985–993.
23. Martin JL, Ballesteros M, Baxter RC. Endocrinology 1992;131:1703–1710.
24. Oh Y, Muller HL, Pham H, Lamson G, Rosenfeld RG. Endocrinology 1992;131:3123–3125.

25. Fowlkes J, Freemark M. Endocrinology 1992;131:2071−2076.
26. Conover CA, Kiefer MC, Zapf J. J Clin Invest 1993;91:1129−1137.
27. Myers SE, Cheung PT, Handwergber S, Chernausek SD. Endocrinology 1993;133:1525−1531.
28. Zhou`J, Dsupin BA, Giudice LC, Bondy C. Insulin-like growth factor, receptor and binding protein gene expression in human endometrium during the menstrual cycle. Soc Gynecol Invest, March 1994; (abstract).
29. Bhaumick F, George D, Bala RM. J Clin Endocrinol Metab 1992;74:1005−1011.
30. Oh Y, Meuller HL, Rosenfeld RG. J Biol Chem 268;14964−14971.
31. Ruoslahti E, Pierschbacher MD. Science 1987;238:491−497.
32. Jones JI, Gockerman A, Busby WH Jr, Wright G, Clemmons DR. Proc Natl Acad Sci USA 1993;90: 10553−10557.
33. Damsky CH, Fitzgerald ML, Fisher SJ. J Clin Invest 1992;89:210−222.
34. Kurman RJ, Main CS, Chen H-C. Placenta 1984;5:349−370.
35. Kliman HJ, Courifaris C, Feinberg RF, Stauss JF III, Haimowitz JE. In: Yoshinaga K (ed) Blastocyst Implantation. Boston: Adams Publishing Group, 1989;83−91.

Insulin-like growth factor-I and the testis target

P.G. Chatelain, M.O. Avallet, A. Clark, F. Chuzel, H. Lejeune, M. Nicolino and J.M. Saez

INSERM U 307 and Department of Pediatrics, Université Claude Bernard, Hôpital DEBROUSSE, 29 rue Soeur Bouvier, 69322, Lyon, France

Abstract. Delayed sexual maturation observed either in isolated growth hormone (GH) deficiency or in GH receptor defect in the human as well as in Snell dwarf mice strongly suggest that GH and/or IGF-I play a role in the testis (T) endocrine function differentiation. IGF-I mRNA and IGF-I-like peptide has been found in the T. In vitro Leydig (LC) and Sertoli (SC) cells express IGF-I transcripts and secrete IGF-I. This secretion can be regulated by the specific hormone, LH and FSH respectively and by other factors including bFGF, EGF and Insulin. IGF-I is required for the maintenance of LC and SC specific functions. It increases the FSH receptor (R) number and the responsiveness of SC to FSH. Without IGF-I cultured LC lose, within a few days, most of their specific functions. Treatment with IGF-I induces in a dose dependent manner hCG R mRNA and number, enhances the coupling of the R to intracellular effectors and increases the activity, the protein and mRNA level of the three main enzymes of steroidogenesis, p450SCC, p450-I7-α and 3-β-hydroxysteroid dehydrogenase. These IGF-I effects result in an 8–10-fold increase in the steroidogenic LC response to hCG. In vivo, treatment of Snell dwarf GH deficient mice by IGF-I or GH, similarly increase hCG R number and potentiate the responsiveness to hCG. These data confirm the IGF-I requirement for LC maturation and suggest that most of GH effects on the T are mediated by IGF-I. Finally recent data indicates that IGF-I also stimulates some steps of spermatogenesis in the rat.

Taken together the results show that the T is the site of production and action of IGF-I and that this peptide might play a crucial role in both the endocrine and exocrine function of the T.

Introduction

Male newborns with congenital severe isolated growth hormone (GH) insufficiency, either idiopathic or due to GH gene deletion, often present with microphallus and later develop very short stature and delayed puberty. Early GH treatment results in normalization of growth, puberty and gonadal steroidogenesis [1]. Normalization of microphallus requires combined testosterone and GH therapy. Patients with GH insensitivity syndrome with GH receptor gene deletion, resulting in GH severe resistance and IGF-I severe insufficiency show a noticeable delayed puberty without gonadotropin insufficiency [2]. In laboratory animals such as Snell dwarf mice, GH deficiency is due to a Pit-1 gene defect [3]. In these male mice puberty is delayed and progresses slowly. Treatment with exogenous GH normalizes pubertal timing and development. These clinical observations, both in the human and laboratory animals, point to the contribution of insulin-like growth factor-I (IGF-I) to normal steroidogenesis in the gonad. We shall summarize data pointing to the male gonad as an IGF-I target since the male gonad is a site of IGF-I binding, secretion and action.

IGF-I binding to the male gonad

IGF-I and its receptor have been documented in rat testis (T) [4]. Both Leydig and Sertoli cells, isolated from porcine and grown in vitro in a serum-free chemically defined medium, bind IGF-I [5,6]. Preincubation of each of these two cell types with increasing concentration of IGF-I, results in the downregulation of about 40% of the type 1 IGF receptors in vitro under our culture conditions [5]. In addition, when Leydig cells are incubated with increasing concentration of hCG, there is an upregulation of type 1 IGF receptors in both pig [7] and rat [8], apart from the classical complete downregulation of hCG receptors [7]. Furthermore IGF-I upregulates in vitro both hCG binding sites on Leydig cell and FSH binding sites on Sertoli cells [5,6,8]. Therefore IGF-I binds to the somatic testicular cells in vitro and IGF type 1 receptors are hormonally regulated by the gonadotrophins. This reciprocal upregulation of IGF-I on the gonadotrophins receptors, and of the gonadotrophins on IGF type 1 receptor, adds evidences to the cooperation between the somatotroph and the gonadotroph functions.

IGF-I secretion by the male gonad

Both IGF-I-like material and IGF-I transcripts have been documented in steroidogenic tissues, that is the gonad and the adrenal [9,10]. IGF-I mRNA are expressed in human tissues during fetal life [11]. Further evidence that differentiated somatic cells from the male gonad are capable of secreting IGF-I in vitro, was obtained in several laboratories. We have shown that porcine Sertoli cells grown in primary culture under chemically defined conditions, secreted immunoreactive IGF-I material [12]. Both Leydig and Sertoli cells isolated from porcine and grown in vitro in a serum-free chemically defined medium secrete IGF-I-like material [13,14]. These data document that IGF-I gene is being expressed in steroidogenic cells and that IGF-I is secreted in steroidogenic tissues. We have shown that when pig Sertoli cells are cultured in bicameral chambers in vitro, there is an opposite secretion of IGF-I and its binding proteins [15]. FSH increases IGF-I secretion at the basal compartment, whereas most of the IGF binding proteins (IGFBPs) with apparent molecular size of 39–43, 34, 29 and 24 kDa are secreted at the apical compartment, IGFBP-3 secretion also being stimulated by FSH [15].

The conditions of IGF-I regulation in steroidogenic cells has been well documented. IGF-I secretion by porcine Leydig cells in vitro is little, if any, stimulated by GH. On contrast both bFGF and EGF, two growth factors that are being expressed by the gonadal tissue, are potent stimulators of IGF-I secretion in vitro. Furthermore, although hCG/LH has no direct effect on IGF-I secretion, it dramatically potentiates the secretion induced by bFGF. Furthermore, when these experiments are conducted in the presence of insulin, there is a further potentiation of IGF-I secretion in vitro. The phenomenon is analogous with FSH and Sertoli cells [14]. In addition, when Sertoli and Leydig cells are cocultured there is a potentiation of IGF-I secreted in vitro, the phenomenon being further stimulated by the gonadotrophins [14]. In the lit/lit mice GH deficient model, Mathews reports no significant in vivo effect of GH treatment on IGF-I mRNA level in the gonad, nor is there any significant decrease of IGF-I mRNA level in the gonad in the GH deficient, compared to the non-GH deficient, lit/lit mice [10]. In contrast GH is clearly controlling the IGF-I mRNA in the liver. These data, combined with our in vitro porcine Leydig and Sertoli cells data, sustain the concept that GH does not seem to be a major IGF-I gene regulator in the male gonad.

These findings provide strong evidence that in the male gonad there is a paracrine regulation and an endocrine modulation of IGF-I secretion, involving local growth factors, trophic hormones LH and FSH and insulin, but seemingly with little direct influence of GH. Still it is possible that the liver production of IGF-I, clearly GH dependent, targets the gonad through the endocrine IGF-I compartment. Whether these experimental observations are relevant to in vivo human situation remains to be clarified.

IGF-I action on the male gonad

IGF-I acts on both porcine Sertoli and Leydig cells in vitro. On Sertoli cells, IGF-I increases FSH receptor number and responsiveness to FSH in vitro, by increasing cAMP response to FSH. IGF-I selectively stimulates spermatogonial DNA synthesis during rat spermatogenesis [16]. It is therefore tempting to postulate that the FSH dependent Sertoli cells produced apically secreted IGF-I contributes to spermatogenesis [15,16].

Pig Leydig cells are sensitive to IGF-I action in vitro and have been used to characterize both IGF-I actions and its molecular mechanisms [5,6,8,17]. When immature pig Leydig cells are cultured in chemically defined serum free medium without insulin at micromolar concentration, they lose within 3 days both hCG receptors and hCG responsiveness. Treatment with nanomolar concentration of IGF-I, results in normalization of these responses [17]. Furthermore when freshly isolated immature pig Leydig cells are cultured for 2 days in primary culture in the presence of nanomolar concentrations of IGF-I, there is a dramatic potentiation of responsiveness to hCG on both cAMP and testosterone [5,6,8]. This IGF-I effect results in an 8–10-fold increase in the steroidogenic Leydig cells response to hCG. IGF-I induces a rapid expression of proto-oncogenes c-*fos* and *jun*-B [18], increases mRNA for hCG receptor and increases hCG receptor number. Treatment with IGF-I seems to increases the activity of the protein and mRNA level of the two main enzymes steroidogenic, p450SCC, p450-I7-α, but has little effect on the 3-β-hydroxysteroid dehydrogenase. These effects of IGF-I result in a final maturation of Leydig cells function, switching under IGF-I action from a prepubertal to a fully mature pattern of response to hCG.

We have verified that a part of these in vitro actions of IGF-I on Leydig cells, were observed in vivo by using the Snell dwarf prepubertal male mice. The Snell dwarf mice present severe GH insufficiency due to Pit-1 gene point mutation. They develop both a severe growth retardation and a delayed puberty. We have treated these mice with either human recombinant GH, IGF-I or saline for 7 days with three subcutaneous injections per day. The mice were then given an acute hCG test on day 8 [19]. Both hGH and IGF-I treatments induced a significant increase in total body weight, T weight and size gain compared to controls. Furthermore IGF-I treatment, as GH, significantly increased both the testosterone response to hCG and the hCG receptor number. These results show that IGF-I, in vivo as in vitro, is inducing and maintaining the differentiated function of Leydig cells and that most GH effects on the T are mediated through IGF-I [19].

The mechanisms by which IGF-I induce these changes are multiple and point to a pleiotropic effect of IGF-I within the steroidogenic cells, involving regulation of specific receptors, potentiation of transduction mechanisms of the signal and control of the level of expression of key steroidogenic enzymes.

Conclusion

The male gonad is a target for IGF-I. IGF-I is a testicular growth factor involved in the final differentiation and maintenance of both somatic male gonadal cells, Leydig and Sertoli cells. IGF-I is probably necessary for a normal expression and maintenance of the endocrine function of the male gonad. It could possibly contribute to the expression of a normal reproductive function as well. IGF-I is acting as an autocrine or paracrine testicular factor, regulated by local growth factors and modulated by the gonadotropins and insulin. This does not exclude the endocrine GH dependent action. These data have potential therapeutic implications. IGF-I treatment will target the endocrine T and possibly spermatogenesis. Although this might open the field wider for potential IGF-I therapy, it should be kept in mind and evaluated in clinical situations where IGF-I treatment could be used in conditions other than substitution therapy, including when it will aim at targeting other organs than the T.

References

1. Laron Z, Sarel R, Fertzelan A. Eur J Pediatr 1980;134:79–83.
2. Kulin HE, Samojlik E, Santen R, Santner S. Clin Endocrinol 1981;15:462–472.
3. Hochereau-de Reviers MT, de Reviers MM, Monet-Kuntz C, Perreau C, Fontaine I, Viguier-Martinez MC. Acta Endocrinol 1987;115:399–405.
4. Handelsman DHJ, Spaliviero JA, Scott CD, Baxter R. Acta Endocrinol 1985;109:543–549.
5. Bernier M, Chatelain P, Mather JP, Saez JM. J Cell Physiol 1986;129:257–263.
6. Perrard-Sapori MH, Chatelain P, Jaillard C, Saez JM. Eur J Biochem 1987;165:209–214.
7. Lin T, Blaisdell J, Haskell JF. Endocrinology 1988;123:134–139.
8. Saez JM, Chatelain P, Perrad-Sapori MH, Jaillard C, Naville D. Reprod Nutr Dev 1988;28:989–

1008.

9. D'Ercole Al, Stiles AD, Underwood LE. Proc Natl Acad Sci USA 1984;81:936–939.
10. Mathews LS, Norstedt G, Palmiter RD. Proc Nat Acad Sci USA 1986;83:9343–9347.
11. Han VKM, D'Ercole AJ, Lund P. Science 1987;236:193–196.
12. Chatelain P, Naville D, Saez JM. Biochem Biophys Res Commun 1987;146:1009–1017.
13. Chatelain P, Naville D, Avallet O, Penhoat A, Jaillard C, Sanchez P, JM Saez. Acta Pediatr Scand 1991;372(suppl);92–95.
14. Naville D, Chatelain P, Avallet O, Saez JM. Mol Cell Endocrinol 1990;70:217–224.
15. Skalli M, Avalet O, Vigier M, Saez JM. Endocrinology 1992;131:985–987.
16. Soder O, Bang F, Wahab A, Farvinen M. Endocrinology 1992;131:2344–2350.
17. Avallet O, Vigier M, Chatelain P, Saez JM. J Steriod Biochem 1991;40:453–464.
18. Hall S, Berthelon MC, Avallet O, Saez JM. Endocrinology 1991;129:1243–1249.
19. Chatelain P, Sanchez P, Saez JM. Endocrinology 1991;128:1857–1862.

The IGF axis in prostatic disease

Pinchas Cohen[1], Donna M. Peehl[4], Ajay Bhala[1], Gangi Dong[1], Raymond L. Hintz[3]
and Ron G. Rosenfeld[2]

[1]*Department of Pediatrics, University of Pennsylvania School of Medicine;* [2]*Department of Pediatrics,
Oregon Health Sciences University; and* [3]*Departments of Pediatrics and* [4]*Urology, Stanford University
Medical Center, Philadelphia, PA 19104, USA*

Abstract. The insulin-like growth factor (IGF) axis is a multi-component network of molecules involved
in the regulation of cell growth. The axis includes two major ligands, (IGF-I and IGF-II), cell surface
receptors, (the type 1 IGF receptor family as well as the type 2 IGF receptor), a family of high affinity
binding proteins which regulate IGF availability to the receptors, (the IGFBPs), and a group of IGFBP
proteases which cleave IGFBPs and modulate IGF action.

We have studied the role of the IGF axis in the autocrine-paracrine control of normal and neoplastic
prostatic cell growth. Human seminal plasma contains IGFs, IGFBPs and IGFBP protease activity. A
prostatic source for these IGF-axis molecules is likely. We have demonstrated the human prostate to
contain all the elements of a functional IGF system. Prostate stromal cells in primary culture (PC-S)
express mRNA for IGF-II and produce high molecular weight (15 kDa) IGF-II peptide in biologically
active concentrations. Prostate epithelial cells in primary culture (PC-E) and PC-S express the type 1 IGF
receptor. PC-E also produce IGFBP-2 and -4, (on both mRNA and peptide levels), while PC-S secrete
IGFBP-2, -3 and -4. PC-E are exquisitely sensitive to the mitogenic effects of IGFs.

Additionally, prostate specific antigen (PSA), secreted from PC-E in vivo and found in seminal
plasma, can function as a potent IGFBP protease. PSA proteolysis reduces the affinity of IGFBP-3 to IGFs
and can remove the inhibitory effects of IGFBP-3 on IGF induced PC-E growth.

We have been able to identify several abnormalities in the IGF axis in the serum of patients with
prostate cancer. Compared to age matched controls, serum from patients with prostate cancer displayed
elevations of IGFBP-2 levels, as well as reduction of intact IGFBP-3 levels associated with a serum
IGFBP-3 protease activity which is distinct from PSA. However, PC-E and PC-S from cancer sources
showed no differences in the expression of IGF axis molecules relative to normal prostate cells.

Finally, when PC-S from patients with benign prostatic hypertrophy (BPH) were compared to normals,
several IGF axis molecules were abnormally expressed. Ten-fold hyper-expression of the mRNA for IGF-
II was noted, but was not associated with increased IGF-II peptide secretion. PC-S BPH IGFBP-2 peptide
and mRNA levels were significantly decreased. CM from BPH PC-S displayed the presence of a 29 kDa
IGFBP-5 doublet not seen in normal PC-S CM. These cells also displayed increased levels of the mRNA
for the type 1 IGF receptor. These observations suggest that alterations to the prostatic IGF axis in BPH
patients may be involved in the pathogenesis of abnormal stromal-epithelial interactions contributing to
the development of BPH.

Address for correspondence: Pinchas Cohen, M.D., Assistant Professor of Pediatrics, Division of
Endocrinology, Department of Pediatrics, University of Pennsylvania, Children's Hospital of Philadelphia,
34th and Civic Center Blvd., Philadelphia, PA 19104, USA. Tel.: +1-215-590-3420. Fax: +1-215-590-
3053.

The insulin-like growth factor (IGF) axis

The IGF axis is a multi-component network of molecules involved in the regulation of cell growth. This axis includes two major ligands, IGF-I and IGF-II [1], cell surface receptors, which include the type 1 IGF receptor family and the type 2 IGF receptor [2], a family of high affinity binding proteins, the IGFBPs, which regulate IGF availability to the receptors [3], a group of IGFBP proteases which cleave IGFBPs and modulate IGF action [4] and cell membrane binding sites for the IGFBPs which may mediate the IGF-independent actions of the IGFBPs. The IGFs, their receptors and their binding proteins participate in endocrine as well as autocrine-paracrine growth processes and may be involved in neoplastic transformation [1–3]. A scheme of this complex systems is shown in Fig. 1.

IGF production and expression by normal prostate cells

The human prostate differs considerably from the prostates of most animals in embryologic development, adult anatomy and spectrum of disease. However, because of these dissimilarities, animal models may be inadequate for the study of human prostate growth and an in vitro culture system for human prostate cells is essential for evaluation of the biological parameters of prostate disease. Pure populations of cultured epithelial (PC-E) or fibroblastic cells (PC-F) obtained from radical prostatectomy specimens have been developed [5].

We have succeeded in identifying endogenous IGF production by cultured prostate

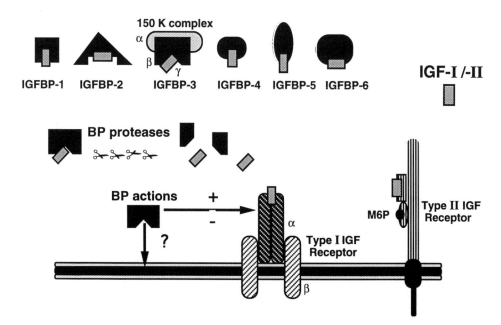

Fig. 1. The IGF axis. Details in text.

cells, employing a variety of experimental approaches. Conditioned media (CM) from PC-E and PC-F obtained from normal prostate tissues and propagated in primary culture under serum-free conditions were acid chromatographed on a G-50 column to remove IGFBPs and then radioimmunoassayed for IGF-I and IGF-II. IGF-I levels were below the limit of detection (<0.05 ng/ml) in both fluids [6].

On the other hand, while IGF-II levels were undetected in CM from PC-E, IGF-II levels of 2–5 ng/ml were present in the CM of the five strains of normal prostate fibroblasts that were tested.

Northern blots of polyA+ RNA from five strains of normal PC-F showed the presence of abundant IGF-II message (not seen in PC-E). Ribonuclease protection assays for IGF-I mRNA were negative regarding its presence in PC-E and PC-F.

Thus, at least within our culture system, IGF-I is not normally produced by prostate cells, but IGF-II is expressed and secreted by prostate stromal cells at physiological active concentrations.

The finding of IGF-II production by adult prostatic fibroblasts is potentially important. Of interest is the fact that the IGF-II produced by prostate fibroblasts appears to be of a high molecular weight (15 kDa) variety. Similar high molecular weight forms have been reported in the sera of patients with tumors associated with hypoglycemia and in several tumor cell lines [7].

IGF receptors in normal PC-E

To evaluate the mechanisms by which IGFs exert their effects in the prostate, we evaluated IGF binding to prostate epithelial cell membranes. Crude membranes preparations were isolated from PC-E and cross-linked to ^{125}I-IGF-I or ^{125}I-IGF-II in the presence (nonspecific binding or NSB) or absence (B_0) of excess peptides, under both reducing and nonreducing conditions. In autoradiographs of a 6% SDS-PAGE the type 2 IGF receptor was not detectable. The type 1 IGF receptor, however, was abundant in PC-E and PC-F membranes [6]. RNAase protection assays for both receptor mRNAs confirmed these findings on the molecular level, with detection of mRNA for the type 1, but not the type 2 receptor.

IGFBPs in normal prostate cells

We further investigated prostate cells for a possible role of IGFBPs in modulating IGF action and bioavailability within the prostate. Conditioned media from PC-E was subjected to Western ligand blotting (WLB), which disclosed the presence of two major IGFBPs of 24 kDa and 31 kDa [8]. These proteins were nonglycosylated and were identified by sizing and immunologic characteristics to be IGFBP-2 and IGFBP-4. Interestingly, these same two IGFBPs were present in seminal plasma and are likely to be of prostatic origin. Northern blots of mRNA isolated from PC-E demonstrated the presence of mRNA for IGFBP-2 and IGFBP-4, but neither IGFBP-1 nor IGFBP-3. In PC-F CM, we have shown, by the WLB technique, that IGFBP-2, IGFBP-4 and IGFBP-3 are present; unlike PC-E, PC-F produce IGFBP-4 in both the glycosylated (28 kDa) and the nonglycosylated (24 kDa) forms [6]. Northern blots of PC-F demonstrated expression of IGFBP-2, IGFBP-4 and IGFBP-3 mRNA, but not IGFBP-1.

Treatment of PC-E cultures with various growth factors and media additives known to stimulate PC-E growth, did not significantly alter IGFBP-2 or IGFBP-4 secretion or induce the production of additional IGFBPs. IGFBPs appear to be constitutively produced by prostate epithelial cells and may modulate IGF action at the cellular level. It is of great interest that in the prostate carcinoma cell line PC-3, we documented serum-free CM to contain only IGFBP-4, but not IGFBP-2. It remains to be determined if this phenomenon has oncological significance.

IGF action in normal PC-E

To evaluate the role of IGFs in stimulating prostate epithelial cell growth, we performed clonal growth assays on PC-E cultures maintained under serum-free conditions, with and without increasing concentrations of insulin, IGF-I or IGF-II. While only superphysiological concentrations of insulin stimulated PC-E growth, IGF-I and IGF-II were effective at concentrations often found in biological fluids. In fact, PC-E were exquisitely sensitive to IGF-I, with a maximal effect reached at 10 ng/ml and a half maximal effect at 0.1 ng/ml. IGF-II was also highly effective in PC-E stimulation, with a half maximal effect at approximately 1 ng/ml [6]. This relative efficacy of the three growth factors which stimulate PC-E growth (IGF-I>IGF-II>>insulin) is identical to the reported affinity of these ligands for the type 1 IGF receptor. It appears, therefore, that IGF stimulation of PC-E occurs through the type 1 IGF receptor and that both IGF-I and IGF-II are capable of performing this task at physiological concentrations.

PSA as a IGFBP-3 protease

Since human seminal fluid contains prostatic secretions, we postulated that the seminal plasma milieu is at least partially a reflection of the in vivo extracellular prostatic environment. We have shown earlier that IGFBP-2 and IGFBP-4 are the two IGFBPs found in seminal plasma and that they are also the ones produced by PC-E. While IGFBP-3 is produced by PC-F, no IGFBP-3 is detectable in seminal plasma by WLB. However, radioimmunoassay for IGFBP-3 in seminal plasma demonstrated significant amounts (approximately 200 ng/ml). Since this situation was analogous to that observed in pregnancy serum, we employed our newly developed IGFBP protease assay to detect any IGFBP-3 protease activity in seminal plasma. ^{125}I-IGFBP-3 was degraded by adding pregnancy serum, seminal plasma or PSA, but not by nonpregnant serum or prostate cell conditioned media [9].

Comparison of the dose response of purified PSA to that of seminal plasma titrated to the same PSA concentrations as the purified PSA, revealed identity of the IGFBP-3 protease activity. IGFBP-3 protease activity was detected in all of the 20 seminal plasma samples tested and was unchanged in azospermic samples. Thus, PSA is an IGFBP-3 protease normally occurring in seminal plasma in high concentrations. Coincubation experiments revealed that PSA has no proteolytic effect on IGFBP-2 and only a minimal effect on IGFBP-1 and IGFBP-4. These and other characteristics clearly distinguished PSA from the pregnancy-associated and other IGFBP proteases recently described [10–12]. PSA is the first chemically-defined IGFBP-3 protease identified in a biological fluid. In addition, using immunoprecipitation with a specific IGFBP-3 antibody developed in our laboratory, followed by SDS-PAGE, we have documented that seminal plasma contains IGFBP-3 fragments with a molecular weight of approximately 25 kDa. These IGFBP-3 fragments are identical to the fragments generated in vitro when recombinant-glycosylated IGFBP-3 is cleaved by PSA and subjected to the same electrophoresis methodology. We therefore conclude that PSA acts as a specific IGFBP-3 protease in vivo. In order to demonstrate a biological role for PSA as an IGFBP-3 protease, we incubated recombinant IGFBP-3 with and without PSA and crossed-linked it to ^{125}I-IGF-I or 125I-IGF-II in the presence or absence of increasing concentrations of each peptide. After subjection to SDS-PAGE and densitometric analysis, displacement curves for IGF-I and IGF-II were generated for both intact and cleaved IGFBP-3. Cleavage of IGFBP-3 by PSA caused a modest decrease in the affinity of IGFBP-3 fragments for IGF-II, but the affinity of IGF-I for the PSA-derived IGFBP-3 cleavage products fell by an order of magnitude.

This represent an important mechanism by which PSA can enhance IGF action, since decreased affinity of a PSA-generated IGFBP-3 fragment for IGFs will result in an increased availability of free IGF to interact with the IGF receptor. In order to test the latter theory at the prostate epithelial cell level, we performed clonal assays for PC-E growth in the presence and absence of IGF, IGFBP-3 and exogenous PSA. It should be noted that PC-E in our culture system do not produce substantial amounts of any of these three proteins. However, in vivo, prostate epithelial cells produce PSA and prostate fibroblasts (based on our in vitro data) presumably secrete IGFBP-3 and IGF-II, which would be available for the epithelial cells.

Compared with cells grown under serum-free conditions without insulin or IGFs for 5 days, cells grown in the presence of submaximally-stimulating concentrations of IGFs doubled their growth rate. The addition of IGFBP-3 at concentrations of 200 ng/ml had no effect when added alone. However, IGFBP-3 completely blocked the stimulatory effects of simultaneously added IGFs. The most noteworthy phenomenon observed in this experiment was that when cells were grown in the presence of PSA, IGFBP-3 and IGFs, PSA was able to reverse the inhibitory effects of IGFBP-3 on IGF stimulated PC-E growth [13]. It appears, therefore, that PSA functions as a PC-E growth enhancer in the presence of IGFs and IGFBP-3 (as found in serum), by a mechanism directly related to its IGFBP-3 protease characteristics. The system of IGF related molecules and their interactions within the prostate are shown in Fig. 2.

374

The IGF axis in prostate cancer

To assess whether patients with prostate carcinoma have alterations in serum IGFBPs related to the production of IGFBPs by their tumors, we performed WLB and IGFBP-2 RIA on serum samples from 32 patients with prostate carcinoma of various degrees of clinical severity and compared them to results in 16 healthy, age-matched controls. We have also measured serum IGF-I and IGF-II by RIA and assessed the presence of IGFBP-3 protease activity in the serum of these subjects. The mean level of IGFBP-2 in the prostate cancer patients was 170% of control levels by WLB analysis and 195% of control levels by RIA (p < 0.01). The degree of elevation of IGFBP-2 was related to the stage of the tumor and to the levels of the serum tumor marker, prostate specific antigen (PSA) [14]. We also noted the presence of an IGFBP-3 protease activity in the serum of three out of five patients with prostate carcinoma and low serum IGFBP-3 by WLB, but no protease activity was noted in patients with intact serum IGFBP-3 by WLB. Of interest is that the cleavage pattern of IGFBP-3 by prostate cancer serum was different than PSA and similar to pregnancy serum and other sera of cancer patients. Others have also shown that IGFBP-2 and IGFBP-3 levels change in prostate cancer serum in relation to the PSA levels [15]. Serum IGF-I, IGF-II and IGFBP-3 levels, measured by RIA, were not different among the subjects with cancer and the normal controls. We concluded that patients with prostate carcinoma showed significant alterations in their serum IGFBPs. We speculated that prostate derived IGF axis molecules may be secreted by prostate tumors.

The IGF axis in BPH

Comparing cultured prostate cells from patients with normal prostate histology and

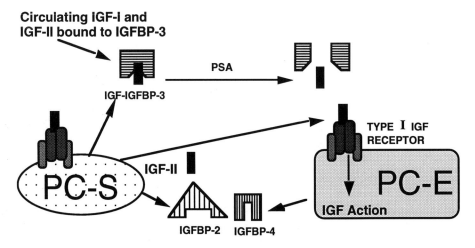

Fig. 2. The IGF axis in the prostate. Details in text.

from patients with benign prostatic hypertrophy (BPH), we evaluated some components of the IGF axis. Preliminary data suggests that prostate epithelial cells from BPH patients respond normally to IGFs. However, prostate fibroblasts appear to harbor IGF axis abnormalities. We evaluated IGF-II mRNA levels in six strains of BPH fibroblasts compared with six normal strains and found the expression of IGF-II mRNA to be 10-fold higher in fibroblasts isolated from BPH tissues as compared to controls [8]. However, the levels of IGF-II peptide in the conditioned media of these cells was not different. When we studied the IGFBPs secreted into the conditioned media of normal PC-S cells we were able to demonstrate IGFBP-2, IGFBP-3, and IGFBP-4. The conditioned media of BPH PC-S was dramatically different. IGFBP-2 was reduced and IGFBP-5 appearing as a 29 kDa doublet was seen instead. The mRNA of these IGFBPs followed a similar pattern [16]. Furthermore, when studying the expression of the type 1 IGF receptor in PC-S, we were able to demonstrate, using RT-PCR methods, that BPH strains expressed 2–3-fold more IGF-R mRNA than normal strains of PC-S. Experiments are in progress to identify further abnormalities in these cells.

These dramatic findings suggests a role for the IGF axis in the pathogenesis of BPH. As seen in Fig. 3, this set of abnormalities in the IGF axis can serve as an autocrine-paracrine loop mediating abnormal growth of prostates in the BPH population. While it is obvious that increased levels of IGF-II and the type 1 IGF-R can mediate an autocrine loop of growth stimulation in BPH, we propose a mechanism by which PC-E, (who themselves do not harbor a molecular defect in the IGF system), are stimulated to grow by the adjacent PC-S abnormally expressing IGF axis components. It should be noted that limited information is available on the biological effects of IGFBPs, but it is clear that IGFBP-2 has inhibitory effects on IGF action. IGFBP-5 on the other hand has recently been reported to be an IGF

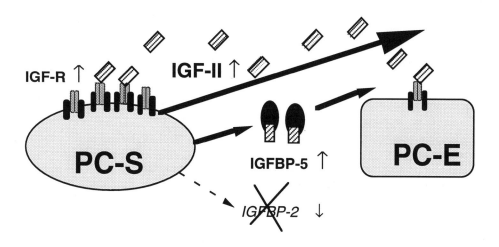

Fig. 3. The IGF axis in BPH. Details in text.

enhancing IGFBP and to promote mitogenesis of osteoblasts in the presence of IGFs [17]. By this scheme, we propose that the IGF-II produced in the BPH PC-S is not only increased in toto, but is bound to IGFBP-5 rather than to IGFBP-2, thus delivering an increased mitogenic message to the PC-E.

Summary

We have established the presence of a fully functioning IGF axis within the prostate. This axis includes the prostate epithelial cells, which bind and respond to IGFs through the type 1 IGF receptor and secrete IGFBP-2 and IGFBP-4. The prostate fibroblasts, in turn, secrete high molecular weight IGF-II, as well as IGFBP-2, -3 and -4. Prostate specific antigen, present in PC-E in vivo, is an IGFBP-3 protease and is capable of stimulating prostate epithelial cell growth in vitro by cleavage of IGFBP-3 and enhancement of IGF action. In addition, prostatic cells are subject to circulating IGF-I and IGF-II, which are transported in serum complexed to IGFBPs, particularly IGFBP-3. We have identified abnormalities in the serum of patients with prostate cancer. Compared to age matched controls, serum from patients with prostate cancer displayed elevations of IGFBP-2 levels, as well as reduction of intact IGFBP-3 levels associated with a serum IGFBP-3 protease activity which is distinct from PSA. Finally, when PC-S from patients with benign prostatic hypertrophy (BPH) where compared to normals, several IGF axis molecules where abnormally expressed including IGF-II, IGF-R and IGFBP-5 which displayed increased mRNA expression and IGFBP-2 which showed decreased gene and peptide expression. These observations suggest that alterations of the prostatic IGF axis in BPH patients may be involved in the pathogenesis of abnormal stromal-epithelial interactions contributing to the development of BPH.

Acknowledgements

Supported in part by Grants 1RO1 DK47591-01 (PC) and 1RO1 CA58110-01 (RGR).

References

1. Rotwein P. Growth Factors 1991;5:3—18.
2. Neely EK, Beukers MW, Oh Y, Cohen P, Rosenfeld RG. Pediatr Scand 1991;372(suppl):116—123.
3. Lamson G, Giudice LC, Rosenfeld RG. Growth Factors 1991;5:19—28.
4. Cohen P, Fielder PJ, Hasegawa Y, Frisch H, Giudice LC, Rosenfeld RG. Acta Endocrinol (Copenh) 1991;124(suppl 2):74—85.
5. Peehl D. Freshney RI (ed) Culture of Specialized Cells. New York; John Wiley & Sons Inc., 1992; 159—180.
6. Cohen P, Peehl DM, Lamson G, Rosenfeld RG. J Clin Endocrinol Metab 1991;73:401—407.
7. Shapiro ET, Polansky KS, Rubinstein AH, Mew MC, Tager HS. J Clin Invest 1990;85:1672—1679.
8. Cohen P, Peele DM, Hintz RL, Rosenfeld RG. Clin Res 1992;40:93a.

9. Cohen P, Graves HCB, Peehl DM, Kamarei M, Giudice LC, Rosenfeld RG. J Clin Endocrinol Metab 1992;73:491—407.
10. Lamson G, Cohen P, Guidice LC, Fielder PJ, Oh Y, Hintz RL, Rosenfeld RG. Growth Reg 1993;3: 91—95.
11. Giudice LC, Farrell EM, Pham H, Lamson G, Rosenfeld RG. J Clin Endocrinol Metab 1990;71:806—816.
12. Davies SC, Wass JA, Ross RJ, Cotterill AM, Buchanan CR, Coulson VJ, Holly JM. J Endocrinol 1991;130:469—473.
13. Cohen P, Peehl DM, Graves HCB, Rosenfeld RG. Biological effects of prostate specific antigen (PSA) as an IGF binding protein-3 (IGFBP-3) protease. J Endocrinol 1994 (in press).
14. Cohen P, Peehl DM, Stamey TA, Wilson K, Clemmons DR, Rosenfeld RG. J Clin Endocrinol Metab 1993;76:830—835.
15. Kanety H, Madjar Y, Dagan Y, Levi J, Papa MZ, Pariente C, Goldwasser B, Karasik A. J Clin Endocrinol Metab 1993;77:229—233.
16. Cohen P, Peele DM, Hintz RL, Rosenfeld RG. Insulin-like growth factor axis abnormalities in cultures of prostate stromal cells from patients with benign prostatic hypertrophy. Proceedings of the Endocrine Society Meetings 1993.
17. Andress DL, Birnbaum RS. J Biol Chem 1992;267:22467—22472.
18. Cohen P, Vu T, Peele DM, Rosenfeld RG, Hoffman AR. Increased expression of the IGF-I receptor in BPH. Proceedings of the ADA Meeting 1993.

In vivo actions

The somatomedin hypothesis revisited: differential effects of growth hormone and IGF-I on skeletal growth of the rat in vivo

J. Zapf[1] and E.B. Hunziker[2]

[1]*Department of Medicine, University Hospital, CH-8091 Zürich; and* [2]*M.E. Müller Institute of Biomechanics, University of Bern, CH-3010 Bern, Switzerland*

Abstract. The extended somatomedin hypothesis postulates that IGF-I mediates GH actions on skeletal growth, via auto/paracrine besides endocrine mechanisms. We have compared the effects of s.c.-infused GH and IGF-I on differentiation of tibial epiphyseal growth plate cartilage in hypophysectomized rats. Both hormones increase cell structural parameters equipotently, but GH reduces cell cycle times and enhances cell productivity more effectively at all differentiation stages. This data supports the extended somatomedin hypothesis. Since infused IGF-I acts on proliferative chondrocytes by shortening cycle time rather than by "clonal expansion", the "dual effector theory" does not hold true in vivo.

The original somatomedin hypothesis [1] postulated that growth hormone (GH) did not act directly to stimulate growth of skeletal tissues, but that its effects were mediated by a serum factor termed somatomedin, and later IGF-I, which is synthesized and secreted by the liver under the influence of GH [2]. Although this concept was supported by many studies [3], experimental evidence has accumulated that GH acts "directly" on peripheral tissues and above all on growth plate chondrocytes to stimulate growth. This has led to a modification and extension of the original somatomedin hypothesis. Besides endocrine effects of circulating IGF-I, the extended hypothesis now includes peripheral effects of GH which are mediated via local production of IGF-I by auto/paracrine mechanisms [4—6]. Further data derived from in vitro investigations using chondrocyte subpopulations have indicated that IGF-I influences chondrocytes principally during the proliferative phase by stimulating "clonal expansion", whereas GH acts selectively upon stem cells as a differentiation factor and that the subsequent effect on proliferation is triggered by local production of IGF-I ("dual effector theory") [7,8].

To date, analyses of IGF-I or GH effects in vivo, have been restricted to the measurement of bulk parameters such as growth plate width, matrix production (^{35}S incorporation) or accumulated bone growth [9—11]. We have therefore tried to analyze the physiological mechanisms by which IGF-I and GH act on growth plate chondrocytes in vivo at various stages of differentiation. To this end, recombinant human (rh) IGF-I or rhGH were continuously infused by subcutaneously implanted mini osmotic pumps. Cell proliferative activity, cell height and volume and net matrix production were investigated for each phase of the chondrocyte life cycle using stereological, autoradiographic and fluorescence microscopic techniques. In addition, the molecular size distribution in serum of infused and endogenous IGF-I and of IGF binding proteins (IGFBPs) was studied and the distribution patterns were compared with the effects of the two hormones on chondrocyte performance and growth.

Materials and Methods

Two weeks after hypophysectomy of 35 day old male Wistar rats, mini osmotic pumps were implanted subcutaneously in the abdominal region and rhIGF-I or rhGH were infused at a rate of 300 µg/rat × day and 200 mU/rat × day, respectively, during 8 days. Saline-infused hypophysectomized (hypox) rats served as controls. After 8 days of infusion, animals were bled by aortic puncture. Serum was stored at –20°C until used for analysis. Growth rate, proliferating cell pool sizes and matrix production as well as cell activities and cell kinetics were determined as described [12]. Stereology, fluorescence microscopy and autoradiography were performed according to established methods [12].

Molecular size distribution of IGF-I and IGFBPs was determined by fractionation of sera on a Sephadex G-200 column at neutral pH. Immunoreactive (ir) IGF-I in pooled serum fractions was measured by radioimmunoassay after SepPak C_{18} chromatography [13], using either rh or rat IGF-I (kindly provided by Dr. M. Kobayashi, Fujisawa, Japan) as standards. IGFBPs were analyzed by Western ligand blotting [13,14].

Results

Serum parameters

Serum levels of glucose, free thyroxine (FT_4), testosterone and immunoreactive (ir) IGF-I were significantly decreased in hypox rats (Table 1). Serum glucose, FT_4 and testosterone did not change during IGF-I or GH treatment. GH treatment raised endogenous IGF-I ~8-fold to 50% of normal, IGF-I infusion caused a 5-fold increase of the total (endogenous rat and rh) IGF-I. The in vitro potencies of rh and rat IGF-I in stimulating methyl-^{3}H-thymidine incorporation in BALB/c3T3 fibroblasts are identical [15].

Bulk parameters

As shown earlier [9,11] IGF-I, like GH, caused a significant increase in body weight. When expressed per 100 g rat, the relative increase in body weight was normalized by GH (0.21), but not by IGF-I (0.13, calculated from Table 2). Similarly, total growth plate height and longitudinal growth rate were stimulated in the hormone-treated animals, but GH was more effective (Table 2). The increase in growth plate height was due to an increase of the height of the proliferative and hypertrophic

Table 1. Serum glucose and hormone levels of normal, saline- and hormone-treated hypophysectomized rats (n = 6/group), from [12]

	Hypophysectomized rats			Normal rats (age-matched)
	NaCl (control)	IGF-I (300 μg/d)	GH (200 mU/d)	
Glucose (mmol/l)	5.8 ± 1.1	5.5 ± 0.6	6.5 ± 0.5	13.2 ± 2.6
Free thyroxine (pmol/l)	3.6 ± 0.5	3.2 ± 0.7	3.2 ± 0.9	48.5 ± 15.2
Testosterone (nmol/l)	<0.4	<0.4	<0.4	1.0 ± 0.5
irIGF (ng/ml)[a]	106 ± 32	412[a] ± 128	887 ± 196	1,771 ± 228

Mean values ± SD for six animals are represented; [a]IGF-I was determined against a rhIGF-I standard in the IGF-I-infused group and against a rat IGF-I standard in the three other experimental groups. Since rat IGF-I does not cross-react in our human IGF-I-RIA, the total IGF-I level in the IGF-I-infused rats is 412 + 106 = 518 ng/ml.

zones, whereas the height of the resting zone was unaltered (Table 2). In contrast, and as observed earlier [11], IGF-I infusion had more pronounced effects than GH on kidney, thymus and spleen weights (Table 3). Liver weight did not increase under IGF-I infusion, but was restored to normal by GH when expressed per 100 g body weight. Thus, IGF-I and GH have differential effects on different organs.

Cell structural characteristics

Mean cell height and cell volume did not differ significantly in the stem cell phase between the four experimental groups (Fig. 1A and B). However, both IGF-I and GH caused a comparable increase in mean cell height and cell volume in the proliferative

Table 2. Body weight, longitudinal growth rate and growth plate height of normal, saline- and hormone-treated hypophysectomized rats (n = 6/group), from [12]

	Hypophysectomized rats			Normal rats (age matched)
	NaCl (control)	IGF-I (300 μg/d)	GH (200 mU/d)	
Body weight				
— onset of exp.	128 (2%)	126 (2%)	123 (3%)	241 (1%)
— End of exp.	121 (2%)	145 (2%)	156 (4%)	302 (2%)
Total growth plate height (μm)	244 (2%)	380 (4%)	484 (2%)	401 (3%)
Longitudinal growth rate (μm/d)	31 (5%)	92 (7%)	163 (2%)	284 (4%)
Height (μm) of				
— resting zone	33 (4%)	27 (11%)	31 (4%)	36 (5%)
— proliferating zone	97 (2%)	146 (3%)	174 (2%)	128 (3%)
— hypertrophic zone	114 (2%)	207 (3%)	279 (1%)	237 (1%)

Mean values for six animals are represented; coefficients of error are given in parentheses.

Table 3. Organ weights of normal, saline- and hormone-treated hypophysectomized rats (n = 6/group)

Organ	Hypophysectomized rats						Normal rats (age-matched)	
	NaCl (control)		IGF-I (300 μg/d)		GH (200 mU/d)			
	g	mg/100 g bw	g	mg/100 g bw	g	mg/100 g bw	g	mg/100 g bw
Heart	0.36 (4%)	2.98	0.45 (3%)	3.10	0.42 (5%)	2.69	0.907 (4%)	3.00
Liver	4.30 (5%)	35.50	5.20 (3%)	35.80	7.20 (4%)	46.10	15.10 (3%)	50.00
Spleen	0.28 (13%)	2.31	0.51 (3%)	3.51	0.40 (5%)	2.56	0.854 (4%)	2.83
Thymus	0.38 (9%)	1.79	0.71 (5%)	4.90	0.64 (4%)	4.10	1.17 (5%)	3.87
Kidneys	0.70 (2%)	5.79	0.96 (2%)	6.62	0.85 (4%)	5.45	2.02 (4%)	6.69

Mean values for six animals are represented; coefficient of error are given in parentheses.

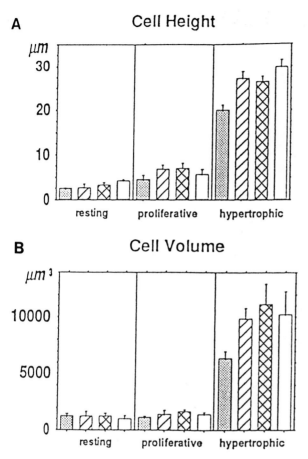

Fig. 1. Mean cell heights (A) and cell volumes (B) in the stem cell, proliferative and hypertrophic phases of growth plate chondrocytes of normal (□) and saline- (■), IGF-I- (▨) and GH- (▨) treated hypox rats (n = 6 for each group). No significant differences exist between the stem cell phases of the four groups. In the proliferative and hypertrophic phases, values for the normal and hormone-treated hypox groups differ significantly from the saline-treated hypox group, whereas no significant difference exists between the normal and the hormone-treated hypox groups (modified from [12]).

and hypertrophic phases. Most strikingly, the final cell height and cell volume in these two zones were the same as in normal age-matched animals (Fig 1A, B and Fig. 2).

In none of the three activity phases did the mean lateral cell diameter or the mean matrix production/cell differ significantly between hypox, hormone-treated hypox and normal animals (not shown). Quantitative ^{35}S-autoradiography of cartilage matrix showed that grain densities, and thus proteoglycan concentration, did not differ significantly between the proliferating and the hypertrophic zones or between the four different experimental groups (not shown).

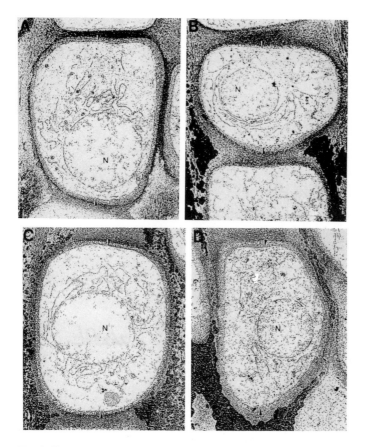

Fig. 2. Electron micrographs of vertical sections through hypertrophic growth plate chondrocytes of the proximal tibia of normal (A) and saline- (B), IGF-I- (C) and GH-treated hypox (D) rats. All pictures are represented at identical magnifications. N = nucleus, modified from [12].

Cell kinetics and cell productivity

In contrast to the steady state structural parameters, conspicuous differences in cell activity levels were found between the various treatment groups. These differences were due, above all, to modulations of the cell cycle time (mitotic activity) (Fig. 3A) and hence the kinetics of an axial column (Fig. 3B).

In normal rats, cell columns produced and eliminated 10 cells/day. Hypophysectomy reduced this number to one cell/day and treatment with IGF-I and GH increased it to three and six cells/day, respectively (Fig. 3B). This means that IGF-I and GH had dramatic effects on cell proliferation and productivity. This effect was most pronounced in the stem cell phase. Here, the cycle time, i.e., the time required for a resting cell to complete one mitosis, was increased from 6 days in normal rats to 50 days in hypox animals. IGF-I and GH shortened the prolonged cycle time to 15 and 8 days, respectively (Fig. 3A). IGF-I thus had a significant stimulatory effect upon

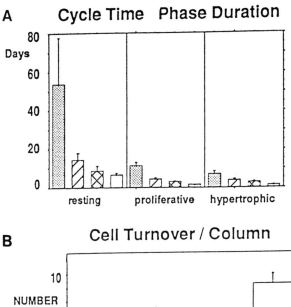

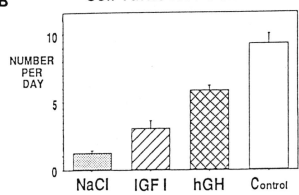

Fig. 3. Cycle time (phase duration) of stem, proliferative and hypertrophic cells (A) and cell turnover per column (number of chondrocytes produced and eliminated per day and per column) (B) of normal and saline-, IGF-I- and GH-treated hypox rats (symbols as in Fig. 1), from [12].

stem cell mitosis. GH nearly normalized this activity. Similar, although less dramatic effects of IGF-I and GH were observed on the cycling activity of the proliferating and on phase duration of the hypertrophic cell pool. In the proliferative phase, cycle time was reduced from 11 days in hypox animals to 4.5 and 3 days after IGF-I and GH treatment, respectively. During hypertrophy, phase duration decreased from 6 days to 4 and 2.8 days, respectively (Fig. 3A). Besides cell kinetics, the other main regulatory pathway subject to significant modulation is cell productivity. The major productivity parameters analyzed were increases in cell height, cell volume and net matrix production per unit of time (shown for cell height in Fig. 4). In the hypox group these values were reduced by a factor of around 10. Treatment with IGF-I and GH significantly increased productivity rates during all phases of differentiation, but again IGF-I was less effective than GH.

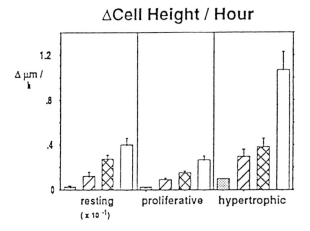

Fig. 4. Cell height increase/h (μm/h) of stem, proliferative and hypertrophic chondrocytes in the tibial growth plate of normal and saline-, IGF-I- and GH-treated hypox rats. All values differ significantly from one another (p < 0.05) in all four treatment groups (from [12]).

Discussion

According to the original somatomedin hypothesis, it should be possible to replace GH by its mediator IGF-I in growth-arrested states due to growth hormone deficiency. This postulate has been challenged by the "dual effector theory" [7,8,16] which states that GH is a prerequisite of cartilage maturation and thus of bone growth. According to this theory, priming of resting chondrocytes in the growth plate by GH is required for IGF-I, to promote "clonal expansion" of growth plate chondrocytes and to stimulate skeletal growth. Our study shows that the dual effector theory, which was derived from in vitro experiments, does not apply to the in vivo situation. Infused IGF-I, in the absence of GH, does not only stimulate longitudinal growth, as reflected by the enhanced growth rate of the proximal tibia, and growth of several organs, but also exerts distinct effects on each of the individual growth plate zones each of which represents a differentiation-specific cell pool. Although IGF-I is less effective than GH in stimulating longitudinal growth rate (Table 2), it restores total growth plate height and the height of the proliferating and the hypertrophic zone towards that of age-matched normal animals. Furthermore, both mean cell height and volume are restored to physiological values in the proliferating and hypertrophic activity phases not only by GH, but also by IGF-I (Fig. 1 and Fig. 2). Under physiological conditions, cell hypertrophy is the most efficient cellular process which contributes to bone elongation by controlled modulation of cell shape [17–19]. The pronounced differences between the growth rates achieved by IGF-I and GH are therefore not attributable to modulations in cell structural characteristics, but rather to differences in cell kinetics and cell productivity.

The relative increases in growth rate induced by IGF-I and GH (Table 2) are paralleled by proportional increases in cell activity not only in the proliferative and hypertrophic, but also in the stem cell phase. Thus, both IGF-I and GH exert their effects at each stage of differentiation rather than acting specifically upon particular subpopulations of cells at certain phases of chondrocyte differentiation, as postulated by the dual effector theory. Altogether, these findings tell us that exogeneously administered IGF-I in the absence of GH at least qualitatively imitates the effects of GH on skeletal growth and that these effects are compatible with an endocrine mechanism of action of the infused IGF-I. In this respect, the results obtained in this study agree with the original somatomedin hypothesis.

Nevertheless, our in vivo study also reveals important differences between the effects of IGF-I and GH on bone growth. These quantitative differences are reflected by the effects of the two hormones on cell kinetics (expressed by cell cycle time and cell turnover) (Fig. 3A and B) and on cell productivity (expressed as cell height, cell volume and matrix production/h, shown for cell height/h in Fig. 4) at each stage of growth plate chondrocyte differentiation. GH clearly completes chondrocyte maturation at each of these stages within a shorter period of time than IGF-I. Furthermore, the cell pool size of the proliferative zone was identical in normal and in saline- and IGF-I-treated hypox rats, but was greater in GH-treated animals (not shown). These quantitative differences between the effects of GH and IGF-I on cell kinetics and cell productivity are not due to the different total serum IGF-I levels attained during IGF-I- or GH-treatment (Table 1): 85% of the total IGF-I in IGF-I-infused hypox rats circulates in the form of the 40 kDa IGFBP complex, whereas in GH-treated animals only 40% of the total IGF-I is associated with this complex and the remainder with the 150 kDa complex (Fig. 5). Since the bioavailability of IGF-I in the 150 kDa form is largely restricted by its limited capillary permeability [20,21], it is only the IGF-I in the 40 kDa form which is bioavailable to tissue receptors and thus biologically active (Zapf in preparation). As shown in Fig. 5, the concentration of IGF-I in the 40 kDa complex is similar or — if anything — less in the GH-infused as compared to the IGF-I-infused group. Therefore, it is unlikely that the quantitative differences between IGF-I and GH on growth kinetics are due to the different total circulating IGF-I levels unless endogenous rat IGF-I is more effective than rhIGF-I.

At least in vitro, both IGF-I species are similarly active on cell growth [15]. It is, therefore, reasonable to assume that IGF-I produced locally under the influence of GH, acts immediately as a "nascent" signalling substance in an auto/paracrine manner and that IGF-I circulating in the 40 kDa form amplifies this action. GH stimulation of local IGF-I production as well as the effects of locally produced and circulating IGF-I on chondrocyte maturation, are compatible with the presence of cell surface receptors for both GH and IGF-I at all stages of differentiation in growth plate cartilage [22–24]. In addition "direct" IGF-independent effects of GH have to be envisaged for tissues which carry GH receptors.

In summary, the results of this study demonstrate that both endocrine and auto/paracrine effects of IGF-I are responsible for GH-stimulated skeletal and organ growth. It appears, however, that tissues differ from each other in their responses to endocrine and auto/paracrine IGF-I. All of the data provide evidence that the

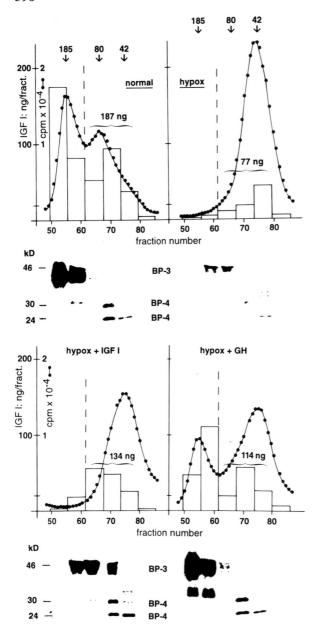

Fig. 5. Radiochromatographic patterns and molecular size distribution of IGF-I and IGF binding proteins in pooled sera from normal and saline-, IGF-I- and GH-treated hypox rats. Radiochromatographic patterns were obtained by gel-filtration on Sephadex G-200 at neutral pH, as described in [13]. To obtain pooled fractions represented in Fig. 5, 0.75 ml of the sera was gel-filtered on a Sephadex G-200 column (2 × 70 cm; pumping rate 10 ml/h) and eluted with Dulbecco's buffer/0.02% NaN$_3$ (pH 7.4). Pooled fractions were dialyzed in Spectrapor (molecular cut-off 3500) against 0.1 M NH$_4$HCO$_3$, lyophilized and dissolved in 0.3 ml of distilled water. Endogenous or rhIGF-I was determined after SepPak C$_{18}$ chromatography of 0.1 ml acid-treated aliquot as described in [13]. 10 µl aliquots were used for Western ligand blotting [13,14].

extended somatomedin hypothesis is valid in vivo. Moreover, since the effects of IGF-I at the proliferative phase of chondrocyte activity are exerted primarily by a shortening of the cycle time rather than by "clonal expansion", i.e., by increasing cell pool size, the dual effector theory on the mechanisms of action of IGF-I and GH on growth plate chondrocytes does not hold true in vivo.

References

1. Daughaday WH, Hall K, Raben MS, Salmon WD, Van den Brande JL. Nature 1972;235:107.
2. Chochinov RH, Daughaday WH. Diabetes 1976;25:994—1007.
3. Daughaday WH. Perspect Biol Med 1989;32:194—211.
4. Schlechter NL, Russell SM, Spencer EM, Nicoll CS. Proc Natl Acad Sci 1986;83:7932.
5. Trippel SB, Hung HH, Mankin HJ. Orthop Trans 1987;11:422.
6. Isgaard J, Muller C, Isaksson OGP, Nilsson A, Matthews LS, Norstedt G. Endocrinology 1988;122:1515.
7. Green H, Morikawa M, Nixon T. Differentiation 1985;29:195—198.
8. Ohlsson C, Nilsson A, Isaksson O, Lindahl A. Proc Natl Acad Sci USA 1992;89:9826—9830.
9. Schoenle E, Zapf J, Humbel RE, Froesch ER. Nature 1982;296:252—253.
10. Isaksson OG, Jansson JO, Gause IA. Science 1982;216:1237—1239.
11. Guler HP, Zapf J, Scheiwiller E, Froesch R. Proc Natl Acad Sci USA 1988;85:4889—4893.
12. Hunziker EB, Wagner J, Zapf J. Differential effects of insulin-like growth factor I (IGF-I) and growth hormone (GH) on developmental stages of rat growth plate chondrocytes in vivo. J Clin Invest 1994 (in press).
13. Zapf J, Hauri C, Waldvogel M, Futo E, Häsler H, Binz K, Guler HP, Froesch ER. Proc Natl Acad Sci USA 1989;86:3813—3817.
14. Hossenlopp P, Seurin D, Segovia-Quinson B, Hardouin S, Binoux M. Anal Biochem 1986;154:138—143.
15. Tamura K, Kobayashi M, Ishii Y, Tamura T, Hashimoto K, Nakamura S, Niwa M, Zapf J. J Biol Chem 1989;264:5616—5621.
16. Isaksson OG, Nilsson A, Isgaard J, Lindahl A. Acta Paediatr Scand 1990;36(suppl):137—141.
17. Hunziker EB, Schenk RK. J Physiol (London) 1989;414:55—71.
18. Breur GJ, VanEnkevort BA, Farnum CE, Wilsman NJ. J Orthop Res 1991;9:348—359.
19. Hunziker EB, Schenk RK, Cruz Orive LM. J Bone Joint Surg (Am) 1987;69:162—173.
20. Binoux M, Hossenlopp P. J Clin Endocrinol Metab 1988;67:509—514.
21. Guler HP, Zapf J, Schmid C, Froesch ER. Acta Endocrinol 1989;121:753—758.
22. Trippel SB, Van Wyk JJ, Foster MB, Svoboda ME. Endocrinology 1983;112:2128—2136.
23. Barnard R, Haynes KM, Werther GA, Water MJ. Endocrinology 1988;122:2562—2569.
24. Werther GA, Haynes KM, Barnard R, Waters MJ. J Clin Endocrinol Metab 1990;70:1725—1731.

The insulin-like growth factors and their regulatory proteins
R.C. Baxter, P.D. Gluckman and R.G. Rosenfeld, editors

393

Immunologic effects of IGF-I

Ross Clark[1] and Paula Jardieu[2]

Departments of [1]Endocrine Research and [2]Immunology, Genentech Inc.,
460 Pt San Bruno Blvd., South San Francisco, California 94044, USA

Abstract. There is a connection between anabolic hormones and the immune system. Mice treated with recombinant human IGF-I (rhIGF-I) show increased lymphoid tissue mass, T-cell and B-cell number and function, and antibody titers following antigen challenge. The administration of rhIGF-I accelerates the rate of cellular repopulation of peripheral lymphoid organs following autologous bone marrow transplantation. These studies show that rhIGF-I enhances T- and B-cell function in mouse models of immune deficiency.

Introduction

The growth hormone (GH) system regulates and coordinates postnatal whole body growth in mammals. In the 1950s some of the effects of GH were shown to be mediated indirectly by "somatomedins" in serum, which led to the "somatomedin hypothesis" [2]. A prediction of that hypothesis was that the administration of the serum factors (somatomedins) would duplicate the effects of GH. It was proven subsequently that the administration of somatomedins (IGFs) purified from human sera, could stimulate whole body growth in the hypophysectomized rat [3]. Initially this data was interpreted as indicating that the growth promoting effects of GH were duplicated when IGF-I was administered [4], although it was known that the metabolic effects of IGF-I and GH could be very different, for example, the insulin-like effects of IGF-I compared to the diabetogenic effects of GH.

With the advent of recombinant DNA technology it was possible to produce and to administer large amounts of recombinant human (rh)IGF [5]. Such studies [6,7] indicated that in rodents the whole body growth response to rhIGF-I is less than that achieved with rhGH. Another significant finding [6,7] of these studies was that rhGH and the rhIGF-I have different relative effects on growth and anabolism in different body organs. An important outcome of these differential anabolic effects of rhIGF-I and rhGH is that their coadministration has an additive effect on whole body size [8] and anabolism [9]. This review focuses on the in vivo growth responses to IGF-I and in particular the growth of the lymphoid organs.

Address for correspondence: Ross Clark, Department of Endocrine Research, Genentech Inc., 460 Pt San Bruno Blvd., South San Francisco, CA 94080, USA.

Experimental results

Organ growth with GH and IGF-I

Among the most obvious organs showing "overgrowth" in response to IGF-I administration (i.e., growth disproportionate to the growth of the rest of the body) were the spleen and the thymus [6]. In rodents the effects of GH and prolactin on the growth of lymphoid organs were well known [10], but in comparison IGF-I administration seemed to produce even larger effects on lymphoid organs [6,7].

Effects of IGF-I on lymphoid organ size in rats

The first experiments to characterize the effects of IGF-I on the immune system, beyond that of simple descriptive effects on organ size, were performed by Froesch's group [11]. Insulin deficient diabetic rats, which have a reduced lymphoid tissue mass, were treated with IGF-I. There was an increased cell number in the spleen and thymus after 7 days of IGF-I treatment, which was similar in effect to insulin replacement. In this model it was debatable whether IGF-I was having direct growth promoting effects or whether it was having an indirect effect by improving glucose metabolism [12,13].

Collaborations between endocrinologists and immunologists were necessary to expand this area of research. What was needed was to extend these studies to immune compromised animals, in which the immune defects did not result primarily from endocrine dysfunction.

Animal models

The immune system shows a reduction in function with age in rodents and humans [14]. In rodents this decline is accelerated in a breeding animal compared to that of a virgin animal. The majority of studies with IGF-I, as can be seen by the above discussion, had been performed in the rat. However the mouse is the best characterized and preferred animal for immunology studies. Therefore we chose to test the efficacy of IGF-I in retired breeder male mice. These animals are readily available allowing us to run a large number of experiments in a defined "naturally" immune impaired population.

IGF-I dosing in normal mice

There is little data [15,16] on the anabolic effects of IGF-I in the mouse. One study, in which IGF-I was administered to young GH-deficient mice, showed that two or more injections of IGF-I per day were necessary to effect body growth [16]. This is presumably due to the short half life of IGF-I which necessitates frequent administration to maintain adequate tissue exposure. For this reason, we chose to administer rhIGF-I by osmotic minipump, which had been shown to be the preferred mode of delivery in the rat [5,6]. We were not aware of data on dosing with IGF-I in adult or "middle-aged" mice with normal pituitary function, so we first established [17] the IGF-I dose response relationships on body weight gain and organ growth in retired breeder mice (Fig. 1). Significant effects of IGF-I on weight gain were seen when 4 mg/kg/day of rhIGF-I was given for 1 week by subcutaneous minipump infusion, so this dose (120 µg/mouse/day) was chosen in all subsequent studies.

Effect of IGF-I on lymphoid organ size and cellularity

In young GH-deficient rats [6–8] the spleen and thymus size increased after treatment with IGF-I for 7 days. This dose increased whole body weight, but had minimal hypoglycemic activity. In retired breeder mice it was unknown what doses of IGF-I or length of treatment would be needed to observe increased thymic and splenic size. We were surprised when our initial studies in mice showed that IGF-I caused a prompt and profound reversal of the involution of the thymus and a doubling of spleen mass [17]. The reproducibility of the effects of rhIGF-I on lymphoid organs was remarkable and allowed groups of four to six mice to be used while maintaining statistically significant effects. These findings are in contrast to the in vivo effects of lymphokines on lymphoid organs which have been difficult to characterize without large numbers of animals.

In our experiments in mice [17–19], rhIGF-I was administered by subcutaneous infusion from osmotic minipumps. After 7 or 14 days the mice were sacrificed, their

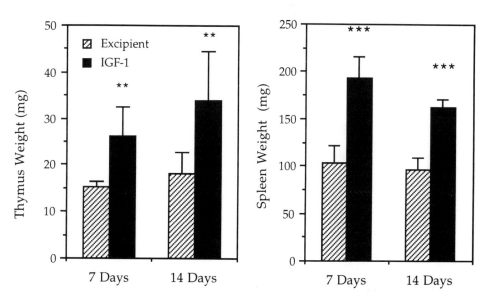

Fig. 1. The weights of thymus (left panel) and spleen (right panel) in adult mice treated with excipient (hatched bars) or rhIGF-I (solid bars). The length of treatment was either 7 days (left) or 14 days (right). Treatment with rhIGF-1 (4 mg/kg/d) dramatically increased both spleen and thymus weight. Treated groups were compared with their respective excipient treated controls (** p < 0.01, *** p < 0.001). Means and standard deviations are shown in all Figures. Reproduced with permission from Clark et al. [17].

spleens and thymuses were removed, dispersed and viable cells counted. Lymphocyte subpopulations were quantitated by FACS analysis using fluorescently tagged antibodies against appropriate cell surface markers. Total lymphocyte number was dramatically increased by treatment with rhIGF-I for 7 or 14 days, compared to excipient treated control mice and was due to increases in both T- and B-lymphocyte cell numbers (Fig. 2). Analysis of T-cell subsets showed that the increase in cell number was due to a general increase in the number of both CD4 (helper) and CD8 (suppressor) cells. The effect of IGF-I on B-cell number was unexpected at the time of our initial studies. Although there were data suggesting that T-cells possessed receptors for IGF-I there was no evidence that IGF-I affected B-cells. It should be emphasized that in these studies the effects of rhIGF-I were to increase the number

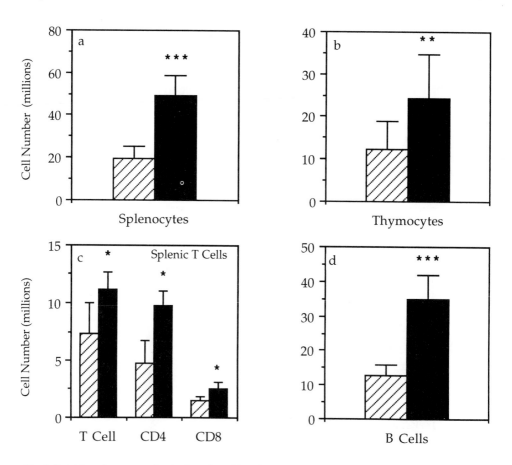

Fig. 2. Total lymphocyte number in the spleen (a) and thymus (b), T-cell subsets in spleen (c) and B-cell subsets in spleen (d) in mice treated with excipient (hatched bars) or rhIGF-I (solid bars) for 7 days. The increased wet weights seen in Fig. 1 were reflected in increased lymphocyte numbers. Treatment with rhIGF-1 (4 mg/kg/d) increased total thymic and splenic lymphocyte number, increased splenic T-cell number, and CD4, CD8, and B-cell number in spleen. Treated groups were compared with their respective excipient treated controls (* $p < 0.05$, ** $p < 0.01$, *** $p < 0.001$). Reproduced with permission from Clark et al. [17].

of cells in lymphoid organs, with little effect on the number of cells circulating in peripheral blood. This presents a challenge to the clinical investigator who does not have the access to lymphoid organs for analysis. To aid clinical investigation the demonstration of functional effects of rhIGF-I was needed.

Lymphocyte function in vitro

In addition to quantitating and characterizing the lymphocyte subsets we also performed in vitro tests of lymphocyte function [17]. Spleen cells were incubated with a T-cell mitogen, Concanavalin A (ConA), B-cell mitogen or pokeweed mitogen (PWM). In mice treated for only 7 days the results were disappointing, since the proliferative responses of lymphocytes taken from rhIGF-I treated mice were decreased compared to controls. Similar results were seen by Froesch's group in the rat [11]. However, cells taken from mice treated with IGF-I for 14 days had an enhanced ability to respond to the mitogens (Fig. 3). The length of treatment, or the time of sampling following IGF-I treatment, clearly influenced the results obtained. This difference between 7 and 14 day treatments could be due to the population of the spleen at 7 days with newly recruited immature cells which are known to show submaximal responses to mitogens. By 14 days the cells would have matured and therefore would regain mitogen responsiveness. Such differences have been reported in ontogenic studies where mitogenic responses continue to increase as an animal matures [20]. It should be noted that the mitogen data are obtained from a fixed number of cells. These in vitro data suggested that IGF-I enhanced immune function, as it increased the number of lymphocytes and on a per cell basis enhanced their

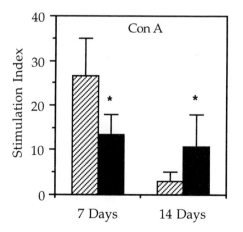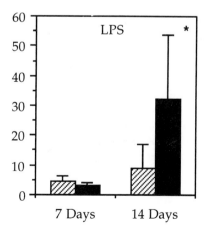

Fig. 3. The stimulation indices are shown for the in vitro mitogen responses of splenocytes harvested from experimental animals. ConA (left panel) stimulates T-cells and LPS (right panel) stimulates B-cells. The mice were treated with excipient (hatched bars) or rhIGF-I (solid bars) for either 7 or 14 days. After treatment with rhIGF-1 for 7 days mitogen responses were reduced. After 14 days mitogen responses were increased. Treated groups were compared with their respective excipient treated controls (* $p < 0.05$). Reproduced with permission from Clark et al. [17].

function. With both the mass and function of lymphoid cells being increased, the net effect on immune function would be expected to be considerable.

Response to immunization

To test directly for enhanced immune function in the whole animal we examined the ability of IGF-I treated mice to mount an in vivo antibody response to antigen challenge [18]. Binz et al. [11] measured the response of IGF-I treated rats to an immunogen, but could detect no treatment effect. As discussed previously, this lack of effect could have been due to inappropriate sampling times or length of IGF-I exposure. In mice we investigated whether rhIGF-I could enhance the ability of mice to mount an immunoglobulin response to a foreign antigen [18]. The responses to graded doses of dinitrophenyl-ovalbumin (DNP_2-OA) were measured, by an antigen specific ELISA, in retired breeder mice given rhIGF-I infusions for 14 days either at the time of a primary or secondary antigen challenge.

In these long-term immunization experiments, primary and secondary responses to antigen, as well as repeated exposures to rhIGF-I were needed, with a 3 week withdrawal between the 2 week exposures. After one exposure to rhIGF-I there was an increase in lymphocyte numbers in peripheral lymphoid organs. This response was maintained for up to 3 weeks after IGF-I exposure. A second administration of rhIGF-I, given when lymphocyte numbers had returned to control values, resulted in similar increases in the peripheral T- and B-cell populations. Remarkably, when rhIGF-I treated mice were immunized with a low, sub optimal, dose of antigen they produced antibody titers which were equivalent to those generated by immunization with optimal doses of antigen. Likewise, in vitro addition of rhIGF-I to splenocyte cultures from antigen primed mice, stimulated immunoglobulin synthesis. These studies [18] demonstrate that the increased lymphocyte numbers had functional significance, because rhIGF-I treated mice had elevated antibody titers after both primary and secondary antigen challenges.

Effect of IGF-I on regeneration of the immune system

The above experiments established that IGF-I could enhance the ability of animals to mount an immune response and suggested that IGF-I might be a normal component of B- and T-cell lymphopoiesis. However, they did not address the site(s) of action of IGF-I. To further investigate the activity of rhIGF-I on immunity we tested its efficacy in a mouse model of bone marrow transplantation. Lethally irradiated (900 rads) male BALB/c mice (6–7 weeks old) were reconstituted with 10^7 bone marrow cells from syngeneic donors and received infusions of rhIGF-I or excipient. Treatment with rhIGF-I reduced the catabolic effect of the radiation, as measured by attenuation of body weight loss, and increased spleen and thymus weight measured at 14 and 23 days following transplantation. Treatment with rhIGF-I also had dramatic effects on lymphoid populations. By day 23, increased splenic T-cell number and function were evident in the rhIGF-I treated mice compared to excipient controls. Moreover, the thymus weight was doubled and there was a tripling of thymic cell count in the hormone treated mice. A series of experiments showed that treatment with rhIGF-I increased the rate of peripheral lymphocyte repopulation after syngeneic bone marrow transplantation by acting directly on bone marrow progenitors and by stimulating entry of peripheral lymphocytes into S phase of the cell cycle. In other studies [21], after chemically destroying lymphoid tissues, Beschorner and colleagues have shown similar restorative effects of rhIGF-I treatment in the rat.

Discussion

It could not have been predicted when IGF-I was discovered as a "somatomedin" or "nonsuppressible insulin-like activity" that it would cause overgrowth of lymphoid organs. We compared the activities of rhGH injections and rhIGF-I infusions on lymphoid mass in rats and mice and found that rhGH injections had much less activity [18]. This is surprising given both that the liver is a major source of IGF-I in the blood and that the somatomedin hypothesis would predict that IGF-I circulating from the liver mediated GH action. However, the discovery of local production of IGF-I in many tissues argues against the idea that IGF-I mediate GH action purely in an endocrine mode and supports the notion of a paracrine mode of action. The relatively weak effects of rhGH on lymphoid tissues might be explained if the autocrine or paracrine induction of IGF-I in lymphoid tissues is regulated by cytokines other than rhGH. IGF-I production can be controlled by a variety of factors in other tissues. For example, in the uterus it is controlled by steroids, in the adrenal by ACTH and in the liver by nutritional status. There is a large literature on the impact of nutrition on immune status [22], yet the role of IGF-I in this setting is poorly characterized.

An aspect of IGF-I biology that has now been clarified is its effects on B-cell production from bone marrow. Dorshkind had shown that bone marrow stromal cells produce a "B-cell differentiation factor" crucial for the progression of B-cells from the pre-B to pro-B stages. Several lines of evidence have led to his conclusion [23] that the factor having this activity is IGF-I. Animal studies have confirmed this conclusion. In IGF-I treated mice, B-cell progenitors (B220+ IgM- cells) are increased in bone marrow (Jardieu, Mortensen, Clark and Dorshkind, unpublished data). Therefore a physiological role and mechanism of action for IGF-I have been established in B-cell development. Less information is available on the role of IGF-I in T-cell development, although the dramatic effects of IGF-I in bone marrow and thymus suggest multiple sites of action.

These findings may be of therapeutic significance if rhIGF-I has similar effects in humans. Short periods of rhIGF-I administration may be of use to enhance antibody responses in patients with impaired immune function. There is a slow restoration of T- and B-lymphocyte number and function following chemotherapy, radiotherapy or bone marrow transplantation. Accordingly, there is a need for therapies such as rhIGF-I that might accelerate this repopulation. The recognition that IGF-I has a role in regulating immune function should lead to further studies and a clearer picture of the physiology and pharmacology of this important growth factor.

Acknowledgements

We wish to thank the staff in several departments at Genentech; without their help these studies would not have been possible.

References

1. Salmon WD, Daughaday WH. J Lab Clin Med 1957;49:825–836.
2. Daughaday WH, Hall K, Raben MS et al. Nature 1972;235:107.
3. Schoenle E, Zapf J, Humbel RE, Froesch ER. Nature 1982;296:252–253.
4. Van Wyk JJ. In: CH Li (ed) Hormonal Proteins and Peptides 12. New York: Academic Press, 1984; 81–125.
5. Froesch ER, Guler HP, Ernst M et al. In: Isaksson O et al. (eds) Growth Hormone Basic and Clinical Aspects. Amsterdam: Elsevier, 1987;321–336.
6. Guler HP, Zapf J, Scheiwiller E, Froesch R. Proc Natl Acad Sci USA 1988;85:4889–4893.
7. Skottner A, Clark RG, Fryklund L, Robinson ICAF. Endocrinology 1989;124:2519–2526.
8. Clark RG, Mortensen D, Carlsson LMS. Proc 74th Annual Meeting of the Endocrine Society, 1992; abstract 1078.
9. Kupfer SR, Underwood LE, Baxter RC, Clemmons DR. J Clin Invest 1993;91:391–396.
10. Ammann A. In: Underwood L (ed) Human Growth Hormone-Progress and Challenges. New York; Marcel Dekker, 1988;243–253.
11. Binz K, Joller P, Froesch P et al. Proc Natl Acad Sci USA 1990;87:3690–3694.
12. Scheiwiller E, Guler HP, Merryweather J et al. Nature 1986;323:169–171.
13. Carlsson LMS, Clark RG, Skottner A, Robinson ICAF. J Endocrine 1989;122:661–670.
14. Simons RJ, Reynolds HY. Sem Resp Infect 1990;5:251–259.
15. Van Buul-Offers S, Ueda I, Van den Brande JL. Pediatr Res 1986;20:825–827.
16. Woodall SM, Breier BH, O'Sullivan U, Gluckman PD. Horm Metab Res 1991;23:581–584.
17. Clark R, Strasser J, McCabe S, Robbins K, Jardieu P. J Clin Invest 1993;92:540–548.
18. Robbins K, McCabe S, Scheiner T, Strasser J, Clark R, Jardieu P. J Clin Exp Immunol 1994;95:337–343.
19. Jardieu P, McCabe S, Robbins K, Strasser J, Clark R. Proc 75th Annual Meeting of the Endocrine Society, 1993;abstract 654.
20. Dzlanski R. Dev Comp Immunol 1985;9:119–130.
21. Beschorner WE, Divic J, Pulido H, Yao X, Kenworthy P, Bruce G. Transplantation 1991;52:879–884.
22. Gershwin ME, Beach RS, Hurley LS. In: Nutrition and Immunity. Orlando; Academic Press, 1985.
23. Landreth KS, Narayanan R, Dorshkind K. Blood 1992;80:1207–1214.

IGF-I and GH: metabolic effects during experimentally induced catabolism

K. Malmlöf, Z. Cortova, H. Saxerholt, V. Arrhenius-Nyberg, E. Karlsson, C. Larsson, G. Klingström and A. Skottner

Department of Pharmacology, Pharmacia, Kabi Peptide Hormones, S-11287 Stockholm, Sweden

Abstract. Metabolic effects of recombinantly manufactured human growth hormone (rhGH) and human insulin-like growth factor I (rhIGF-I) were compared during experimentally induced catabolism. In surgically traumatized pigs hind limb net balances of amino acids were significantly ($p < 0.05$) increased by both rhGH and rhIGF-I. Accordingly, both peptides increased significantly ($p < 0.05$) the nitrogen balance of dexamethasone treated pigs. In rats given the same drug, only rhIGF-I was effective. In pigs, rhGH significantly ($p < 0.05$) increased circulating levels of most amino acids and glucose compared with rhIGF-I. We conclude that increases in skeletal muscle amino acid retention is an integrated part of the nitrogen sparing effect of both rhGH and rhIGF-I. It is however, uncertain whether the same pathway is used, since we observed that the effects of rhGH on amino acid metabolism were not dependent on increases in circulating IGF-I.

Introduction

Surgical intervention, mechanical injury, burns or severe infections are all examples of conditions associated with dramatic alterations in hormone physiology and metabolism of nutrients. Typically, the circulating levels of the stress hormones cortisol, catecholamines and glucagon [1] are elevated and those of insulin-like growth factor I (IGF-I) depressed [2]. These changes are seen in parallel with an accelerated breakdown of proteins from skeletal muscles and transport of amino acids to visceral organs [3]. Although a fraction of these amino acids is used for synthesis of immune proteins [3], the remainder is converted to glucose and the nitrogen moiety synthesized into urea which later is excreted via the urine [4]. Therefore the catabolic process can be followed by an increase in circulating urea and urinary nitrogen excretion and a substantial decrease in nitrogen balance, which in severe cases often becomes deleteriously negative [5].

It has been demonstrated that nutritional support alone does not stop the peripheral efflux of amino acids [6] and hence does not reverse the negative nitrogen balance [7]. However, the recombinant DNA technique has made growth factors available for use as adjuncts to total parenteral nutrition (TPN). So far, recombinant human growth hormone (rhGH) has proven to be a safe and efficient agent in the improvement of nitrogen economy in critically ill patients [5]. The protein anabolic effects of recombinant human insulin-like growth factor I (rhIGF-I) are less established [8] even though experimental data show that this peptide can also improve nitrogen balance during experimentally induced catabolism in man [9] and animals [10].

Although rhGH and rhIGF-I, by direct comparison, have been found to have similar effects on nitrogen balance in food restricted humans [9], knowledge as to their specific effects on nitrogen economy as well as peripheral amino acid metabolism in various other types of catabolic states is incomplete. The present studies, were undertaken with the purpose of such direct comparisons between rhGH and rhIGF-I. In the following, results from experiments performed in surgically traumatized and dexamethasone treated pigs, as well as dexamethasone treated rats will be presented.

Methods and experimental designs

Surgically traumatized and dexamethasone treated pigs

Following a 24 h fast, 18 female pigs weighing on average 52.2 kg (SD 3.5) went through major surgery during which catheters and flow probes were implanted to allow intravenous infusion and measurements of hind limb fluxes. On the next day the animals were evenly assigned (n = 6) to receive intravenous infusion of either vehicle, rhIGF-I (0.36 mg/kg/day) or rhGH (0.47 IU/kg/day). Vehicle or peptides were infused together with total parenteral nutrition providing 31 kcal/kg/day of nonprotein calories and 0.35 g nitrogen/kg/day. Of the nonprotein calories 75% was provided as glucose and 25% as lipids. Infusions were maintained during 10 h, between 8.00 am and 6.00 pm, for 2 successive postoperative days. Here fluxes of amino acids and hormones, as well as circulating levels during the first postoperative day are presented.

In a subsequent study five pigs weighing on average 44.1 kg (SD 3.6) were fitted with arterial (carotid) and venous (jugular) cannulas. Intravenous 48 h infusions of dexamethasone (0.27 mg/kg/day) were combined with either saline, rhIGF-I (0.8 mg/kg/day) or rhGH (0.9 IU/kg/day). Each pig received all three treatments in rotation, together with a higher level of total parenteral nutrition than in the first experiment; 74 kcal/kg/day of nonprotein calories and 0.8 g nitrogen/kg/day. Between the infusion periods the animals were allowed a standard pig diet. Here plasma glucose 48 h profiles and nitrogen balances, calculated as the difference between amounts of nitrogen infused and excreted in urine, are presented.

Dexamethasone treated rats

In an experiment with growing Sprague-Dawley rats weighing approximately 200 g, the effects of rhGH (360 µg/day) and rhIGF-I (500 µg/day) were compared with saline at three doses of dexamethasone (Dex, 26, 13 or 6.5 µg/day). Six animals were included in each of the nine groups. Infusions of peptides and dexamethasone were performed subcutaneously via osmotic mini-pumps and were maintained for 8 days.

During this time, the rats were placed individually in metabolic cages which allowed quantitative collection of urine and faeces, as well as registration of feed intake and weight changes. The rats were on a 12/12 h light-dark cycle and had free access to water and a milled feed, which comprised 222 g crude protein/kg and 3.6 Mcal/kg of metabolizable energy. Nitrogen balances were calculated as the difference between nitrogen intake and the sum of feacal- and urinary-nitrogen excretions.

Surgically traumatized pigs

The average baseline concentration of total IGF-I before infusions was approximately 75 µg/l whole blood, which was a 50% reduction from preoperative values. Infusion of vehicle or rhGH as adjuncts to TPN did not significantly increase circulating IGF-I from baseline, whereas preoperative levels were more than restored by administration of rhIGF-I (Fig. 1). However, when the net fluxes of IGF-I over the hind limbs were analyzed they always appeared negative. Thus all treatments seemed to be associated with a net release of IGF-I, if analysed as total IGF-I after acid ethanol extraction (Fig. 2). Although none of the treatments were found to differ significantly from a statistical point of view, there was a trend for rhGH to increase and rhIGF-I to decrease the net efflux of IGF-I.

Infusions of rhIGF-I were also associated with a significantly ($p < 0.05$) lower mean blood level of insulin (0.98 µg/l) in comparison with vehicle (2.41 µg/l) and rhGH (2.21 µg/l, pooled SE 0.2). In parallel with the depression of circulating insulin, rhIGF-I also produced a significant ($p < 0.05$) decrease in the rate of insulin uptake over the hind limbs if compared with rhGH. Despite these effects on peripheral insulin uptake, rhIGF-I was found to decrease and rhGH to increase the 10 h mean level of glucose in comparison to vehicle (data not shown).

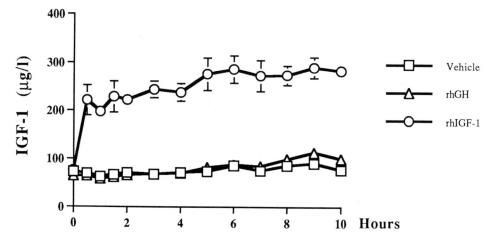

Fig. 1. Arterial blood levels of IGF-I in pigs given i.v. infusions of TPN together with either vehicle, rhIGF-I or rhGH for 10 h on the first day following abdominal surgery. Data represent means of six observations together with error bars (±SE).

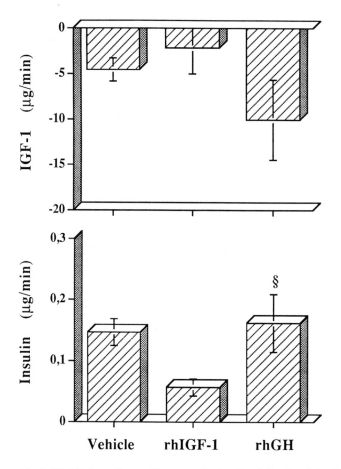

Fig. 2. Hind limb net fluxes of hormones in pigs that, following abdominal surgery, were given infusions of TPN together with either vehicle, rhIGF-I or rhGH. Data represent the average flux over and integrated time of 10 h on the first postoperative day and are means of six independent observations together with error bars (±SE). § = rhGH differ significantly (p < 0.05) from rhIGF-I.

The same differential effect of rhIGF-I and rhGH as seen with glucose was also seen with blood levels of total amino acids (data not shown). Despite this, both hormones significantly (p < 0.05) increased the hind limb balance of total amino acids. Thus, net fluxes of –44.2, +69.5 and +100,9 µmol/min (pooled SE 35.3) were associated with infusion of vehicle, rhIGF-I and rhGH, respectively (Fig. 3).

Dexamethasone treated pigs

The combination of dexamethasone and rhGH produced a dramatic increase in plasma glucose and insulin levels reaching approximately 20 mmol/l and 35 µg/l, respectively, by the end of the 48 infusion period. In contrast, both rhIGF-I and saline infusions

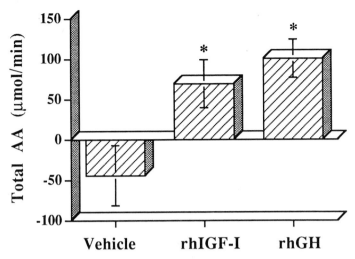

Fig. 3. Hind limb net fluxes of total amino acids in pigs that, following abdominal surgery, were given infusions of TPN together with either vehicle, rhIGF-I or rhGH. Data represent the average flux over and integrated time of 10 h on the first postoperative day and are means of six independent observations together with error bars (±SE). * = rhGH or rhIGF-I differ significantly (p < 0.05) from vehicle.

were associated with a more stable glycemic response (Fig. 4). Both rhIGF-I and rhGH significantly depressed circulating levels of urea in comparison with saline (data not shown). The urea depressing effects of the peptides emerged successively from 12 h and onwards and were associated with significantly (p < 0.05) increased nitrogen balances (Fig. 5).

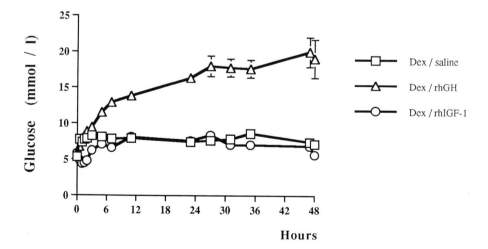

Fig. 4. The mean concentration of plasma glucose and insulin in pigs receiving intravenous infusion of dexamethasone and TPN together with either saline, rhGH or rhIGF-I. Data represent means of five observations together with error bars (±SE).

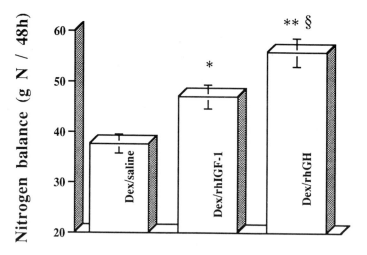

Fig. 5. The cumulative nitrogen balance of pigs receiving intravenous infusion of dexamethasone and TPN together with either saline, rhGH or rhIGF-I for 48 h. Data represent means of five observations together with error bars (±SE). rhGH or rhIGF-I differ significantly (* $p < 0.05$, ** $p < 0.01$) from vehicle. § = rhGH differ significantly ($p < 0.05$) from rhIGF-I.

Dexamethasone treated rats

It was observed that the general effect of dexamethasone was to retard body weight gain in a dose dependent manner. However, at all doses of dexamethasone, 26, 13 or 6.5 µg/day, body weight gain as measured after 8 days of study was significantly (p < 0.05) increased by rhIGF-I when compared with saline, whereas rhGH had the opposite effect. Nitrogen retention followed a similar pattern although not showing statistical significance in all instances (Fig. 6).

Conclusions

From the studies in pigs presented here it could be concluded that both rhIGF-I and rhGH have a potential to prevent the erosion of muscle protein and increase the efficacy of total parenteral nutrition, as shown by significantly higher hind limb net balances of amino acids. Both rhIGF-I and rhGH were also observed to progressively decrease plasma urea and increase nitrogen balance in dexamethasone treated pigs. However, when this synthetic corticoid was given to rats, rhIGF-I, but not rhGH, it was found to improve nitrogen balance. The effect of rhIGF-I is in accordance with previous findings in dexamethasone treated rats [10], whereas the results obtained with rhGH is at variance with what we found in pigs and what has been found in prednisolone treated humans [11]. However, if prednisolone is given to rats, rhGH does not mediate any anabolic effects [12]. In contrast, such positive effects of rhGH were observed in methylprednisolone treated rats [13]. Taken together these variable

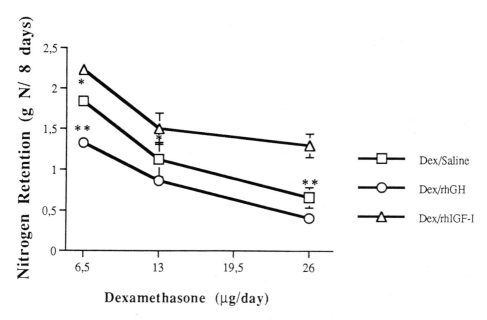

Fig. 6. The cumulative nitrogen retention in rats subcutaneously infused with either saline, rhGH (360 μg/day) or rhIGF-I (500 μg/day) for 8 days at three doses of dexamethasone (Dex). Data represent means of six observations together with error bars (± pooled SE). Significant differences between Dex/saline and other groups are shown, * (p < 0.05), ** (p <0.01).

results indicate the possible limitations of the rat as a model for man in studies of the interaction between rhGH and corticoids and it cannot be excluded that this is related to the fact that rats have corticosterone and not cortisol as the principal glucocorticoid [14] in contrast to both humans and pigs.

In the present studies with dexamethasone treated pigs, the nitrogen sparing effect of rhGH was paid at the price of marked hyperglycemia and insulin resistance. This was prevented by administration of rhIGF-I, a fact that might be of clinical importance.

Although the effects were similar on peripheral net flux of amino acids, the differential effect of rhGH and rhIGF-I on circulating levels of amino acids seems to imply that their mode of action at some other site or level of amino acid metabolism may differ. The peptides had very different effects on circulating glucose levels, but we have shown that the hyperglycemic effect of rhGH is not associated with a decrease in peripheral insulin uptake.

Finally, and perhaps most intriguing observation made in the present studies was that the net fluxes of total IGF-I were generally negative. Although not statistically verified, these net fluxes appeared less negative with rhIGF-I and more so with rhGH. This finding seems to underline the importance of local IGF-I production [15] and it would be tempting to speculate that the main effect of rhGH was to stimulate this process, whereas that of rhIGF-I would be to slow down the entry of endogenous

IGF-I into the circulation. However, in the absence of any firm evidence our findings on this point can only be taken as a further illustration as to the complexity of GH and IGF-I action.

References

1. Alberti KGMM, Phil D, Batstone GF, Foster KJ, Johnston DG. J Parenternal Enterol Nutr 1980;4: 141–146.
2. Ross RJM, Miell JP, Freeman E, Jones J, Matthews D, Preece M, Buchanan C. Clin Endocrinol 1991;35:47–54.
3. Rosenblatt S, Clowes GHA, George BC, Hirch E, Lindberg B. Arch Surg 1983;118:167–175.
4. Wilmore DW. J Am Coll Nutr 1983;2:3–13.
5. Wilmore DW. N Engl J Med 1991;325:695–670.
6. Finley RJ, Inculet RI, Pace R, Holliday R, Rose C, Duff JH, Groves AC, Woolf LI. Surgery 1986;99: 491–499.
7. Streat SJ, Beddoe AH, Graham LH. J Trauma 1987;27:262–266.
8. Mauras N, Horber F, Haymond MW. J Clin Endocrinol Metab 1992;75:1192–1197.
9. Clemmons DR, Smith-Banks A, Underwood LE. J Clin Endocrinol Metab 1992;75:234–238.
10. Ballard FJ, Tomas FM, Read LC, Knowles SE, Lemmey AB, Martin AA. In: Mornex R, Jaffiol C, Leclère J (eds) The Proceedings of the Ninth International Congress of Endocrinology Nice 1992. New York: Parthenon Publishing Group, 1993;268–275.
11. Horber FF, Haymond MW. J Clin Invest 1990;86:265–272.
12. Örtoft G, Kelly C, Brüel A-M, Smith A, Carter N, Oxlund H. Eur J Musculoskel Res 1993;2:135–142.
13. Kovàcs G, Fine RN, Worgall S, Schaefer F, Hunziker EB, Skottner-Lundin A, Mehls O. Kidney Int 1991;40:1032–1040.
14. Shimizu K, Amagaya S, Ogihara Y. J Chromat 1983;272:170–175.
15. D'Ercole AJ, Stiles AD, Underwood LE. Proc Natl Acad Sci 1984;81:935–939.

©1994 Elsevier Science B.V. All rights reserved
The insulin-like growth factors and their regulatory proteins
R.C. Baxter, P.D. Gluckman and R.G. Rosenfeld, editors

In vivo effects of IGF-I on gut growth and function

Leanna C. Read, Gordon S. Howarth, Corinna-B. Steeb and Andrew B. Lemmey

Cooperative Research Centre for Tissue Growth and Repair, Child Health Research Institute, North Adelaide, SA 5006, Australia

Abstract. Infusion of IGF-I, and particularly LR³IGF-I, into adult or newborn rats induces a marked increase in small bowel absorptive surface area through the combined effects of a proliferative response in the mucosal epithelium, together with enhanced linear growth of the small bowel. The accompanying reduction in fecal nitrogen excretion also suggests an improvement in absorptive function in IGF-treated rats. Other evidence is emerging that IGF-I can accelerate regeneration of the resected small bowel and possibly also enhance repair of intestinal damage induced by chemotherapy agents. Taken together, these results suggest therapeutic applications for IGF-I in gut disorders characterised by compromised absorptive function, with the expected dual benefit of reducing weight loss and improving gut growth and repair.

Introduction

Over the last few years, the effects of subcutaneous IGF-I infusion in rats on growth of the gastrointestinal tract, have been determined under a range of catabolic conditions including dexamethasone treatment, diabetes or gut resection [1–6]. These studies have identified the gastrointestinal tract as one of the most sensitive target tissues for IGF-I, so that fractional gut weight is increased by up to 30% above normal with only 7 days' IGF-I infusion. The gut response to IGF-I is generalised throughout the gastrointestinal tract, with responses apparent in both the mucosal and muscularis layers. A modulating role for IGF binding proteins (IGFBPs) has been suggested by the consistently higher potency of IGF-I analogs with low affinity for IGFBPs, including des(1–3)IGF-I and LR³IGF-I, an analog with a 13 amino acid N-terminal extension [1–4,7].

These findings suggest an important role for IGF-I and IGFBPs in the growth and repair of the gastrointestinal tract and point towards therapeutic applications for IGF-I in the treatment of gastrointestinal disease. For this reason, recent studies have examined in more detail the mechanisms of IGF-I induced intestinal growth in normal animals and have begun to address the possible roles of IGF-I in gut disorders.

Address for correspondence: LC Read M.D., Child Health Research Institute, 72 King William Road, North Adelaide, SA 5006, Australia.

IGF-I enhances proliferation and absorptive function of the small bowel mucosa

A number of gastrointestinal disorders, including infection, short bowel, inflammatory bowel diseases, necrotizing enterocolitis, radiation or chemotherapy damage cause loss of mucosal absorptive capacity, either through epithelial ablation or loss of small bowel length [8–13]. Since many of these conditions are lacking effective therapies, the consistent increase in mucosal mass of the small bowel in response to IGF-I infusion is potentially important to the development of new treatments for gut disease. Accordingly, we have examined the mechanisms of IGF-I induced small bowel growth, initially in normal rats.

Normal 120 g female rats (6/group) were maintained in metabolism cages and infused continuously for 14 days with 0, 44, 111 or 278 µg/day IGF-I via subcutaneous osmotic mini-pumps. On a body weight basis, these doses of IGF-I were equivalent to 0.3–2.0 mg/kg/day. For comparison, other groups of rats were treated with the same doses of the IGF-I analog, LR³IGF-I, which binds poorly to IGF-IBPs [7].

As observed in other rat models, infusion of IGF-I or LR³IGF-I induced dose-dependent increases in body weight and fractional gut weight, without affecting food intake. The small bowel represented the most responsive region, showing proportional increments in the weight of the mucosal and muscularis layers so that total small bowel weight increased by up to 36% and 47% above control values for IGF-I and LR³IGF-I treated rats, respectively [7]. The effect on small bowel weight resulted from a dual action of IGF peptides to increase length by up to 18% and cross-sectional mass by 8–26% above control values (Fig. 1).

These changes were associated with marked increases in the cellularity of the mucosal epithelium. In the crypt compartment of the duodenum, 278 µg/day IGF-I or LR³IGF-I increased the total number of epithelial cells by at least 30% due to the combined effect of greater crypt length with a proportional increment in cell number, amplified by an increased circumferential cell count (Fig. 2). This was accompanied

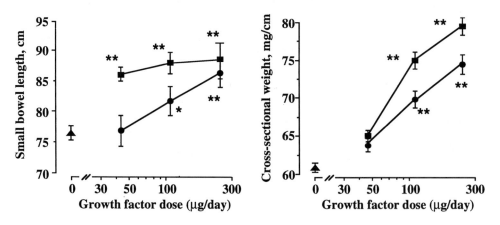

Fig. 1. Length (left) and cross-sectional weight (right) of the small intestine in normal rats infused subcutaneously for 14 days with vehicle (▲), IGF-I (●) or LR³IGF-I (■). Values are means ± SEM for six rats per group. Significance by ANOVA from the vehicle group is shown by: * ($p < 0.05$); ** ($p < 0.01$).

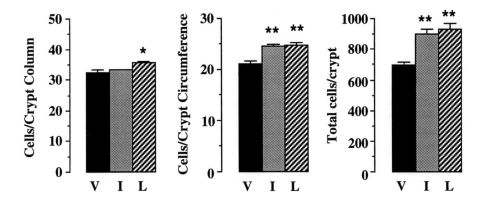

Fig. 2. Treatment of normal rats with 278 µg/day IGF-I (I) or LR³IGF-I (L) stimulates duodenal crypt proliferation compared with vehicle-infused controls (V), as illustrated by the number of epithelial cells per crypt column (left), the circumferential crypt cell count (middle) and the total number of epithelial cells per crypt (right). Values are means ± SEM for six rats per group. Significance by ANOVA from the vehicle group is shown by: * ($p < 0.05$); ** ($p < 0.01$).

by an increased number of proliferative cells, as indicated by a significantly higher number of crypt cells expressing PCNA, the auxiliary protein for DNA polymerase (results not shown). However, in contrast to uncontrolled growth situations such as cancer, the percentage of cells expressing PCNA increased only in proportion to crypt length, indicating maintenance of a normal balance between the proliferative and maturation compartments of the crypt.

The enhanced crypt cell proliferation in the duodenum of IGF-treated rats was accompanied by markedly longer villi and a more than 25% increase in the number of absorptive epithelial cells per villus. In addition, the epithelial cells of the villus compartment were much more densely packed than in vehicle-treated control rats, perhaps reflecting a change in migration rate of epithelial cells up the villus (Fig. 3). The marked increase in absorptive cell number in the small intestine of IGF-treated rats would predict an enhanced absorptive capacity. To test this, we took advantage of the fact that rats were maintained in metabolism cages for accurate measurement of food intake and quantitative collection of fecal output. Calculation of fecal fat excretion, as a percentage of intake, indicated that over 95% of dietary fat was absorbed in control rats and accordingly no significant improvement with IGF treatment was demonstrable (results not shown). Nitrogen was also absorbed efficiently, with less than 8% excreted in control rats, but nevertheless treatment with 278 µg/day LR³IGF-I significantly reduced fecal nitrogen output with IGF-I showing similar, but nonsignificant trends (Fig. 4).

Can IGF-I accelerate intestinal regrowth following small bowel resection?

The ability of IGF-I and LR³IGF-I to enhance mucosal proliferation, linear growth

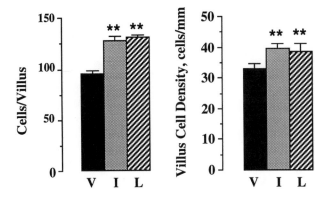

Fig. 3. Villus epithelial cell number is increased in the duodenum of normal rats infused with 278 µg/day IGF-I (I) or LR³IGF-I (L) compared with vehicle-treated controls (V). Data show the number of epithelial cells per villus column (left) and the density of villus cells (right). Values are means ± SEM for six rats per group. Significance by ANOVA from the vehicle group is shown by: ** ($p < 0.01$).

and absorptive function of the small bowel suggests therapeutic applications in the treatment of short bowel resulting from surgical removal of diseased or nonfunctioning intestine or from congenital disorders. Although resection itself is one of the most powerful stimuli for mucosal proliferation, recovery of bowel function can be inadequate in cases of massive gut resection. Since there are no therapies available to enhance intestinal regrowth, patients with massive gut resection may face a lifetime of parenteral nutrition.

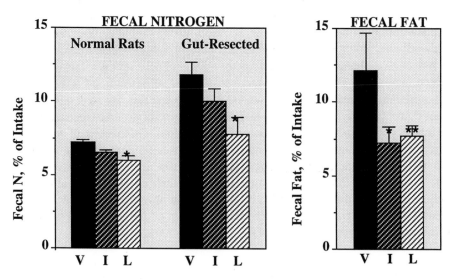

Fig. 4. Fecal nitrogen (left) and fat excretion (right) as a percentage of intake in normal rats or rats with 70% jejuno-ileal resection. Rats were infused with vehicle (V) or 278 µg/day IGF-I (I) or LR³IGF-I (L) for 14 days (normal rats, six per group) or 7 days (resected rats, nine per group). Significance by ANOVA from the vehicle group is shown by: * ($p < 0.05$); ** ($p < 0.01$).

We and others have now shown that 7-day infusion of IGF-I into rats with 70–80% jejuno-ileal resection improves body weight gain and enhances mucosal proliferation as well as linear regrowth of the proximal small bowel [2–4]. The gut resection studies also provided the opportunity to test the effects of IGF peptides on gut function in a model of compromised absorptive capacity. Gut resection induced mild diarrhea, together with a marked increase in fecal nitrogen and fat excretion compared with normal rats (Fig. 4). Under these circumstances, the improvement in gut function was much more evident than in normal animals, so that IGF-I infusion markedly reduced fat excretion while LR³IGF-I nearly halved both fat and nitrogen excretion (Fig. 4).

IGF-I therefore has considerable potential in the treatment of gut resection, firstly for its anticatabolic action to improve nitrogen balance and weight gain and secondly to improve intestinal regeneration and gut absorptive capacity.

The immature gut is especially sensitive to the analog, LR³IGF-I

A number of gastrointestinal disorders are prevalent in infancy, notably infectious diarrhea, necrotizing enterocolitis, short bowel and a range of congenital abnormalities. We therefore determined whether IGF-I is capable of stimulating small bowel growth in neonatal animals in a comparable manner to the adult.

Suckling 12-day old rats were infused subcutaneously for 6 days with vehicle or 2–12 mg/kg/day IGF-I or LR³IGF-I via osmotic mini-pumps. Qualitatively, responses to IGF peptides in the neonatal gut were similar to those in the adult, with dose-dependent increments in small bowel weight and length (Fig. 5). On the other hand, the potency difference between LR³IGF-I and the native peptide was markedly enhanced in the neonates, particularly for small bowel weight, where IGF-I at doses up to 12 mg/kg/day failed to achieve the stimulation seen at the lowest dose of LR³IGF-I (2 mg/kg/day). This difference may reflect increased binding protein

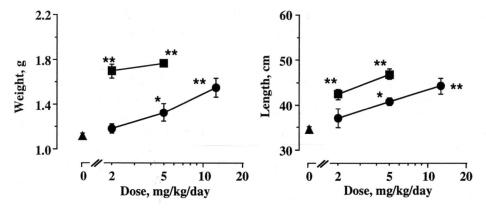

Fig. 5. Total weight (left) and length (right) of the small intestine in suckling rats infused subcutaneously for 6 days with vehicle (▲), IGF-I (●) or LR³IGF-I (■). Values are means ± SEM for six rats per group. Significance by ANOVA from the vehicle group is shown by: * (p < 0.05); ** (p < 0.01).

expression in the immature gut [14] since the enhanced potency of LR³IGF-I appears to reflect its reduced affinity for IGFBPs [15].

Can IGF-I enhance repair of the intestinal mucosa?

While the marked growth response to IGF peptides in the intestinal mucosa of adult and neonatal rats suggests therapeutic applications for IGF-I in the treatment of mucosal disease, little direct evidence has been accumulated to date. We have recently examined the potential role for IGF-I in the prevention of mucosal damage associated with chemotherapy. Chemotherapy or radiation enteritis is a major side-effect of tumour therapy, to the extent that intestinal damage can be the limiting factor in choosing the radiation or chemotherapy dose [9,10].

As a model of small bowel enteritis, we injected 140 g rats for 3 consecutive days with 2.5 mg/kg of the chemotherapy agent, methotrexate [16], resulting in marked atrophy and disruption of the small bowel mucosa, loss of appetite and reduced body weight gain. Intestinal damage was assessed by measurements of crypt depth and villus height, or in the early phases of recovery where damage was too severe to apply standard histological measures, we used a histological "surface area index", which estimates the length of intact crypt or villus epithelium per unit length of intestinal circumference. IGF-I, infused subcutaneously for 5 days starting coincident with the first methotrexate injection, had no effect on body weight gain or mucosal regeneration, as indicated by the surface area index of the crypt and villus fraction of the ileal mucosa (Fig. 6).

On the other hand, a significant increase in mucosal regeneration was apparent if the 5-day IGF-I infusion was not started until 24 h after the last methotrexate injection (Fig. 6, sequential IGF-I treatment). At this timepoint, where mucosal repair of methotrexate damage was sufficiently advanced for standard histological analysis, sequential IGF-I treatment increased crypt depth and villus height in the ileum by more than 30% compared with methotrexate-treated rats receiving no IGF infusion (Fig. 6). It would appear, therefore, that IGF-I may accelerate regrowth of the methotrexate-damaged small bowel when administered after, but not simultaneously with the chemotherapy agent.

Other evidence that IGF-I accelerates repair of the damaged mucosa was reported recently by Huang et al. [17] in a study measuring bacterial translocation in rats with severe topical burns. Bacterial translocation across the gut wall, associated with mucosal atrophy and increased permeability, is characteristic of major trauma such as burns and sepsis. Huang et al. found that subcutaneous infusion of 3 mg/kg/day IGF-I in burned rats improved body weight, attenuated mucosal atrophy and reduced bacterial translocation. Treatment of traumatised patients with IGF-I could therefore have dual benefit: an anabolic action to prevent catabolic weight loss and an improvement in gut barrier function to reduce infectious morbidity. The study may also be relevant to the treatment of conditions such as AIDS in which opportunistic infection across the gut presumably contribute to the pathogenesis.

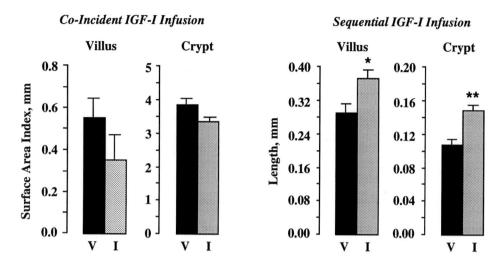

Fig. 6. Effects of 700 µg/day IGF-I on repair of the ileum in rats with methotrexate-induced small bowel mucosal damage. IGF-I (I) or vehicle (V) was infused s.c. for 5 days, starting (left) coincident with the first methotrexate injection or (right) starting 24 h after the third and final methotrexate injection (sequential infusion). Mucosal damage in the ileum was assessed in the coincident infusion study by a "surface area index" which estimates the amount of intact epithelium in the villus or crypt per unit circumference length, or in the sequential infusion study by standard measures of crypt and villus length. Data show means ± SEM for six rats per group. Significance by ANOVA from the vehicle group is shown by: * (p < 0.05); ** (p < 0.01).

The role of IGF-I in the pathogenesis and treatment of inflammatory bowel diseases, such as Crohn's disease and ulcerative colitis, is not yet clear. Reduced plasma IGF-I has been demonstrated in children with inflammatory bowel disease, suggesting that IGF-I therapy may be useful in prevention of the growth retardation associated with these conditions [18,19]. On the other hand, IGF-I has recently been implicated in the development of intestinal fibrosis and strictures in Crohn's disease [20,21]. Clarification of the therapeutic potential for IGF-I in inflammatory bowel disease must therefore await studies in appropriate animal models.

Conclusions

Considerable evidence is now emerging to support the therapeutic application of IGF-I for the treatment of several gut disorders, particularly short bowel and loss of barrier function, while the role of IGF-I in other disorders, such as inflammatory bowel disease, remains to be defined. In view of the fact that plasma IGF-I concentrations are depressed in many of these conditions, IGF-I therapy could be viewed as addressing an IGF deficiency and is likely to have the dual benefit of reducing weight loss as well as improving gut function. The risks in using IGF-I for treatment of gut diseases, particularly precancerous conditions such as ulcerative

416

colitis, have not been addressed adequately at this stage. However, it is encouraging that although IGF-II is synthesised by many tumours, no clear link has been established between IGF-I and human tumours [22].

Acknowledgements

This work was supported by a Cooperative Research Centre grant from the Australian Government, as well as funding from the Channel 7 Children's Research Foundation of SA. The assistance of Jo Cool, Anna Mercorella and Kerry Penning is gratefully acknowledged.

References

1. Read LC, Tomas FM, Howarth GS, Martin AA, Edson KJ, Gillespie CM, Owens PC, Ballard FJ. J Endocrinol 1992;133:421–431.
2. Lemmey AB, Martin AA, Read LC, Tomas FM, Owens PC, Ballard FJ. Am J Physiol 1991;260: E213–E219.
3. Lemmey AB, Ballard FJ, Martin AM, Tomas FM, Howarth GS, Read LC. Treatment with IGF-I peptides improves function of remnant gut following small bowel resection in rats. Growth Factors (in press).
4. Vanderhoof JA, McCusker RH, Clark R, Mohammadpour H, Blackwood DJ, Harty RF, Park JHY. Gastroenterology 1992;102:1949–1956.
5. Read LC, Howarth GS, Lemmey AB, Steeb C, Trahair J, Tomas FM, Ballard FJ. Proc Nutr Soc NZ 1992;17:136–142.
6. Read LC, Lemmey AB, Howarth GS, Martin AA, Tomas FM, Ballard FJ. In: Spencer EM (ed) Modern Concepts of Insulin-Like Growth Factors. Amsterdam: Elsevier Science Publishing Co, 1991; 225–234.
7. Steeb C-B, Trahair JF, Tomas FT, Read LC. Prolonged administration of IGF peptides enhances growth of gastrointestinal issues in normal rats. Am J Physiol (in press).
8. Selby WJ. Gastroenterol Hepatol 1993;8:70–83.
9. Russell N, Rogers S, Hunter A. Blood 1993;81:1972.
10. Debraud F, Bajetta E, Dibartolomeo M, Colleoni M. Tumori 1992;78:228–234.
11. Stringer MD, Spitz L. Arch Dis Child 1993;69:269–271.
12. Labrooy JT. J Acq Immun Def Syndrome 1993;6:S16–S19.
13. Rutgeerts P, Peeters M, Geboes K, Vantrappen G. Endoscopy 1992;24:565–567.
14. Orlowski CC, Brown AL, Ooi GT, Yang YWH, Tseng LY-H, Rechler MM. Endocrinology 1990;126: 644–652.
15. Francis GL, Ross M, Ballard FJ, Milner SJ, Senn C, McNeil KA, Wallace JC, King R, Wells JRE. J Mol Endocrinol 1992;8:213–223.
16. Vanderhoof JA, Park JHY, Mohammadpour H, Blackwood D. Gastroenterology 1990;98:1226–1231.
17. Huang KF, Chung DH, Herndon DN. Arch Surg 1993;128:47–54.
18. Kirschner BS, Sutton MM. Gastroenterology 1986;91:830–836.
19. Thomas AG, Holly JMP, Taylor F, Miller V. Gut 1993;34:944–947.
20. Zimmerman EM, Sartor RB, McCall RD, Pardo M, Bender D, Lund PK. Gastroenterology 1993;105: 399–409.
21. Cohen JA, Zimmerman EM, Sartor RB, Lund PK. Gastroenterology 1993;105:A683 (abstract).
22. Daughaday WH. Endocrinology 1990;127:1–4.

Insulin-like growth factors and the kidney

Allan Flyvbjerg and Hans Ørskov

Institute of Experimental Clinical Research, Departments of Medicine M and V, Aarhus Kommunehospital, DK-8000 Aarhus, Denmark

Abstract. Several lines of evidence indicate that insulin-like growth factors (IGFs) modulate the nephron in normal and diseased kidney, both in respect to function and size. Virtually all members of the IGF axis are present in the kidney, comprising of: 1. IGF-I and IGF-II mRNA; 2. distinct receptors for IGFs: the IGF-I receptor and the IGF-II/Mannose-6-phosphate receptor; and 3. specific binding proteins (IGFBPs), indicating that IGFs may affect the kidney in both an endocrine and autocrine/paracrine fashion. IGFs modulate renal metabolism and the kidney plays an important role in the metabolism and degradation of circulating IGFs. IGFs exert a number of actions on renal tissues at a cellular level, having both proliferative and differentiative effects. In addition, renal growth and renal repair following various pathophysiological conditions (e.g., reduction in renal mass, diabetes mellitus, ischemic renal injury) are preceded by an increase in endogenous renal IGF-I. Furthermore, there is indirect evidence that IGF-I and growth hormone (GH) may be involved in long-term renal changes in renal scarring and experimental diabetes mellitus. Given the ability of IGF-I to stimulate various functions in the kidney, the potential use of IGF-I as a therapeutic agent in the setting of both acute and chronic renal failure (CRF) has been suggested.

Introduction

Increasing evidence suggests that the insulin-like growth factor (IGF) system plays an important role in various physiological and pathological processes in the kidney. The present review will focus on a description of the expression of the IGFs in normal kidney and the physiological actions of IGFs on kidney known today. Furthermore, it summarizes the most recent studies on the possible pathophysiological role of the IGF system in kidney diseases, with emphasis on diabetic kidney disease and renal failure.

Expression of IGFs in the kidney

Virtually all members of the IGF-system are present in the kidney, ranging from messenger RNA (mRNA) expression for IGF-I and IGF-II [1–10], their respective receptors: the IGF-I receptor and the IGF-II/Mannose-6-phosphate receptor (IGF-

---

Address for correspondence: Allan Flyvbjerg M.D., Institute of Experimental Clinical Research, Aarhus Kommunehospital, University of Aarhus, DK-8000 Aarhus, Denmark.

II/Man-6-P receptor) [11—18], to the presence of six different classes of specific binding proteins (IGFBPs) for IGF-I and IGF-II [18—21]. As will be described below each member of the IGF system has specific localization in the nephron and constitutes thereby a unique system in which IGFs in the circulation and in the kidney may affect the nephron in both an endocrine and autocrine/paracrine fashion.

IGF-I and IGF-II

IGF-I and IGF-II mRNAs have been detected in rat and human kidney [1—6] indicating the capacity in kidneys to synthesize IGF-I and IGF-II. Furthermore, IGF-I and IGF-II are found in high concentrations when extracted from the kidney [8,9]. By immunohistochemistry IGF-I has been localized to the thin limb of Henle's loop, the distal convoluted tubule and cortical and medullary collecting ducts [1,7], thereby corresponding to the distribution of the IGF-I mRNA by in situ hybridization [1]. By immunohistochemical staining in rats, IGF-II has been reported to be located predominantly in the collecting ducts [10].

IGF-I- and IGF-II/Man-6-P receptors

Some of the biological actions of IGFs are thought to be mediated via two classes of specific cell surface receptors. The IGF-I receptor is a heterotetrameric glycoprotein with a primary structure which is highly homologous to the insulin receptor, consisting of two α and to β subunits linked by disulfide bridges. The IGF-I and insulin receptors belong to a family of tyrosine kinases. The IGF-I receptor has been identified in the kidney on the basis of competitive binding experiments, Northern blotting and in situ hybridization [11—14]. The IGF-I receptor mRNA in rat and human kidney has been localized in glomeruli and in the tubular epithelium of the medulla and barely detectable in the proximal tubules [18]. It is evident from various studies, however, that IGF-I receptors are widely distributed in the proximal tubules, present at both the luminal and basolateral portions of the tubular cell [11—14]. The IGF-II/Man-6-P receptor is structurally unrelated to the IGF-I and insulin receptors, consisting of a single-chain transmembrane glycoprotein lacking tyrosine-kinase activity [17]. In rat and human kidney the IGF-II/Man-6-P receptor mRNA has a localization similar to the IGF-I receptor, although not found in the glomeruli [18]. The IGF-II/Man-6-P receptor has, in competitive binding experiments in rats, been found to be abundant in both glomeruli and the proximal tubule [11,13,15—18]. In a recent immunohistochemical study the IGF-II/Man-6-P receptor has been found to be localized solely to the proximal tubule [16].

IGFBPs

IGF-I and IGF-II are bound to specific IGFBPs in the circulation and in the extracellular space. To date, six different IGFBPs have been cloned and designated IGFBP-1 to -6 [19,20]. Under normal circumstances IGFBP-3 is the predominant carrier of IGFs in the circulation and one of its roles is to function as a carrier protein for IGFs, thereby protecting IGFs from degradation and sequestration and ensure a sufficient supply to target tissues. It seems evident today, however, that IGFBPs may also act as modulators of IGF actions at a cellular level, both by enhancing and inhibiting the biological actions of IGFs. All six IGFBPs are expressed in the kidney tissue [18–21]. IGFBP-1 and its mRNA has been localized to the medullary thick ascending limbs of Henle's loop and in the collecting ducts [18,21]. IGFBP-2 mRNA in both rat and human kidney has been demonstrated in glomeruli, the medullary interstitium and collecting ducts [18,19]. Studies on the distribution of IGFBP-3 to -6 in the nephron have not yet been published. Finally, it is noteworthy that the abundance of IGFBP-5 mRNA in rat kidney is greater than in any other tissue [19].

IGFs in renal physiology

Metabolism of IGFs in the kidney

It is generally believed that the kidney plays an important role in the metabolism of IGFs. IGF-I and IGF-II are removed from the circulation and exposed to proximal tubular handling, degradation and urinary excretion as has been shown for IGF-I [11,14,22] and IGF-II [16,23]. Very little is known today about the renal handling of IGFBPs in respect to the degree of proximal tubular handling and degradation. It is noteworthy, however, that a significant inverse correlation between the elevated circulating IGFBPs (IGFBP-1, -2 and -3) and glomerular filtration rate (GFR) has been reported in patients with chronic renal failure and furthermore that the elevated IGFBP levels normalize after renal transplantation [24–26]. Urinary excretion of some of the smaller IGFBPs has been reported [23,27], but it is still unknown whether these IGFBPs are filtered from the circulation or secreted from the distal parts of the nephron [28].

Effects of IGFs on renal metabolism

IGF-I and IGF-II exert distinct actions on various metabolic and transport processes in the kidney in vitro. IGF-I has been shown to enhance gluconeogenesis in the proximal tubule [29] while neither IGF-II [29] nor insulin [30] has similar actions. In addition, IGF-I has been shown to stimulate reabsorption of phosphate through the Na^+-dependent phosphate transporter in the brush-border membrane [31,32]. Finally, IGF-I has been shown to stimulate renal transepithelial Na^+ transport by the toad bladder, a model of the mammalian nephron [33]. IGF-II has been shown to stimulate the Na^+/H^+ antiport across the brush border of proximal tubular cells, suggesting a potential regulatory role in the proximal tubule [34]. Studies on the possible effects of IGFBPs on renal metabolism have not yet been published.

Effects of IGFs on renal function

Compelling evidence exists that IGF-I and GH are implicated as mediators of renal function. Originally it was shown in 1965 by Falkheden and Wickbom, that GH-deficient patients have abnormally low GFR and renal plasma flow (RPF), both of which normalize after GH-administration [35]. Hirschberg et al. [36] demonstrated that a single intramuscular injection of GH in adults did not affect GFR or RPF acutely, but both functions were increased within 24 h in parallel with a rise in serum IGF-I. Infusion of IGF-I in animals [37] and man [38] acutely (within hours) increases both GFR and RPF, pointing at a direct effect of IGF-I on kidney function independently of primary changes in kidney size. The action of IGF-I on glomerular hemodynamics may be direct or mediated through prostaglandins [37] or nitric oxide (EDRF)[39], as the stimulatory effect of IGF-I on kidney function can be abrogated by coinfusion of indomethacin [37] or N-nitro-L-arginine methyl ester (a specific inhibitor of nitric oxide synthesis) [39].

Effects of IGFs on kidney growth

IGF-I exerts a number of growth promoting actions on renal tissues at a cellular level, having both proliferative and differentiative effects. In glomerular mesangial cells in mice [40] and rats [41], and in rabbit renal cortical tubular [42] and proximal tubule epithelial cells [43], IGF-I has mitogenic actions. In human fetal mesangial cells, IGF-I stimulates protein and proteoglycan synthesis [44]. The growth-promoting effect actions of GH in many tissues, including the kidney, are thought to be mediated mainly through IGF-I. The GH dependence of the kidney IGF-I content has been confirmed by the finding of reduced kidney IGF-I levels in hypophysectomized rats [45] and in dwarf rats with isolated GH deficiency [46,47]. In both conditions, kidney IGF-I concentration and renal size rose in response to GH-administration [45–47]. Furthermore, studies have shown that IGF-I infusion in hypophysectomized [48], GH-deficient dwarf [46] and pituitary intact animals [49] induces renal growth within days to weeks. Apart from playing a role in GH-induced kidney growth, further evidence for a general renotropic action of IGF-I arises from the observation that endogenous kidney IGF-I accumulation takes place in at least three other conditions characterized by rapid renal growth [2,7,13,45,47,50–60]: experimental diabetes (see below), unilateral nephrectomy and potassium (K^+) depletion.

IGFs in renal pathophysiology

It has become increasingly evident over the past years that IGFs, in addition to playing an important role in renal physiology, are also involved in various pathological processes in the kidney. Accordingly IGFs (and GH) have been suggested to play a role in diabetic nephropathy [2,13,47,50–52,54–61], nondiabetic glomerulosclerosis [62–64] and in regeneration of postischemic damage of the proximal tubule [65–67]. Furthermore, the potential use of IGF-I and GH as therapeutic agents in the setting of renal failure has been suggested [68–75]. In the following, recent evidence will be emphasized for IGFs playing a role in diabetic kidney disease and renal failure.

IGFs in diabetic kidney disease

Diabetic kidney disease is characterized by an early increase in kidney size, glomerular volume and kidney function and later by the development of mesangial proliferation, accumulation of glomerular extracellular matrix (ECM), increased urinary albumin excretion (UAE) and glomerular sclerosis. The search for significant pathogenic mechanisms in diabetic kidney disease has focused on the early events, at the point in time when the above mentioned pathophysiological changes take place. Accordingly, the IGF system has attracted attention in several areas of diabetes research including conceivable effects on the renal changes seen in experimental and human diabetes. Several metabolic, functional and structural renal changes in streptozotocin (STZ)-diabetic rats have fundamental similarities to those occurring in diabetic patients and this model has accordingly been used extensively in diabetes research aiming to elucidate the possible role of the IGF system in the pathogenesis of diabetic kidney disease.

It is evident today from different groups that the rapid increase in renal growth and function seen in STZ-diabetes is preceded by a rise in renal tissue concentration of IGF-I reaching a peak 24–48 h after the induction of diabetes and returning to basal levels after about 4 days [2,47,50–52,54]. In addition, IGF-I infusion into diabetic rats commencing after the initial rapid growth rate has abated, with restoration of the initial high kidney IGF-I levels, reaccelerates diabetic renal hypertrophy [56]. Concomitantly with the rise in endogenous kidney IGF-I a transient increase in kidney IGFBP species is seen, supporting the notion that IGFBPs may modulate the renotropic action of IGF-I in diabetic renal enlargement [57]. This finding is corroborated by the finding of IGF-I binding in the diabetic kidney to low-molecular weight material that may represent IGFBPs [13,55]. Diabetic dwarf rats with isolated GH and IGF-I deficiency exhibit slower and lesser initial renal and glomerular hypertrophy as well as a smaller rise in kidney IGF-I than diabetic controls with intact pituitary, indicating that GH per se may be involved in the modulation of renal enlargement [47]. Strict insulin treatment abolishes both the increase in kidney IGF-I and renal hypertrophy [50] and a long-acting somatostatin analogue (octreotide) equally inhibits kidney IGF-I accumulation and growth without affecting the blood glucose levels (51).

At present there is no direct evidence that IGF-I is also involved in maintaining diabetic kidney hypertrophy and function. However, in view of the evidence that octreotide may directly inhibit IGF-I synthesis independently of GH inhibition [58], it is intriguing that 6 months administration of octreotide to diabetic rats reduces diabetic UAE, renal hypertrophy and serum and kidney IGF-I without affecting metabolic control [59]. Furthermore, reduction in renal size and hyperfunction is seen in type 1 diabetic patients treated with octreotide for a period of 3 months without discernible reductions in serum GH, glucagon or HbA_{1C}, but with pronounced reductions in circulating IGF-I levels [61]. Finally, long-term diabetic dwarf rats, with a diabetes duration of 6 months, display a smaller degree of renal and glomerular hypertrophy and rise in UAE, when compared to the changes observed in pituitary intact diabetic rats [60].

These results indicate that IGF-I through a complex IGF system comprising IGF ligands, IGFBPs and the influence of GH, acts as an initiating growth factor for the early diabetic renal enlargement in experimental diabetes. As mentioned above there is only indirect evidence for an involvement of the IGF system in long-term diabetic renal changes and studies elucidating a possible participation are presently in progress.

IGFs in renal failure

Little is known about the changes in local IGFs in the kidney in acute and chronic renal failure. Matejka and Jennische [65,66] have, however, recently reported that immunoreactive IGF-I, IGF-I binding and IGF-I mRNA increase in a transient manner in regenerative cells in the distal (S3) segment of the proximal tubule in the postischemic experimental rat model of acute renal failure (ARF). Similarly, increased levels of both IGF-I mRNA and renal IGF-I content are seen in the remnant kidney tissue following partial kidney infarction [67]. It seems evident, however, that a tremendous amount of questions are still to be answered, before an exact picture of the local autocrine/paracrine changes in kidney IGFs in both acute and chronic renal failure is achieved.

It is interesting, however, that recent studies based on the ability of GH and IGF-I to stimulate various functions in normal kidney, have suggested the potential use of GH or IGF-I in the setting of both acute and chronic renal failure. Encouraged by the observation that endogenous IGF-I increases locally in the kidney in experimental models of ARF [65–67], a single study has so far focused on the effect of IGF-I as a therapeutic agent in ARF [68]. Miller et al. [68] showed that exogenous IGF-I infusion during the first 7 days after acute ischemic renal injury in rats accelerated the recovery of normal renal function and the regeneration of damaged proximal tubular epithelium.

Due to the ability of GH to chronically stimulate kidney function and kidney growth in experimental models and in man, it was expected that GH would also be capable of enhancing kidney function in the setting of chronic renal failure (CRF). However, the data available today relating to this possibility have been disappointing. The administration of GH to experimental animals with reduced functional renal mass has no effect on kidney function [69]. Furthermore, the administration of GH to children with CRF and growth failure has been found to have no significant effect on renal function, despite the well-known effect on longitudinal growth [70–72]. Finally, GH-administration has no effect on kidney function in adult patients with CRF [73]. Until recently the use of IGF-I as a therapeutic agent in CRF was as disappointing as the lack of an GH effect when judged from experimental models of CRF. Administration of IGF-I to rats that had undergone 1⅔ [69] and 1½ renal ablation [74] did not enhance kidney function, despite beneficial effects on growth and catabolism. On the basis of the above mentioned negative effects of GH and IGF-I to stimulate kidney function in CRF, it was suggested that the uremic state per se induces a relative resistance to the renal actions of GH and IGF-I. O'Shea et al. [75] have, however, recently reported that short-term (4 days) administration of IGF-I to adult patients with moderate CRF (inulin clearance between 22 and 55 ml/min/1.73 m^2) enhances glomerular filtration rate, renal plasma flow and kidney volume. The potential use of short-term or long-term administration of IGF-I in children with CRF has not yet been conducted. Future research should be directed at elucidating the long-term clinical effects of IGF-I administration alone and in combination with GH, on kidney function and somatic growth.

Conclusions and outlook

Although it is only little more than 2 decades since the characterization of IGFs began in earnest, knowledge of this group of peptide growth factors in relation to renal physiology and pathology is expanding rapidly. This is mainly due to a extensive worldwide interest in the IGF system in relation to the kidney and the availability of modern molecular/cellular techniques and biosynthetically produced peptides. IGFs have a variety of effects on renal physiology and their implication in a number of pathophysiological processes in the kidney has become increasingly obvious over the past few years. In view of the complexity of the IGF system, it will be a tremendous challenge for the coming years to fully characterize the renal effects of IGFs. There is no doubt, however, that information on this topic will occur with increasing pace in the near future.

Acknowledgements

The Danish Diabetes Association, the Danish Medical Research Council, the Aage Louis-Hansen Memorial Foundation, the Novo Foundation, the Nordic Insulin Foundation, the Novo-Nordisk A/S and the Ruth König Petersen Foundation are thanked for financial support.

References

1. Bortz JD, Rotwein P, DeVol D, Bechtel PJ, Hansen VA, Hammerman MR. J Cell Biol 1988;107: 811–819.
2. Flyvbjerg A, Bornfeldt KE, Marshall SM, Arnqvist HJ, Ørskov H. Diabetologia 1990;33:334–338.
3. Murphy LJ, Bell GI, Frisen HG. Endocrinology 1987;120:1279–1282.

424

4. Bell GI, Gerhard DS, Fong NM, Sanchez-Pescador, Rall LB. Proc Natl Acad Sci USA 1985;82: 6450–6454.
5. Han VKM, Lund PK, Lee DC, D'Ercole AJ. J Clin Endocrinol Metab 1988;66:422–429.
6. Hammerman MR, Miller SB. Am J Physiol 1993;265:F1–F14.
7. Flyvbjerg A, Marshall SM, Frystyk J, Rasch R, Bornfeldt KE, Arnqvist HJ, Jensen PK, Pallesen G, Ørskov H. Am J Physiol 1992;262:F1023–F1031.
8. D'Ercole JA, Stiles AD, Underwood LE. Proc Natl Acad Sci USA 1984;81:935–939.
9. Lee W-H, Bowsher R, Apathy M, Smith MC, Henry DP. Endocrinology 1991;128:815–822.
10. Lee W-H, Evan AP, Summurlin PB, Henry DP. Immunocystochemical localization of insulin-like growth factor II (IGF-II) in adult rat kidney (abstract). 2nd International Symposium on Insulin-like Growth Factors/Somatomedins, January 12–16th 1991, San Francisco (USA).
11. Hammerman MR, Rogers SA. Am J Physiol 1987;253:F841–F847.
12. Pillion DJ, Haskell JF, Meezan E. Am J Physiol 1988;255:E504–E512.
13. Werner H, Shen-Orr Z, Stannard B, Burguera B, Roberts CT, LeRoit D. Diabetes 1990;39:1490–1497.
14. Flyvbjerg A, Nielsen S, Sheikh MI, Jacobsen C, Ørskov H, Christensen EI. Am J Physiol 1993;43: 796–807.
15. Haskell JF, Pillion DJ, Meezan E. Endocrinology 1988;123:774–780.
16. Cui S, Flyvbjerg A, Nielsen S, Kiess W, Christensen EI. Kidney Int 1993;43:796–807.
17. Nissley SP, Kiess W, Sklar MM. In: LeRoit D (ed) IGFs: Molecular and Cellular Aspects. Boca Raton; CRC Press, 1991;111–150.
18. Chin E, Bondy C. J Clin Endocrinol Metab 1992;75:962–968.
19. Shimasaki S, Shimonaka M, Zhang HP, Ling N. J Biol Chem 1991;266:10646–10653.
20. Shimasaki S, Gao L, Shimonaka M, Ling N. Mol Endocrinol 1991;4:1451–1458.
21. Kobayashi S, Clemmons DR, Venkatachalam MA. Am J Physiol 1991;261:F22–F28.
22. Hizuka N, Takano K, Asakawa K, Fukuda I, Ohta T, Shizume K, Demura H. In: Spencer EM (ed) Modern Concepts of Insulin-like Growth Factors. New York; Elsevier Science Publishers B.V., 1991; 607–615.
23. Zumkeller W, Hall K. Acta Endocrinol (Copenh) 1990;123:499–503.
24. Blum WF, Ranke MB, Kietzmann K, Tönshoff B, Mehls O. Pediatr Nephrol 1991;5:539–544.
25. Blum WF, Horn N, Kratzsch J, Jørgensen JOL, Juul A, Teale D, Mohnike K, Ranke MB. Growth Reg 1993;3:100–104.
26. Schwander J, Mary JL. Growth Reg 1993;3:104–108.
27. Cohen P, Fielder PJ, Hasegawa Y, Frisch H, Giudice LC, Rosenfeld RG. Acta Endocrinol (Copenh) 1991;124:74–85.
28. Aron DC, Saadi HF, Nye CN, Douglas JG. Kidney Int 1991;39:27–32.
29. Rogers SA, Karl IE, Hammerman MR. Am J Physiol 1989;257:E751–E756.
30. Chobanian MC, Hammerman MR. Am J Physiol 1987;253:F1171–F1177.
31. Hammerman MR, Karl IE, Hruska KA. Biochim Biophys Acta 1980;603:322–335.
32. Caverzasio J, Faundez R, Fleisch H, Bonjour JP. Endocrinology 1990;127:453–459.
33. Blazer-Yost BL, Cox M. Am J Physiol 1988;255:C413–C417.
34. Mellas J, Gavin JR III, Hammerman MR. J Biol Chem 1986;261:14437–14442.
35. Falkheden T, Wickbom I. Acta Endocrinol (Copenh) 1965;48:348–354.
36. Hirschberg R, Rabb H, Bergamo R, Kopple JD. Kidney Int 1989;35:865–870.
37. Hirschberg R, Kopple JD. J Clin Invest 1989;83:326–330.
38. Guler H-P, Schmid C, Zapf J, Froesch ER. Proc Natl Acad Sci USA 1989;86:2868–2872.
39. Haylor J, Singh I, El Nahas AM. Kidney Int 1991;39:333–335.
40. Conti FG, Striker LJ, Lesniak MA, MacKay K, Roth J, Striker GE. Endocrinology 1988;122:2788–2794.
41. Arnqvist HJ, Ballerman BJ, King GL. Am J Physiol 1988;254:C411–C416.
42. Kanda S, Nomata K, Saha PK, Nishimura N, Yamada J, Kanatake H, Saito Y. Cell Biol Int Rep 1989;13:687–699.

425

43. Zhang G, Ichimura T, Wallin A, Kan M, Stevens JL. J Biol Chem 1991;265:14892–14898.
44. Moran A, Brown DM, Kim Y, Klein DJ. Diabetes 1990;39:70A.
45. Stiles AD, Sosenko IRS, D'Ercole AJ, Schmith BT. Endocrinology 1985;117:2397–2401.
46. Skottner A, Clark RG, Fryklund L, Robinson ICAF. Endocrinology 1989;124:2519–2526.
47. Flyvbjerg A, Frystyk J, Østerby R, Ørskov H. Am J Physiol 1992;262:E956–E962.
48. Guler H-P, Zapf J, Scheiwiller E, Froesch ER. Proc Natl Acad Sci USA 1988;85:4889–4893.
49. Mathews LS, Hammer RE, Behringer RR, D'Ercole AJ, Bell GI, Brinster RL, Palmiter RD. Endocrinology 1988;123:2827–2833.
50. Flyvbjerg A, Thorlacius-Ussing O, Naeraa R, Ingerslev J, Ørskov H. Diabetologia 1988;31:310–314.
51. Flyvbjerg A, Frystyk J, Thorlacius-Ussing O, Ørskov H. Diabetologia 1989;32:261–265.
52. Flyvbjerg A, Ørskov H, Nyborg K, Frystyk J, Marshall SM, Bornfeldt KE, Arnqvist HJ, Jørgensen KD. In: Spencer EM (ed) Modern Concepts of Insulin-like Growth Factors. New York; Elsevier Science Publishers, 1991;207–218.
53. Lajara R, Rotwein P, Bortz JD, Hansen VA, Sadow JL, Betts CR, Rogers SA, Hammerman MR. Am J Physiol 1989;257:F252–F261.
54. Bach LA, Jerums G. Diabetes 1990;39:557–562.
55. Bach LA, Cox AJ, Mendelsohn FAO, Werther G, Jerums G. Diabetes 1992;41:499–507.
56. Flyvbjerg A, Bornfeldt KE, Ørskov H, Arnqvist HJ. Diabetologia 1991;34:715–720.
57. Flyvbjerg A, Kessler U, Dorka B, Funk B, Ørskov H, Kiess W. Diabetologia 1992;35:589–593.
58. Flyvbjerg A, Jørgensen KD, Marshall SM, Ørskov H. Am J Physiol 1991;260:E568–E574.
59. Flyvbjerg A, Marshall SM, Frystyk J, Hansen KW, Harris AG, Ørskov H. Kidney Int 1992;41:805–812.
60. Grønbæk H, Bjørn SF, Østerby R, Ørskov H, Flyvbjerg A. Effect of specific GH/IGF-I deficiency on long-term renal and glomerular hypertrophy and urinary albumin excretion in diabetic dwarf rats (abstract). 3rd International Symposium on Insulin-like Growth Factors, February 6–10th 1994, Sydney (Australia).
61. Serri O, Beauregard H, Brazeau P, Abribat T, Lambert J, Harris AG, Vachon L. JAMA 1991;265:888–892.
62. Doi T, Striker LJ, Quaife C, Conti FG, Palmiter R, Behringer R, Brinster RL, Striker GE. Am J Pathol 1988;131:398–403.
63. Doi T, Striker LJ, Gibson CC, Agodoa LYC, Brinster RL, Striker GE. Am J Pathol 1990;137:541–552.
64. El Nahas AM, Bassett AH, Cope GH, Le Carpentier JE. Kidney Int 1991;40:29–34.
65. Andersen GL, Jennische E. Acta Physiol Scand 1988;132:453–457.
66. Matejka GL, Jennische E. Kidney Int 1992;42:1113–1123.
67. Rogers SA, Miller SB, Hammerman MR. Am J Physiol 1993;264:F963–F967.
68. Miller SB, Martin DR, Kissane J, Hammerman MR. Proc Natl Acad Sci USA 1992;89:11876–11880.
69. Miller SB, Hansen VA, Hammerman MR. Am J Physiol 1990;259:F747–F751.
70. Koch VH, Lippe BM, Nelson PA, Boechat MI, Sherman BM, Fine RN. J Pediatr 1989;115:365–371.
71. Tönshoff B, Mehls O, Heinrich U, Blum WF, Schauer A. J Pediatr 1990;116:561–566.
72. Fine RN. Kidney Int 1992;42:188–197.
73. Haffner D, Zacharewicz S, Mehls O, Heinrich U, Ritz E. Clin Nephrol 1989;32:266–269.
74. Martin AA, Tomas FM, Owens PC, Knowles SE, Ballard FJ, Read LC. Am J Physiol 1991;261:F626–F633.
75. O'Shea MH, Miller SB, Hammerman MR. Am J Physiol 1993;264:F917–F922.

The insulin-like growth factors and their regulatory proteins
R.C. Baxter, P.D. Gluckman and R.G. Rosenfeld, editors

The role of IGF-I in the response to organ injury — studies in the central nervous system

P.D. Gluckman, C.E. Williams, J. Guan, E. Beilharz and B.M. Johnston
Research Centre for Developmental Medicine and Biology, University of Auckland, Private Bag 92019, Auckland, New Zealand

Abstract. After hypoxic ischemic injury to the central nervous system, there is a rapid induction of IGF-I, IGFBP-2 and IGFBP-3 at the sites of injury. Administration of IGF-I into the lateral cerebral ventricle of rats following hypoxic-ischemic injury or fetal sheep following ischemic injury, markedly ameliorates the degree of neuronal loss. This effect of IGF-I is not mimicked by des(1–3) IGF-I and is antagonised by IGF-II suggesting a role for IGFBPs in determining the neuroprotective effect of IGF-I. In addition preliminary evidence suggests that some neuroprotective activity is due to IGF-I acting as a prohormone for the production of the terminal tripeptide GPE. The neuroprotective effect of IGF-I may be via inhibition of asphyxial induced apoptosis. The effect of IGF-I is exhibited when administered after the asphyxial insult. This distinguishes IGF-I from most other neuroprotective therapies and suggests an important clinical application.

Introduction

The paracrine IGF system is clearly a key component in the regulation of normal organ development and for the maintenance of tissues such as the gut where there is a high rate of cell turnover. However, IGFs and their BPs are expressed to varying extent in all tissues throughout life, even in the brain where the rate of cell turnover is very low. Limited evidence shows that the paracrine IGF system is affected by tissue injury suggesting that IGF-I plays a role in tissue repair. IGF-I and/or IGF receptor induction has been shown within 1–5 days of injury in skeletal muscle [1–3], vascular smooth muscle [4], skin [5], kidney [6] and brain (see below). As well as playing a role in repair, evidence, at least in the brain, suggests that IGF-I can inhibit the injury process. This paper reviews our studies of the induction of the IGF system after injury to the central nervous system (CNS).

Processes of cell loss after brain injury

Hypoxic-ischemic injury (HII) is the most common form of brain injury. It is now recognised that a number of mechanisms are involved in neuronal and glial cell loss following HII and that there are distinct phases to the timing of post-HII cell death when different processes are operative [7]. During the period of HII, the consequences of energy failure include intracellular edema and calcium accumulation: these processes are partially driven by asphyxia-induced excitotoxic amino acid (aspartate and glutamate) release. The NMDA subtype of glutamate receptor is linked to calcium channels and kainic acid subtype to sodium channels. Free radical production, particularly at the time of reversal of the HII, leads to lipid peroxidation and to cell membrane rupture. However, it is increasingly recognised, that unless the injury is very prolonged or irreversible, most neurones that die do not do so during this primary phase. Instead after some hours of relative neural depression a secondary phase occurs over several days during which neuronal (and glial) death is apparent. While seizures are often associated with the secondary event, excitotoxic mechanisms appear not to be the dominant processes of delayed neuronal death. Inappropriate activation of apoptotic mechanisms may be a key element in delayed cell death. However, not all delayed cell death is classically apoptotic: in many areas, random DNA degradation is observed suggesting a necrotic death − however, this is also delayed and not observed until hours after the injury [8]. Whether apoptotic and necrotic patterns of DNA degradation represent fundamentally different patterns of cell death is not clear. In addition the activation of microglia (which are macrophage like cells) and recruitment of haematogenous macrophages and neutrophils may play a role in delaying neuronal death.

However, because postasphyxial neuronal loss is largely a delayed process, there is a "window of therapeutic opportunity" after the injury, but before the neurones are irreversibly committed to delayed cell death in which intervention may be possible.

Experimental approach

For the majority of our studies we developed a defined, repeatable and gradable model of reversible HII [9,10] in either 21 day old or adult rats. Following unilateral carotid artery ligation, the animals are subjected to a defined period of inhalational hypoxia, the length and degree of which defines whether selective neuronal loss in the cortex and hippocampus is seen or whether cortical necrosis (defined as loss of neurones and glia) and extensive neuronal loss throughout the cerebrum is observed. Cell loss is unilateral and is restricted to the side of ligation. The injury occurs because while the Circle of Willis is adequate under basal conditions to deliver oxygen to the ligated hemisphere, it is not so under asphyxial conditions. Histological outcome is assessed by blinded observers. An acid fuschin stain is used to detect dead neurones 5 days after injury; infarct size is also scored [10].

Growth factor induction

Nieto-Sampedro et al. [11] were the first to suggest the induction of neurotrophic activity in the brain after traumatic injury. We therefore examined after mild or severe HII in the 21 day old rat the induction of growth factors using in situ hybridisation techniques. Neither nerve growth factor (NGF) or brain derived neurotrophic factor (BDNF) were induced in the region of injury: there was a small degree of induction in the contralateral hippocampus presumed secondary to seizures which occurred at the end of the asphyxial phase [12]. A number of early intermediate transcription factors were induced in the brain in association with the BDNF including c-*fos*, c-*jun* and Krox. In less severe injuries, induction of IEGPs could be seen in the ipsilateral (injured) hippocampus and cortex within 1 h of injury. Prolonged expression of c-*jun* was also detected in neurons undergoing delayed cell death.

IGF-I was induced in astrocytic cells. Induction was apparent by 72 h and maximal by 120 h [10]. The most intense induction was in the lateral cortex, hippocampus, striatum, thalamus and pyriform cortex. In marked contrast IGF-II was not induced until 7 days after injury and induction was limited to the one area of cortical infarction and presumably to macrophages. The expression of IGF-I and IGF-II was confirmed by immunohistochemistry.

IGFBP-1 induction was not affected. IGFBP-4 was suppressed on the side of injury within 24 h. IGFBP-5 was induced in white matter, but only 7 days after injury, perhaps suggesting some role in the late glial repair response [13]. IGFBP-2 [14] and IGFBP-3 [10] were both induced in the area of neuronal loss, but with a different but overlapping spatial and temporal distribution. For example whereas IGFBP-2 was at 72 h expressed on the edge of the cortical infarct and in the thalamus, IGFBP-3 was at that time induced throughout the infarct and in the striatum, but not in the thalamus. Induction of these two IGFBPs occurred in parallel with IGF-I. By Northern analysis changes in IGFBP-2 induction were apparent within 6 h of injury [15].

Similarly it has been reported that with a focal ischemic injury IGF-I and IGF-II are induced within days of injury in astrocytes and microglia respectively [16]. Ligand binding studies suggest induction of IGF receptors in the injured hippocampus [17,18]. In vivo microdialysis shows increased CNS production of IGF-I after brain injury [19].

Interventional studies

The degree of neuronal loss after HII is a function of the interaction between those mechanisms leading to cell loss and those endogenous protective responses as modulated by a number of sensitising factors (e.g., metabolic status, degree of cardiovascular compromise, developmental status, maturation and the temporal pattern of the insult [20]). Endogenous protective responses include the release of inhibitory neuromodulators such as GABA and adenosine, brain cooling and potentially the release of endogenous neurotrophic factors. We speculated that induction of IGF-I might be part of the endogenous neuroprotective response [10].

Using the unilateral hypoxic-ischemic rat preparation we investigated the effect of IGF-I administered via the lateral cerebral ventricle on histological outcome following HII [10,21]. Following unilateral carotid artery ligation the rats (300 g male) were subjected to 10 min of 6% oxygen at $90 \pm 5\%$ humidity at $34 \pm 0.5°C$. By day 5 this produced marked infarction in the cerebral cortex and extensive neuronal loss in the thalamus, striatum and hippocampus. A number of studies are summarised below.

Time of administration

IGF-I (20 µg/rat) administered at 2 h after injury significantly reduced the degree of neuronal loss throughout the hemisphere except the hippocampus and reduced the infarct rate. The same dose of IGF-I administered 1 h prior to the inhalational asphyxia had no effect on the outcome [10]. This suggested that IGF-I acted on processes initiated by the HII to prevent delayed neuronal death and did not affect the primary phase of neuronal loss. This timing effect is in marked contrast to most classical approaches to neuroprotection such as calcium channel antagonists that are active prior to, but not after, the injury [7]. However, because IGF-I is active in the window of opportunity, the therapeutic potential is considerable.

Dose

Over the range 5–50 µg IGF1/rat a dose dependent increase in neuroprotection was observed [21]. At 50 µg/rat the incidence of infarction was reduced from 87% to 26% ($p < 0.05$) and neuronal loss was reduced ($p < 0.05$) in the cerebral cortex, striatum, hippocampus, thalamus and amygdala. The degree of protection was most marked in the lateral cortex. The degree of protection was somewhat variable between experiments in the hippocampus and appeared to depend on whether the IGF-I was administered in a low or high volume — the latter perhaps promoting greater diffusion of the IGF-I.

Specificity of action

Previously it has been reported that at high dose, insulin confers some degree of neuroprotection and that this effect is independent of hypoglycaemia. Generally the doses used of insulin have been an order of magnitude greater than that of IGF-I used in our studies and multiple doses have been given [22,23]. We compared 20 µg IGF-I to 20 µg IGF-II to 20 µg insulin 2 h postinjury. No protection was conferred by either insulin or IGF-II suggesting an action via the IGF-I receptor [21].

The role of the IGF binding proteins

We speculated that the local induction of IGFs in the regions of damage might be important to the action of IGF-I. We therefore compared the effect of 20 µg IGF-I to the combination of 20 µg IGF-I plus 30 µg IGF-II, reasoning that the higher affinity of IGF-II for IGFBP-2 and IGFBP-3 might reduce the bioavailability of IGF-I. IGF-II completely blocked the effects of IGF-I in promoting neuronal rescue. In the thalamus and dentate gyrus there was a significant effect of IGF-II alone or in combination with IGF-I to increase damage compared to vehicle treated controls [24]. We also examined the effect of des(1–3) IGF-I, because of its low affinity for IGFBP-3 and IGFBP-2, and observed no neuroprotective effect at either 2 or 20 µg/rat compared to clear neuroprotection with 20 µg IGF-I [24]. The absence of an effect of des IGF-I at low doses might either reflect reduced affinity for IGFBPs or that the terminal tripeptide, GPE, is of biological significance. Because IGF-I receptors are apparently induced after brain injury [18] and because insulin, which does not share the same terminal tripeptide, has some neuroprotective activity [22], we speculate that at least in part the action of IGF-I is mediated via the IGF-I receptor.

The effect of the terminal tripeptide

We administered the N terminal tripeptide GPE at a molar equivalent dose to IGF-I to the adult rat. Significant neuroprotection was conferred, although not with identical spectrum of protection to IGF-I. GPE was markedly neuroprotective in the CA1-2 region of the hippocampus, whereas IGF-I was not − this might reflect simply different diffusion properties from the ventricular space. Conversely GPE appeared not to be neuroprotective in the dentate gyrus in contrast to molar equivalent doses of IGF-I. This might suggest that in this region the only neuroprotective action of IGF-I is via the IGF-I receptor.

It has been reported that IGF-I and GPE are both able to affect GnRH release from hypothalamic explants by antagonist actions at the NMDA receptor [25]. We therefore examined whether the effect of GPE was comparable to the effect of the non-NMDA receptor antagonist MK801. MK801 given 2 h after injury had no effect on neurological outcome − this is compatible with other studies which show that NMDA blockade is neuroprotective if administered close to or before the injury, but not by some hours after. Thus the mode of the neuroprotective action of GPE is not known.

Other observations in the rat

There is considerable evidence that some neuroprotective therapeutic effects are due to hypothermia [26]. We measured brain temperature by implanted thermistors using telemetry; IGF-I therapy did not alter brain temperature.

To assess whether IGF-I improved functional outcome, we performed the bilateral sticky patch test for tactile somatosensory function. An observer blind to the experiment measured the time the rat took to notice a sticky patch placed on each paw. In the absence of damage the ratio between sides is unity, in the presence of a unilateral injury, the ratio deviates from unity. Compared to vehicle treated controls, the IGF-I levels had significantly closer values to unity over the days immediately after injury; although by 1 week control values also normalise because of the plasmic response.

Studies in the fetal sheep

However, because of the obvious clinical potential of these observations, we have extended these studies to a second species. The chronically instrumented late gestation fetal lamb offers particular advantages; at 125/147 days gestation its degree of neural maturity is comparable to the term neonate. We have developed techniques for monitoring neural function in utero and for applying reversible cerebral ischemic episodes to the fetus in the absence of anaesthesia. Thirty min of cerebral ischemia was induced by inflating cuffs placed around each carotid artery some days earlier. At that time the vertebral-occipital anastoses, the source of the vertebral, supply were ligated. Such an insult produces bilateral infarction of the parasaggital cortex and severe neuronal loss throughout the cerebrum [27,28]. Using cerebral impedance to monitor cytotoxic edema two clear phases of neuronal death are observed — immediately associated with the insult and a delayed phase commencing 6—12 h after the ischemic insult and lasting some 48 h. The secondary phase is associated with postasphyxial seizures [27,29]. Using a lateral cerebral ventricular cannula also implanted at surgery, the animals were treated with vehicle or IGF-I administered over a 1 h infusion starting 2 h after injury. Considerable neuroprotection was conferred in most regions of the brain with a single dose of 100 ng (n = 6) compared to vehicle (n = 6) and all regions showed significant improvement with a 1 μg dose of IGF-I (n = 6). The effect was most marked in the dentate gyrus, thalamus and amygdala and least in the parasaggital cortex. We suspect that with this severe HII preparation, considerable primary neuronal loss occurs in this region. Higher doses of IGF-I (>10 μg) did not confer protection. At 1 μg/sheep, the secondary event, as measured by the delayed rise in cerebral impedance, was delayed and attenuated reflecting the reduced secondary neuronal death. Retrospective comparison to the effect of use of a calcium channel antagonist, flunarazine [30] or the NMDA receptor antagonist MK801 [31] showed the degree of protection with IGF-I was greater. There were no signs of systemic toxicity with IGF-I until at least 50-fold higher doses were used, in contrast to the narrow efficacy/toxicity range for the classical neuroprotectants [32].

Discussion

These studies suggest that IGF-I has a relatively unique role both as an endogenous and exogenous neural rescue agent. The mode of action of IGF-I remains to be fully elucidated. It may be that there is a dual mode of action. IGF-I may act directly at the IGF-I receptor and as well act as a prohormone for GPE which has an independent mode of action. IGF-I has been shown to interfere with apoptotic processes in thyocytes [33]. Recent studies in the chick embryo also suggest IGF-I can prevent physiological apoptosis of primary motor neurones [34]. In addition IGF-I has been shown to be a potent trophic agent for embryonic cortical neurones in culture [35] — it is not clear whether this action is as a trophic factor or as a survival factor (preventing cell death). In the rat preparation used in this study there is considerable evidence of apoptotic DNA degradation starting from 6—24 h after the injury; the timing of onset being spatially dependent [8]. The mode of action of GPE remains to be resolved.

IGF-I has been shown to promote repair of the damage peripheral nervous system.

IGF-I is induced in the Schwann cells of surrounding nerve injury [36]. IGF-I has entered clinical trials for peripheral neuropathy in motor neuron disease. Whether such actions of IGF-I reflect analogous actions to that of IGF-I in the central nervous system is not clear.

We have shown the neuroprotective action of IGF-I both in rats and sheep and in both asphyxial and ischemic injury. The much lower dose of IGF-I required for neuroprotection in the sheep presumably reflects the essential identity of structure between the recombinant hIGF-I used in these studies and ovine IGF-I, whereas rat IGF-I has a considerably different primary structure. Similarly the dose of IGF-I required for anabolic/somatogenic effects is much larger in rats than in sheep or man where comparable doses are active. This low dose (100 ng-1 µg/150 g brain) suggests that IGF-I acts as an endogenous neuroprotectant. Whether systemic administration of either IGF-I or GPE will allow sufficient brain entry is currently under study.

Although IGF-II has been suggested to play a particular role in the CNS, largely because neural expression of IGF-II persists after birth in the rat whereas it does not peripherally, our data do not suggest analogous actions between IGF-I and IGF-II in brain injury. IGF-II does not play a role in the early survival response. The late induction of IGF-II largely in areas of white matter and in macrophages might suggest a possible role in gliosis.

Other neurotrophic factors have been shown to have some neuronal rescue activity. We and others have shown a protective effect of TGFβ when given after HII [37,38]. The effect is essentially comparable to IGF-I. As TGFβ has been shown to increase both IGF-I and IGFBP-3 expression in other cell types, the modes of action may be inter-related. Similarly the neurotrophic action of basic FGF are modified by coadministration of antiserum to IGF-I [39].

Hypoxic-ischemic injury is a major clinical problem — the most important categories including perinatal HII stroke, trauma and cardiac arrest. Therapeutic options at the present time are essentially limited to support measures. IGF-I in contrast to calcium channel antagonists, free radical scavenges and NMDA receptor antagonists exerts its effects when administered well after injury. Further experimental studies may well lead to consideration of IGF-I as a therapeutic neural rescue agent.

Acknowledgements

This work was funded by a Programme Grant of the Health Research Council of New Zealand and by grants from the Neurological Foundation of NZ and the NZ Lotteries Board. We thank Dr K Nikolics of Genentech Inc for his assistance.

References

1. Levinovitz A, Jennische E, Oldfors A, Edwall D, Norstedt G. Mol Endocrinol 1992;6:1227–1234.
2. Edwall D, Schalling M, Jennische E, Norstedt G. Endocrinology 1989;124:820–825.
3. Jennische E, Matejka GL. Acta Physiol Scand 1992;146:79–86.

434

4. Khorsandi MJ, Fagin JA, Giannella ND, Forrester JS, Cercek B. J Clin Invest 1992;90:1926–1931.
5. Antoniades HN, Galanopoulos T, Neville-Golden J, Kiritsy CP, Lynch SE. Am J Pathol 1993;142: 1099–1100.
6. Matejka GL, Jennische E. Kidney Int 1992;42:1113–1123.
7. Gluckman PD, Williams CE. Dev Med Child Neurol 1992;34:1010–1014.
8. Beilharz EJ, Williams CE, Dragunow M, Sirimanne E, Gluckman PD. J Neurosci 1993 (submitted).
9. Sirimanne E, Guan J, Williams CE, Gluckman PD. J Neurosci Meth 1993 (submitted).
10. Gluckman PD, Klempt ND, Guan J, Mallard EC, Sirimanne E, Dragunow M, Klempt M, Singh K, Williams CE, Nikolics K. Biochem Biophys Res Commun 1992;182:593–599.
11. Nieto-Sampedro M, Lewis ER, Cotman CW, Manthorpe M, Skaper SD, Barbin G, Longo FM, Varon S. Science 1982;217:860–861.
12. Dragunow M, Beilharz E, Sirimanne E, Lawlor P, Williams C, Bravo R, Gluckman P. Mol Brain Res 1994 (in press).
13. Beilharz EJ, Klempt ND, Klempt M, Sirimanne E, Dragunow M, Gluckman PD. Mol Brain Res 1993;18:209–215.
14. Klempt ND, Klempt M, Gunn AJ, Singh K, Gluckman PD. Mol Brain Res 1992;15:55–61.
15. Klempt M, Klempt ND, Gluckman PD. Mol Brain Res 1993;17:347–350.
16. Lee WH, Clemens JA, Bondy CA. Mol Cell Neurosci 1992;3:36–43.
17. Kar S, Baccichet A, Quirion R, Poirier J. Neuroscience 1993;55:69–80.
18. Bergstedt K, Wieloch T. J Cereb Blood Flow Metab 1993;13:895–898.
19. Yamaguchi F, Itano T, Miyamoto O, Janjua NA, Ohmoto T, Hosokawa K, Hatase O. Neurosci Lett 1991;128:273–276.
20. Williams CE, Mallard C, Tan W, Gluckman PD. Clin Perinatol 1993;20:305–326.
21. Guan J, Williams C, Gunning M, Mallard EC, Gluckman PD. J Cereb Blood Flow Metab 1993;13:609–616.
22. Voll CL, Auer RN. J Cereb Blood Flow Metab 1991;11:1006–1014.
23. Voll CL, Auer RN. Neurology 1991;41:423–428.
24. Gluckman PD, Guan J, Williams CE, Beilharz E, Klempt ND, Miller O. Proc Endocrine Soc 1993 (abstract).
25. Bourguignon JP, Gerard A, Alvarez Gonzalez ML, Franchimont P. Neuroendocrinology 1994 (in press).
26. Busto R, Dietrich WD, Globus MY, Ginsberg MD. Stroke 1989;20:1113–1114.
27. Williams CE, Gunn AJ, Gluckman PD, Synek B. Pediatr Res 1990;27:561–565.
28. Williams CE, Gunn AJ, Mallard EC, Gluckman PD. Ann Neurol 1992;31:14–21.
29. Williams CE, Gunn AJ, Gluckman PD. Stroke 1991;22:516–521.
30. Gunn AJ, Williams CE, Mallard EC, Tan WKM, Gluckman PD. Am J Obstet Gynecol 1993 (in press).
31. Tan WKM, Williams CE, Gunn AJ, Mallard EC, Gluckman PD. Ann Neurol 1992;32:677–682.
32. Gluckman PD, Williams CE. Dev Med Child Neurol 1992;34:1015–1018.
33. Rodriguez-Tarduchy G, Collins MKL, Garcia I, Lopez-Rivas A. J Immunol 1992;149:535–540.
34. Neff NT, Prevette D, Houenou LJ, Lewis ME, Glicksman MA, Yin Q-W, Oppenheim RW. J Neurobiol 1993;24:1578–1588.
35. Nielsen FC, Wang E, Gammeltoft S. J Neurochem 1991;56:12–21.
36. Kanje M, Skottner A, Lundborg G, Sjoberg J. Brain Res 1991;563:285–287.
37. McNeill H, Williams C, Guan J, Dragunow M, Lawlor P, Sirimanne E, Nikolics K, Gluckman PD. Neuro Rep 1993 (in press).
38. Prehn JHM, Backhauss C, Krieglstein J. J Cereb Blood Flow Metab 1993;13:521–525.
39. Drago J, Murphy M, Carroll SM, Harvey RP, Bartlett PF. Proc Natl Acad Sci USA 1991;88:2199–2203.

Clinical studies

In vivo use of recombinant human IGF-I: studies in type 1 diabetes

T.D. Cheetham[1], K.L. Clayton[1], J.M. Holly[2], A.M. Taylor[1], M. Connors[1] and D.B. Dunger[1]

[1]*Department of Paediatrics, John Radcliffe Hospital, Headington, Oxford, OX3 9DU, UK;* [2]*Department of Medicine, Bristol University, Bristol, UK*

Abstract. The elevated GH concentrations which lead to insulin resistance in adolescents with insulin-dependent diabetes mellitus (IDDM) are associated with reduced IGF-I levels and IGF bioactivity. The reversal of these abnormalities with rhIGF-I could lead to improved glycaemic control. In subjects with IDDM, rhIGF-I (40 µg/kg/s) results in a rise in IGF-I concentrations which decline with an estimated half-life of 12.1–22.2 h. In controlled studies (five male, 13 female, HbA1 range 8.4–17.0%, duration of diabetes 3–16 years) the mean IGF-I SDS increased from –1.6 to +0.4 and there was a fall in mean overnight GH levels from 23.7 ± 3.3 to 16.3 ± 2.1 mU/l. Insulin requirements for euglycaemia were reduced from 0.33 ± 0.03 mU/kg/min to 0.25 ± 0.02 mU/kg/min (p < 0.001).

In a longer-term study, rhIGF-I was administered to six males with IDDM for a total of 28 days. Sustained increases in IGF-I and IGFBP-3 levels were observed and mean overnight GH levels were reduced at the beginning and the end of the study. Despite reductions in the long-acting insulin requirements (9–26%, median 18%) there was a fall in HbA1c concentrations during the period of rhIGF-I administration.

No adverse effects were noted during these studies and rhIGF-I may have a useful role as an adjunct to standard insulin therapy in adolescents with IDDM.

Introduction

Abnormalities of the GH/IGF-I axis have been well documented in adolescents and young adults with insulin dependent or type 1 insulin-dependent diabetes mellitus (IDDM). Overall mean GH levels in subjects with IDDM are increased at all puberty stages and overnight GH profiles are characterised by an increase in both pulse amplitude and baseline GH concentrations [1]. GH clearance may be prolonged in IDDM [2], but even allowing for this, deconvolution analysis indicates that GH secretion is increased and subjects with IDDM tend to have more overnight GH secretory episodes [3,4]. The diabetogenic effects of GH are well recognised [5,6] and the GH hypersecretion in IDDM has been directly linked with the "dawn phenomena" of increasing overnight insulin requirements [7,8]. In adolescents with IDDM the elevated GH concentrations also lead to accelerated ketogenesis [9] and may be

Address for correspondence: Dr D.B. Dunger, Department of Paediatrics, John Radcliffe Hospital, Headington, Oxford, OX3 9DU, UK.

implicated in the pathogenesis of microangiopathic complications [10].

Whereas levels of GH are increased in adolescents with IDDM, circulating concentrations of IGF-I [11] and the main IGF carrier protein IGFBP-3 tend to be low or in the low normal range [12]. IGF bioactivity is also reduced [13] in part, because of the inhibitory effects of high circulating levels of IGFBP-1 [14].

These abnormalities of the GH/IGF-I axis are thought to arise, because of relative GH insensitivity. GH receptor activity is in part insulin dependent [15] and in subjects with IDDM inadequate portal delivery of insulin is thought to lead to reduced hepatic GH receptor activity, as reflected by reduced levels of GH binding protein [16]. IGFBP-1 is also insulin dependent and the high levels observed in IDDM are also a direct consequence of the failure to achieve appropriate insulin delivery [17]. Improving insulin delivery using continuous subcutaneous insulin infusion systems (CSII) has invariably led to an increase in IGF-I levels [11], but it does not necessarily lead to reductions in GH levels [18,19]. The peripheral hyperinsulinaemia which is inevitable with CSII therapy may in fact lead to a paradoxical increase in GH secretion [20]. The undoubted advantages of portal rather than subcutaneous insulin delivery in improving metabolic control and restoring GH and IGF-I levels to within the normal range has been recently demonstrated [21]. Even if CSII therapy could be improved it is still doubtful whether this mode of therapy would be acceptable in adolescents.

We have explored the alternative strategy of using recombinant human IGF-I (rhIGF-I) to restore IGF-I levels in IDDM, with the expectation that this would lead to reductions in GH secretion and insulin resistance.

Material and Methods

Subjects

Overnight studies. Data are presented which summarise our findings from two sets of overnight studies in a total of 18 subjects, where rhIGF-I (Pharmacia, Stockholm, Sweden) was administered in a dose of 40 µg/kg at 6 pm and compared with a control night when either no injection or placebo was given at the same time. All of the subjects had developed diabetes at least 2 years before the studies or were C-peptide negative. Their ages ranged between 13.5—18.9 years (median 15.3 years) and they were all in mid to late puberty (Tanner Stage 3—5). There were five males and 13 females. All of the subjects studied were in good health. They were nonobese (median BMI 22.3, range 18.8—29.4 kg/m^2), had normal hepatic and renal function and had no signs of preproliferative or proliferative retinopathy on fundoscopy. Prior to the study all subjects were using combinations of short and intermediate acting insulin administered 2 or 4 times daily (range of insulin doses 0.56—1.50 U/kg, median 1.07 U/kg). The median HbA1 of the study group was 13.4% (range 8.4—17.0%; reference range 5.6—7.5%).

Long-term study. Data are also reported from six subjects who received repeated subcutaneous injections of rhIGF-I in a dose of 40 µg/kg over a period of 28 days. These subjects were all males who were in late puberty, aged 13.6–19.4 years (median 15.6 years). They were nonobese (Body mass index <27 kg/m²; range 18.8–25.9, median 23.6 kg/m²,) and their initial HbA1c values ranged between 8.8–15.6% (median 10.8%). These subjects also had no evidence of proteinuria or retinopathy, and they were on multiple injection therapy (three injections of soluble insulin and intermediate acting insulin last thing at night).

The Central Oxford Research Ethics Committee gave ethical approval for all the described studies.

Study protocols

Overnight studies. All intermediate acting insulin was withdrawn at least 36 h before admission and blood glucose concentrations controlled with regular injections of soluble insulin; the last dose being given at the time of the midday meal on the day of admission. Subjects were admitted on two occasions, 1–2 weeks apart. rhIGF-I (Pharmacia) was given in a dose of 40 µg/kg body weight at 6 pm (s.c. into the anterior aspect of the left thigh). Placebo injections were given at the same time.

In the eight subjects who underwent placebo controlled studies, overnight changes in insulin requirements were studied in detail using a continuous insulin infusion, with a rate designed to maintain a blood glucose of 5 mmol/l calculated by a computer programme and portable bedside Apple IIE computer from 15 min blood glucose concentrations [22]. In the other subjects, insulin was either given as an insulin infusion to achieve less stringent normoglycaemia, or the patients were studied on their normal insulin regimen with or without the addition of rhIGF-I. Any subject who became hypoglycaemic during these studies (defined as a blood sugar of <3.0 mmol/l) has been excluded, as this is known to have an effect on GH secretion and insulin sensitivity.

During the overnight profiles, continuous blood sampling was carried out through a heparinised cannula inserted into a distal forearm vein. The forearm of the limb used for sampling was maintained in a heated box to "arterialize" the venous blood.

Basal samples were taken before the injection of rhIGF-I or placebo and thereafter at 15 min (Glucose and GH) 30 min (IGF-I) and 60 min (free insulin, IGFBP-1, ketones and lactate) and 180 min (IGFBP-3) for the subsequent 14 h. IGF-I half-life data are based on samples taken over 22 h in the eight subjects who were part of the placebo controlled study.

Long-term studies. After a run-in period of 1 month during which blood glucose control was optimised, rhIGF-I (Pharmacia) in a dose of 40 µg/kg body weight was administered subcutaneously by the patient for 28 successive days between 6–8 pm each evening. They remained on their multiple injection therapy and were instructed to "float" their intermediate acting insulin according to the results of fasting home blood glucose tests. Overnight sampling profiles (as above) were conducted in hospital, during the run-in period (week 1), during the first night after rhIGF-I administration (week 0) and after the final injection of rhIGF-I (week 4). Glomerular filtration, urinary albumin/creatinine ratios (three consecutive overnight urines), renal size (ultrasonography), fundoscopy, general haematological and biochemical indices, were assessed before and after 28 days of rhIGF-I administration.

Assays

Whole blood glucose was determined by Yellow Spring's instrument analyser (Clandon Scientific Limited, Farnborough, Hants, UK). The samples for GH assay were centrifuged, separated and the plasma frozen at $-20°C$ until assay. Plasma GH concentrations were measured by immunoradiometric assay (NETRIA) as previously described [1]. For plasma free insulin, 1 ml of whole blood was added immediately to 0.6 ml ice cold 25% polyethylene glycol (PEG) m.w. 6,000; (Sigma Limited, Poole, Dorset, UK). Samples are stored at $0°C$ then separated and centrifuged within 13 h. Plasma was stored at $-20°C$ and assayed by a double antibody RIA (Guildhey Antisera Limited, Guildford, Surrey, UK). Intra-assay coefficients variation at 12.2 and 47.2 mU/l were 5.5% and 8.6% respectively.

Plasma samples for IGF-I determination were acid ethanol extracted and IGF-I concentrations determined by RIA as described previously [13]. Serum IGFBP-1 levels were determined by RIA as previously described [23], using antisera and purified antigen kindly provided by Dr H Bohn (Behringwerke, Marburg, Germany). The limit of detection of the assay was 6 µg/l. The intra-assay coefficients of variation were 10.3% and 9.1% at 9 ng/ml and 353 ng/ml respectively. Interassay coefficients of variation were 10.6% and 7.0% at 106 ng/ml and 253 ng/ml respectively. Serum IGFBP-3 levels were determined using a double antibody RIA. IGFBP-3 antiserum (SCH-2/5) was used at a final concentration of 1:8,000. Recombinant glycosylated IGFBP-3 (kindly provided by Dr. C. Maack, Celtrix Pharmaceuticals, Santa Clara, CA) was used for standards. Bound and free ^{125}I-labelled glycosylated IGFBP-3 were separated using a donkey antirabbit SAC-CEL second antibody. The interassay coefficient of variation was 4.28% at 5 mg/l and the intra-assay coefficient of variation was 5.14% at 5 mg/l. Serum IGF-II concentrations were also determined after acid ethanol extraction in the laboratory of Prof. W. Blum (Tubingen, Germany) using a radioimmunoassay which utilises excess IGF-I to block interference from IGFBPs [24]. The interassay CV at 50% B/Bo was 12.2% and the minimum detection limit was 0.018 ng. IGF bioactivity was determined by uptake of [35]SO$_4$ by porcine costal cartilage as previously described [13]. Using this technique the bioactivity of serum is compared to a pooled standard serum. Statistical parameters for the assay are: index of precision (Fiellers Y) 0.06 and the index of variation (Lambda) 0.18.

At the time of the controlled studies, glycosylated haemoglobin (HbA1) was measured by agar electrophoresis using the Ciba-Corning (Halstead, UK) system. The interassay CV at an HbA1 concentration of 7.5% was 8.2% and at a concentration of 17.1% was 5.2%. During the longer-term study of rhIGF-I administration, glycosylated haemoglobin (HbA1c) levels were measured by HPLC (Diamat, BioRad Laboratories Ltd, UK). The intra-assay coefficients of variation were 1.9% and 2.2% at HbA1c levels of 6.9 and 11.5% respectively. The interassay coefficients of variation were 2.7 and 2.3% at HbA1c levels of 7.0 and 11.6% respectively.

Samples for ketones and lactate were taken directly into ice-cold 10% perchloric acid and after separation they were assayed by standard techniques. Glomerular filtration was estimated by an inulin clearance method. Urinary albumin was measured using ELISA. Other haematological and biochemical indices were assessed using standard methods.

Statistical analysis

Data are expressed as means ± SEM, unless otherwise stated. A pulse detection programme, (pulsar) and time series analyses were used to analyse GH profiles. Blood glucose and insulin infusion data were generally normally distributed. Log transformation normalised the ketone and plasma free insulin data and therefore parametrical statistical tests were used for the analysis of these parameters. Nonparametric techniques have been used for the comparison of IGF-I and IGFBP-3 levels and for analysis of data from the study of longer-term rhIGF-I administration.

Results

Short-term overnight studies

Plasma levels of IGF-I and IGFBPs. The administration of rhIGF-I in a dose of 40 µg/kg s.c. led to a prompt rise in IGF-I concentrations which peaked at 5 h after the injection, declining with an estimated half-life of 16.9 h (range 12.1–22.2 h). Overall mean levels overnight were 391 ± 23 ng/ml after rhIGF-I and 231 ± 18 on the control nights ($p < 0.001$) (Fig. 1). Expressed as IGF-I SDS (based on normal data for sex and pubertal stage), the mean IGF-I SDS was –1.6 (range –4.37 to –0.51) on the control nights and +0.4 (range –1.92 to +2.35) after rhIGF-I administration.

Following rhIGF-I administration mean IGFBP-3 levels were elevated in 13 out of the 18 subjects when compared with the control night. Mean levels were 4.8 ± 0.2 µg/ml on the control night and 5.2 ± 0.2 µg/ml ($p = 0.01$) following rhIGF-I (Fig. 1). IGFBP-1 levels showed the characteristic nocturnal surge on both rhIGF-I and control nights, and there were no significant differences. In those subjects where the blood glucose levels were maintained within a tight euglycaemic range (n = 8) the normal inverse relationship between mean plasma insulin levels and IGFBP-1 was similar after rhIGF-I administration (r = –0.76, $p = 0.01$) and on control nights (r = –0.78, $p = 0.01$).

Serum IGF-II levels fell following rhIGF-I administration, reaching a nadir at 4 am. Overall mean levels were 531 ± 33 ng/ml after rhIGF-I and 599 ± 43 ng/ml on the control night ($p < 0.05$).

442

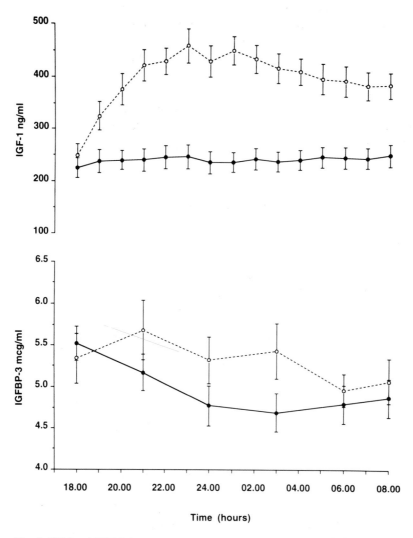

Fig. 1. IGF-I and IGFBP-3 levels after administration of rhIGF-I (--O--) or on the control night (—●—).

IGF bioactivity data are available in four of the subjects studied. In these subjects, bioactivity was 50% of the serum standard on the control night and increased to 89% (0.89 U/ml, range 0.75–1.01 U/ml) after rhIGF-I.

GH secretion. Mean overnight GH levels in the 18 subjects studied fell after rhIGF-I from 23.7 ± 3.3 mU/l to 16.3 ± 2.1 mU/l (p = 0.01) (Fig. 2). In the eight subjects whose blood glucose was clamped in the normal range overnight, detailed pulsar, deconvolution and time series analyses were carried out. These analyses indicated that the administration of recombinant IGF-I did not lead to any change in the dominant

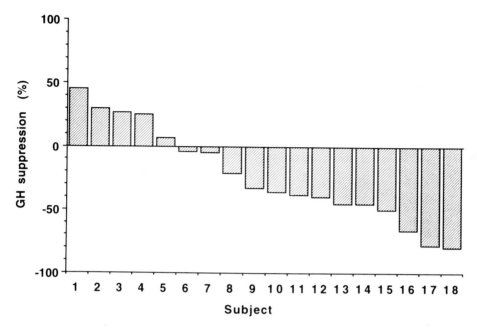

Fig. 2. The percentage reduction in overnight (8 pm to 8 am) GH levels after administration of rhIGF-I, when compared to the control night.

pulse periodicity of GH secretory episodes, but it did lead to a sustained decrease in the amount of GH secreted. The effects on GH secretion were maintained for 22 h and there was no suggestion of any rebound GH secretion.

Overnight insulin requirements. In the eight subjects whose blood sugar was maintained within the euglycaemic range overnight using a variable rate insulin infusion, mean blood glucose concentrations were not significantly different from 2 to 8 am, but insulin requirements were reduced from 0.31 ± 0.04 to 0.25 ± 0.02 mU/kg/min ($p = 0.03$) after rhIGF-I administration. There was also a corresponding fall in mean plasma free insulin levels from 67.9 ± 16 mU/l to 31.9 ± 2.7 mU/l ($p = 0.01$).

In the larger group of 18 subjects, blood glucose concentrations overnight did not differ significantly between the rhIGF-I and control nights from 3.30 am to 7.30 am, but insulin requirements for euglycaemia were 0.33 ± 0.3 mU/kg/min on the control night and 0.25 ± 0.02 mU/kg/min ($p \leq 0.001$) after rhIGF-I (Fig. 3).

Levels of β-hydroxybutyrate and lactate, were not significantly different in these paired studies but overnight concentrations of acetoacetate were significantly lower at 2 am (93 ± 22 μmol/l after rhIGF-I administration when compared with the control night (162 ± 33 μmol/l, $p < 0.05$) (Fig. 3).

Effects of glycaemic control. Mean overnight GH levels on the control nights correlated with HbA1 ($r = 0.62$, $p < 0.01$).

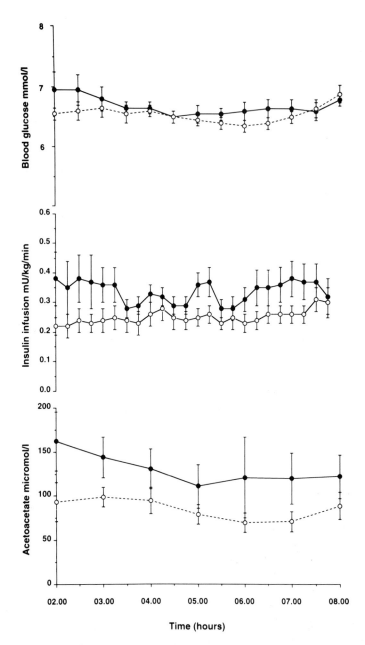

Fig. 3. Insulin infusion requirements and acetoacetate levels during the euglycaemic period (2–8 am) after administration of rhIGF-I (--O--) or on the control night (—●—).

445

Those subjects with the highest GH levels showed the greatest reductions in GH secretion following rhIGF-I. No direct correlation could be identified between the degree of reduction in GH secretion and reductions in insulin requirements in individual subjects.

Long-term rhIGF-I administration

Repeated rhIGF-I administration in an identical dose of 40 µg/kg body weight over a period of a month was well tolerated and did not lead to an increased incidence of hypoglycaemia. Overall mean overnight IGF-I levels were sustained at the end of the 1-month period of treatment in the range 367–485 ng/ml (median 422 ng/ml). Sustained increases in IGFBP-3 concentrations were observed in five of the six subjects with mean levels increasing from 4.5 ± 0.03 µg/ml on the initial baseline night to 5.1 ± 0.4 µg/ml at the end of the 28th day period of treatment.

Overnight mean GH levels were reduced in five out of six subjects on the first night of rhIGF-I administration and in four out of six subjects on the final night, when compared with baseline values. Mean levels were 14.0 ± 3.1 mU/l, 9.2 ± 2.0 mU/l and 7.6 ± 1.7 mU/l from profiles − 1 week, 0 week and +4 weeks, respectively.

Subjects were instructed to reduce the dose of intermediate acting insulin on the first night of rhIGF-I to avoid nocturnal hypoglycaemia. The mean basal insulin requirement remained low throughout the period of rhIGF-I administration (0.41 ± 0.02 U/kg, vs. 0.5 ± 0.02 U/kg during the run-in period, p < 0.05). It increased again to 0.47 ± 0.02 U/kg (p < 0.05) when compared with the treatment period) during the run-out.

Despite reductions in the insulin dose, a significant reduction in HbA1c levels was observed during the treatment period (from 10.4 ± 1.9% to 9.4 ± 1.9%, p < 0.05) (Table 1). HbA1c levels then increased in four subjects during the run-out period. Fructosamine levels were also reduced between week 0 (425 ± 21 µmol/l) and week 4 (400 ± 29 µmol/l).

There were no overall changes in β-hydroxybutyrate and acetoacetate levels, during the overnight profiles. GFR and urinary albumin excretion were not affected by rhIGF-I administration and no changes were observed on retinal examination. No adverse haematological or biochemical changes were noted.

Discussion

With the advent of rhIGF-I therapy there was considerable interest in defining the glucose lowering and insulin-like potential of this peptide. Experimental studies indicated that rhIGF-I had between 6–11% of the glucose lowering effect of insulin [25]. Preliminary studies also indicated that high doses of rhIGF-I may have a role in the treatment of patients with severe insulin resistance either by acting through the IGF-I or even the IGF-II receptor [26,27]. However, the rationale for the use of rhIGF-I in IDDM is quite different. We have argued that restoration of physiological levels of IGF-I in IDDM might lead to normalisation of GH secretion and thus, indirectly to improvements in insulin resistance and the deteriorating glycaemic control which is often observed particularly during adolescence [28].

Our preliminary studies have been very encouraging, in that the restoration of IGF-I levels to the normal range did lead to a sustained reduction in GH secretion. Although the reduction in GH levels was not observed in all cases, significant reductions in GH secretion were noted in those patients with the highest baseline concentrations of GH. Along with the reductions in GH levels overnight, we also noted a concomitant reduction in insulin requirements for euglycaemia. There was a loss of the normal dawn rise in insulin requirements which is generally associated with overnight GH secretion [7,8]. However, we could not detect any direct correlation between reductions in insulin requirements and reductions in GH secretion. This may be due to methodological problems and the relatively small numbers of subjects that we have studied, but we cannot exclude the possibility that rhIGF-I in the dose used may be having direct affects on glucose homeostasis.

Comparable doses of subcutaneous rhIGF-I do not lead to reductions in glucose levels in normal subjects [29], but in those subjects there is a reduction in endogenous insulin secretion which may ameliorate any direct effect of IGF-I on glucose homeostasis. Free levels of IGF-I may be higher after rhIGF-I administration in subjects with IDDM, as they have reduced levels of IGFBP-3 and thus reduced overall IGF binding capacity [12]. IGFBP-3 levels increased following both short-term and long-term rhIGF-I administration in our studies. Data from normal subjects and patients with laron-type dwarfism is, however, conflicting [30–34]. The rise in IGFBP-3 in our subjects is likely to be due to an increase in the formation of ternary complexes, comprising IGFBP-3 and ALS, and thus the half-life of circulating IGFBP-3. These changes occurred despite reductions in GH secretion. ALS production is largely controlled by GH and it generally circulates in excess [35]. Increased ternary complex formation is likely to result from the increased IGF-I levels. IGFBP-1 has been shown to be inhibitory in many bioassay systems and it has been suggested that the overnight rise in IGFBP-1 may exert significant effects on glucose homeostasis [36]. However, in our studies, no significant changes in IGFBP-1 and the relationship between this binding protein and insulin were noted following rhIGF-I administration. Further study will be required to differentiate direct effects of rhIGF-I on glucose homeostasis from those which may result from reductions in GH secretion.

Repeated administration of rhIGF-I in six subjects was well tolerated and led to sustained increases in IGF-I and IGFBP-3. Sustained reductions in GH secretion were observed in four subjects and, although the study design was primarily aimed to look at the safety of repeated rhIGF-I administration, reductions in insulin requirements and in HbA1c levels were also observed. The initial reduction in HbA1c could be attributed to treatment effects as the studies were not controlled, but the rise in HbA1C and insulin requirements with the cessation of IGF-I therapy does suggest an effect of rhIGF-I on blood glucose levels.

Longer-term rhIGF-I therapy must balance beneficial effects on glycaemic control with any possible deleterious effect on diabetic complications. Elevated GH levels have been implicated in the pathogenesis of diabetic microangiopathic complications [10] whereas the IGF-I levels are low in subjects developing these complications [37]. Nevertheless, high IGF-I levels have been noted in some studies of subjects with established complications [38]. There is considerable experimental evidence from animal studies that paracrine production of IGF-I may be implicated in the aetiology of diabetic retinopathy and nephropathy [39]. Reductions in GH and insulin might reduce paracrine production of IGF-I and thus ameliorate complications, but this is yet to be proven.

Further studies of the effects of rhIGF-I in IDDM will have to carefully weigh the obvious benefits inherent in reductions in HbA1c against possible direct adverse effects on microangiopathic complications.

Acknowledgements

TDC was supported by a grant from Pharmacia, Stockholm, Sweden. We would like to thank Pharmacia for providing the rhIGF-I and Professor Werner Blum for undertaking the IGF-II assays. In addition, we would like to thank Sally Strang, Dot Harris and Paul Griffiths for their help with the studies.

References

1. Edge JA, Dunger DB, Matthews DR, Gilbert JR et al. J Clin Endocrinol Metab 1990;71:1356–1362.
2. Mullis PE, Pal BR, Matthews DR, Hindmarsh PC et al. Clin Endocrinol 1992;36:255–263.
3. Pal BR, Matthews DR, Edge JA, Mullis PE et al. Clin Endocrinol 1993;38:93–100.
4. Nieves-Rivera F, Rogol AD, Veldhuis JD, Branscom DK et al. J Clin Endocrinol Metab 1993;77: 638–643.
5. Rizza RA, Mandarino L, Gerich JE. Diabetes 1982;31:663–669.
6. Bratusch-Marrain PR, Smith D, De Fronzo RA. J Clin Endocrinol Metab 1982;55:973–982.
7. Beaurfrere B, Beylot M, Metz C, Reutton A et al. Diabetologia 1988;31:607–611.
8. Edge JA, Matthews DR, Dunger DB. Clin Endocrinol (Oxford) 1990;33:729–737.
9. Edge JA, Harris DA, Phillips PE, Pal BR et al. Diabet Care 1993;16:1011–1019.
10. Gerich JE. N Engl J Med 1984;310:848–849.
11. Amiel SA, Sherwin RS, Hintz RL, Gertner JM et al. Diabetes 1984;33:1175–1179.
12. Batch JA, Baxter RC, Werther G. J Clin Endocrinol Metab 1991;73:964–968.
13. Taylor AM, Dunger DB, Grant DB, Preece MA. Diabet Res 1988;9:177–181.
14. Taylor AM, Dunger DB, Preece MA, Holly JMP et al. Clin Endocrinol 1990;32:229–239.
15. Baxter RC, Bryon JM, Turtle JR. Endocrinology 1980;107:1176–1181.
16. Menon RK, Arslanian S, May B, Cutfield WS et al. J Clin Endocrinol Metab 1992;74:934–938.
17. Holly JMP, Dunger DB, Edge JA, Smith CP et al. Diabet Med 1992;7:618–623.
18. Arias P, Kerner W, de la Fuenta A, Pfeiffer EF. Endocrinologica 1984;107:250–255.
19. Tamborlane WV, Sherwin RS, Koivisto V, Hendler R et al. Diabetes 1979;28:785–788.
20. Press M, Tamborlane MV, Thorner MO, Vale W et al. Diabetes 1984;33:804–806.
21. Shisko PI, Kovaler PA, Goncharov VG, Zajarny IU. Diabetes 1992;41:1042–1049.
22. Matthews DR, Edge JA, Dunger DB. Diabet Med 1990;7:246–251.
23. Holly JMP, Biddlecombe RA, Dunger DB, Edge JA et al. Clin Endocrinol 1988;29:667–675.

24. Blum WF, Ranke MB, Bierich JR. Acta Endocrinol (Copenhagen) 1988;118:374–380.
25. Giacca A, Gupta R, Efendic S et al. Diabetes 1990;39:340–347.
26. Quin JD, Fisher BM, Paterson KR, Inone A et al. N Engl J Med 1990;323:1425–1426.
27. Usala A-L, Madigan T, Burgvera B et al. N Engl J Med 1992;327:853–857.
28. Dunger DB, Cheetham TD, Holly JMP, Matthews DR. Acta Paediatr Suppl 1993;388:49–52.
29. Wilton P, Sietnieks A, Gunnarsson R, Berger L et al. Acta Paediatr Scand 1991;377(suppl):111–114.
30. Young SCJ, Underwood LE, Celniker Ab, Clemmons DR. J Clin Endocrinol Metab 1992;75:603–608.
31. Lieberman SA, Bukar J, Chen SA, Celnicker AC et al. J Clin Endocrinol Metab 1992;75:30–36.
32. Baxter RC, Hizuka N, Takano K, Holman SR et al. Acta Endocrinol 1993;128:101–108.
33. Kanety H, Karasik A, Klinger B, Silbergeld A et al. Acta Endocrinol 1993;128:144–149.
34. Fielder PJ, Gargosky SE, Vaccarello M, Wilson K et al. Acta Paediatr Suppl 1993;388:40–43.
35. Baxter RC. J Clin Endocrinol Metab 1988;67:265–272.
36. Lewitt MS, Denyer GS, Cooney GJ, Baxter RC. Endocrinology 1991;129:2254–2256.
37. Arner P, Sjöberg S, Gjötterberg M, Skottner A. Diabetologia 1989;32:753–758.
38. Merimee TJ, Zapf J, Froesch ER. N Engl J Med 1983;309:527–530.
39. Hammerman MR, Miller SB. Am J Physiol 265 (Renal Fluid Electrolyte Physiol 34):F1–F14.
40. Guler HP, Schmid C, Zapf J, Froesch ER. Proc Natl Acad Sci 1989;6:2868–2872.

Prospects of therapy with IGF-I for catabolic conditions

Louis E. Underwood and David R. Clemmons

Departments of Pediatrics and Medicine, University of North Carolina at Chapel Hill, Chapel Hill, NC 27599, USA

The ability of IGF-I to promote growth in various animal models and in humans with growth hormone insensitivity syndrome [1] indicates that this peptide is anabolic in vivo. Whether IGF-I might be useful as a therapeutic agent for catabolic conditions has not been determined.

Attention has been focused on growth hormone (GH) as a means of reversing catabolic states, as in patients who are unable to ingest adequate calories [2], adults with chronic lung disease [3], patients with burns and in elderly adults. There are reasons to believe, however, that GH alone may have limited usefulness in such conditions: first, GH has been shown to be ineffective in individuals with severe catabolism due to burns [4]. Secondly, in some studies large amounts of GH are required to produce small anabolic effects. Thirdly, GH administration to stressed patients may aggravate insulin resistance and promote hyperglycemia. Finally, there is evidence that anabolic effects of GH attenuate with time, at least in diet-restricted volunteers [5].

This paper will review studies that indicate that IGF-I, used therapeutically, has anabolic actions other than promotion of statural growth. We also will attempt to define some of the conditions under which IGF-I exerts these anabolic actions.

Use of IGF-I in animals made catabolic

Several reports show that IGF-I has anabolic actions when administered in vivo to animals made catabolic. Douglas et al. [6] showed that short-term infusions of IGF-I into fasted lambs reduce net protein loss by 11% using 2.0 nmol IGF-I/kg/h for 5 h; and by 15% using 6.7 nmol IGF-I. The higher dose of IGF-I also significantly increased the rate of protein synthesis in skeletal muscle, cardiac muscle, and liver. In a more long-term (8 weeks) study on castrated yearling sheep, Cottam et al. [7] showed that IGF-I (50 µg/kg q 8 h, s.c.) has minimal effects on body weight gain and no effect on carcass weight or long bone length. In starved mice IGF-I impedes the rate of protein loss [8] and produces a similar effect in lambs infused with tumor necrosis factor [9].

IGF-I in diet-restricted human volunteers; comparison with GH

We have examined the short-term anabolic effects of IGF-I in normal volunteers who are diet-restricted and have compared the effects of IGF-I with those of GH [10]. We produced a state of moderate catabolism in six normal young adult volunteers by restricting their caloric intake to 20 kcal/kg/day for a period of 2 weeks. The test diet contained 1 g protein/kg ideal body weight and nonprotein calories provided as 50% carbohydrate and 50% fat. During the last 6 days of diet restriction, each subject received either human recombinant IGF-I (given intravenously at the rate of 12 μg/kg/h between 4.00 pm and 8.00 am; total daily dose = 182 μg/kg) or 0.05 mg/kg human recombinant GH, given subcutaneously at 4.00 pm. Both the IGF-I and GH were gifts of Genentech, Inc., South San Francisco, CA. Body weight was recorded daily and was used as one of the means for monitoring dietary compliance. Measurements of urea nitrogen and creatinine were made on daily 24 h urine collections. After the completion of each 2-week period of diet-restriction and IGF-I or GH treatment, subjects were permitted to eat a normal diet for 2 weeks. Following this, they resumed dietary restriction for an additional 2 weeks and received the alternate therapy with IGF-I or GH.

IGF-I improved nitrogen balance from –236 ± 45 mmol/day (± SE) during diet restriction alone, to –65 ± 40 mmol/day (p < 0.001) during the last 4 days of IGF-I infusion (Fig. 1).

GH produced a similar effect, such that there was no difference in nitrogen balance between GH and IGF-I during the last 4 days of administration of these hormones. Both IGF-I and GH caused prompt and significant decrements in serum urea nitrogen compared with the period of diet restriction alone (p < 0.001). However, because of its direct insulin-like effects, IGF-I infusions caused fasting

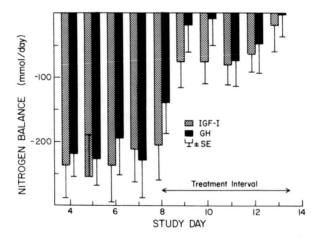

Fig. 1. Changes in nitrogen balance in response to IGF-I and GH. Results are derived from measurements of urea and ammonia nitrogen in 24 h urine collections, which are subtracted from the daily nitrogen intake. Estimated stool and integument losses of nitrogen (245 mmol/day) are added to the urinary values. With permission from [10].

blood glucose levels obtained at the end of each 16-h infusion period to decline (from 4.9 ± 0.91 mmol/l to 3.13 ± 0.44 mmol/l; $p < 0.001$). On the other hand, GH raised fasting glucose values (5.4 ± 1.00 mmol/l during GH treatment). Despite the effects of IGF-I and GH on blood glucose, IGF-I infusions reduced serum insulin and C-peptide while GH raised these indices of carbohydrate metabolism. Infusions of IGF-I caused serum IGF-I concentrations to increase from a basal value of 294 ± 52 µg/l during the period of diet-restriction to 1184 ± 269 µg/l on the last 4 days of IGF-I infusion ($p < 0.001$). Injections of GH increased serum IGF-I values to about 40% of that produced by IGF-I infusions.

This study indicates that our model of caloric restriction produces a state of moderate, controlled catabolism and that IGF-I infusions attenuate this nitrogen wasting. The effects of IGF-I were prompt and were sustained for the duration of the infusions. The magnitude of the IGF-I effects were equivalent to those produced by GH, but because each agent was tested at only a single dose, it is not possible to draw conclusions about the relative potency of the two hormones. The fact that the serum IGF-I levels during IGF-I infusion were nearly 3 times those of GH, suggest that GH might be more potent than IGF-I. Measurement of serum concentrations, however, do not provide information on the IGF-I that might act by autocrine or paracrine mechanisms in response to GH injections. Reports on the relative anabolic effects of IGF-I and GH in rodents suggest that GH is the more potent in hypophysectomized rats, where an 8–10 times greater dose of IGF-I is required to produce an anabolic response equivalent to GH [11,12].

There are several possible mechanisms by which GH might be more potent anabolically than IGF-I or exert slightly different anabolic effects. First, GH is thought to be essential for the stimulation of undifferentiated mesenchmal cells to differentiate into more mature cells such as chondrocytes. These differentiated cells are then capable of responding to IGF-I. Secondly, direct actions of GH on carbohydrate or fat metabolism may be required for an optimal anabolic response. GH enhances insulin secretion and mobilizes free fatty acids. These responses are not produced by IGF-I. Thirdly, because IGF-I is believed to act by autocrine or paracrine mechanisms, large amounts may be needed parenterally to achieve tissue IGF-I concentrations equal to those that occur in response to injections of GH. Finally, GH alters IGF binding protein concentrations by direct mechanisms and in this way may facilitate IGF-I action.

The infusion of IGF-I caused significant increases in IGFBP-1 and IGFBP-2 and a small, but significant, increase in IGFBP-3 [13]. The magnitude of increase in total IGF-I in serum of IGF-I infused patients exceeded the modest increase in IGFBP-3. While the increase in IGFBP-1 and IGFBP-2 might have compensated partially for the small change in IGFBP-3, they were not adequate to provide binding for all the IGF-I infused. This presumption is supported by the disproportionate increase in free IGF-I (from 4.8 ± 2.1 ng/ml basally, to a maximum of 55.5 ± 29 ng/ml during infusion). Baxter and Martin [14] have proposed that IGFBP-3 in the circulation is normally present in amounts that are equimolar with the sum of IGF-I plus IGF-II. A disproportionate increase in IGF-I would therefore perturb this relationship and would cause an increase in free IGF-I unless the change in IGFBP-1 and IGFBP-2 were sufficient to compensate. However, because IGFBP-1 and IGFBP-2 cross intact capillary barriers, whereas IGFBP-3 is bound to the 150 kDa complex and does not exit the circulation, IGF-I that is bound to IGFBP-1 and IGFBP-2 may still equilibrate freely with IGF-I in the extracellular space. Therefore, increases in free IGF-I and changes in the distribution of IGF-I among various IGFBPs could alter the access of IGF-I to tissues.

Combined use of IGF-I and GH in catabolism induced by diet restriction

As the anabolic effects of infusion of IGF-I did not appear to exceed those of injections of GH and hypoglycemia occurred when IGF-I was infused into diet-restricted volunteers, we carried out a second study in which we attempted to determine whether additional GH would enhance the anabolic effect and counterbalance the hypoglycemic effect of IGF-I [15]. We subjected seven normal young adult volunteers to the same calorie-restricted diet under the same experimental protocol as in our previous study. Subjects were given a 20 kcal/kg, 1 g protein/kg diet for two 2-week periods separated by a 2 week interval of normal dietary intake. In the 2nd week of one period of diet restriction, each subject received intravenous infusions of IGF-I for 6 days at the same dose as used in the previous study (12 µg/kg/h for 16 h/day). In the other treatment period the subjects received IGF-I + subcutaneous injections of GH (0.05 mg/kg q day for 6 days).

The effects of IGF-I infusion were virtually identical with those observed in our previous study (Fig. 2). A more pronounced effect, however, was observed with combined IGF-I and GH. The GH/IGF-I combination caused significantly greater

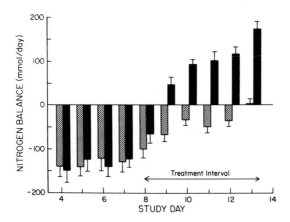

Fig. 2. Changes in nitrogen balance in response to infusion of IGF-I (stippled bars) or combined treatment with GH and IGF-I (solid bars). IGF-I was given by continuous infusion (12 µg/kg IBW/h) for 16 h on days 8–12 between the hours of 4.00 pm and 8.00 am. On day 13 the infusion was given between 8.00 am and 12.00 pm. GH was given by subcutaneous injection (0.05 mg/kg IBW) at 4.00 pm on days 8–12 and at 8.00 am on day 13. Daily nitrogen balance was calculated as in Fig. 1. With permission from [15].

nitrogen retention (262 ± 43 mmol/day) than IGF-I alone (108 ± 28 mmol/day; p < 0.001). In keeping with the evidence for retention of nitrogen was a decrease in serum urea nitrogen. On IGF-I alone the serum urea nitrogen fell from 5.54 ± 0.93 mmol/l (mean ± SD) to 2.35 ± 0.44 (p < 0.001). With combination GH + IGF-I, serum urea nitrogen fell to 1.35 ± 0.33 mmol/l and the mean value for the combination was significantly lower than for IGF-I alone (p < 0.001). GH/IGF-I treatment also caused greater conservation of potassium than IGF-I alone (GH + IGF-I, 34 ± 3 mmol/day, mean ± SE; p < 0.001 compared with IGF-I, which produced no significant potassium conservation) (Fig. 3).

As more than 80% of body potassium is derived from skeletal and connective tissue [16,17] measurement of potassium balance is believed to be an index of protein accretion in these compartments. Our findings, therefore, suggest that a considerable portion of the presumed protein anabolic effect we observed is on nonvisceral protein.

The addition of GH to the IGF-I regimen also attenuated the hypoglycemia observed with IGF-I alone. Capillary blood glucose concentrations measured during IGF-I infusions were consistently higher on GH/IGF-I (4.3 ± 1 mmol/l; mean ± SD) than on IGF-I alone (3.8 ± 0.8 mmol/l; p < 0.001). Additionally, only half as many glucose values were below 3.05 mmol/l (55 mg/dl) on GH/IGF-I as on IGF-I alone, and symptomatic hypoglycemia did not occur with GH/IGF-I after the first day of treatment. Finally, addition of GH attenuated the fall in serum insulin and C-peptide caused by IGF-I alone. The GH/IGF-I regimen produced very high levels of IGF-I in serum (a maximum value of 1854 ± 708 µg/l, 7 times basal). This elevation which is nearly twice that achieved with IGF-I alone is explained in part by the effects of

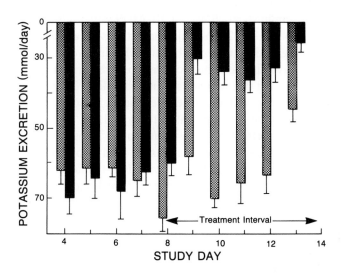

Fig. 3. Changes in urinary potassium excretion in response to infusion of IGF-I (stippled bars) or combined treatment with GH and IGF-I (solid bars). IGF-I and GH were administered as indicated in Fig. 2. Daily urinary potassium excretion was measured from 24-h urine collections. The results are expressed as the mean ± SE for seven subjects. Differences in urinary potassium excretion between treatment groups were significant (p < 0.01) on days 9–13. With permission from [15].

the treatments on IGFBP-3 and the acid labile subunit (ALS) of the 150K circulating IGFBP-3 complex. IGF-I alone suppressed GH secretion, thereby causing the GH-dependent ALS to decline. Replacement of GH caused a modest increase in ALS, an increase in IGFBP-3 and presumably greater sufficiency of each of the components of the 150K IGF-I-IGFBP-3-ALS complex.

These results suggest that GH/IGF-I in combination may be more useful as an anticatabolic regimen than either GH or IGF-I alone. The mechanism(s) for these greater anabolic effects might include: 1. higher tissue concentrations of IGF-I as a result of higher serum values; 2. reversal by GH of the insulin suppressive effect of IGF-I and the possible enhancement of IGF-I's anabolic effect by insulin; 3. the possibility that GH and IGF-I exert their protein anabolic effects by different mechanisms, thereby producing a net additive effect; 4. the increase in ALS and IGFBP-3 almost undoubtedly produced a more stable IGF-I pool in serum and this might improve the availability of IGF-I to tissues. Regardless of the mechanism(s) involved, the results suggest that further study of combined GH/IGF-I therapy in patients with catabolic conditions is warranted.

Use of IGF-I in patients with catabolic conditions

Studies from other laboratories support the possibility that IGF-I might have a therapeutic role in the treatment of the catabolic condition. A study of humans with AIDS-associated cachexia [18] showed that such patients have a smaller increment in serum IGF-I than normal controls in response to injection of GH, suggesting partial GH resistance. Lieberman et al. administered IGF-I to 10 AIDS patients who had average pretreatment weight loss of 15.8 ± 2.1% [18]. The patients received either a low (4 µg/kg/h) or high (12 µg/kg/h) dose of recombinant IGF-I intravenously for 12 h each day for 10 days. Cumulative nitrogen retention was positive during the first 7 days of treatment (+9.52 ± 4.09 g), but this was not so during the final 3 days. The investigators did not observe a significant difference between the high and low doses of IGF-I and expressed concern about the development of tachyphylaxis. Chen et al. [19] also observed signs of a transient effect of IGF-I treatment in 13 patients with catabolism secondary to head trauma. IGF-I treatment was by intravenous infusion at a dose of 10 µg/kg/h for 14 days. Patients treated with IGF-I retained 1.3 g nitrogen/day during the 1st week of treatment. During the 2nd week these patients lost on the average of 4.9 g/day. This decline in their capacity to retain nitrogen was accompanied by a decline in IGF-I serum levels from maximal values early in the infusion, a decline in IGFBP-3 and an increase in IGFBP-2. A pertinent question with regard to these results is whether administration of GH along with IGF-I will prevent the decline in IGFBP-3 and IGF-I, and the loss of nitrogen retaining capacity.

There is also preliminary evidence that IGF-I might have a beneficial effect on bone turnover in patients with osteoporosis. Johannson et al. [20] have reported low plasma concentrations of IGF-I in young men with osteoporosis. This in addition to the evidence that IGF-I has anabolic effects on osteoblasts [21—23] led to a pilot study in which a man with idiopathic osteoporosis was injected with 160 µg IGF-I/kg body weight daily for 7 days. These investigators observed that serum markers of bone formation increased (bone specific alkaline phosphatase increased by 40%, osteocalcin increased by 50% and carboxyl terminal peptide of procollagen type 1 increased by 100%). Markers of bone resorption also increased (i.e., urinary hydroxyproline/creatinine ratio, calcium/creatinine ratio and carboxyl terminal telopeptide of collagen type 1). By 4 weeks after treatment was stopped the markers of bone formation remain elevated, while markers of bone resorption declined. Eberling et al. [24] carried out a multiple dose subcutaneous injection trial of IGF-I in 18 postmenopausal female women over a period of 6 days and observed a dose-dependent increase in serum type 1 procollagen (an index of collagen synthesis) and urinary excretion of deoxypyridinoline (an index of bone collagen breakdown).

Side effects of IGF-I

As with any therapeutic agent, IGF-I has undesirable effects. The dosage that can be administered is limited by the hypoglycemic effect of the peptide. Parotid tenderness and edema of the extremities and face is observed frequently in IGF-I treated adults. Finally, carpal tunnel syndrome has also been reported.

Conclusions

Studies of the potential uses of IGF-I for catabolic conditions are limited, but the results obtained suggest that this peptide will be therapeutically useful. Observations in diet-restricted volunteers suggest that combining IGF-I with GH may produce an additive anabolic effect. IGF-I treatment may also ameliorate the undesirable effects of GH, which raises blood sugar and promotes insulin resistance.

Acknowledgements

Much of the work reported in this manuscript was performed in the General Clinical Research Center of the University of North Carolina. This Center is supported by the General Clinical Research Centers Program of the Division of Research Resources of the National Institutes of Health (Grant RR 00046). The work was also supported by NIH grants HD 26871 and HL 26309 and by a gift from Genentech Inc. The authors acknowledge the assistance of Ms. Vinnie G. Duncan in preparing the manuscript.

456

References

1. Underwood LE, Backeljauw P. J Int Med 1993;234:571–577.
2. Snyder DK, Underwood LE, Clemmons DR. Am J Clin Nutr 1990;52:431–437.
3. Pape GS, Freidman M, Underwood LE, Clemmons DR. Chest 1991;99:1495–1500.
4. Belcher HJ, Mercer D, Judkins KC, Shalaby S, Wise S, Marks V, Tanner NSB. Burns 1989;15:99–107.
5. Snyder DK, Clemmons DR, Underwood LE. J Clin Endocrinol Metab 1988;67:54–61.
6. Douglas RG, Gluckman PD, Ball K, Breier B, Shaw JHF. J Clin Invest 1991;88:614–622.
7. Cottam YH, Blair HT, Gallaher BW, Purchas RW, Breier BH, McCutcheon SN, Gluckman PD. Endocrinology 1992;130:2924–2930.
8. O'Sullivan U, Gluckman PD, Breier BH, Woodall S, Siddiqui RA, McCutcheon SN. Endocrinology 1989;125:2793–2794.
9. Douglas RG, Gluckman PD, Breier BH, McCall JL, Parry B, Shaw JHF. Am J Physiol 1991;261:E606–612.
10. Clemmons DR, Smith-Banks A, Underwood LE. J Clin Endocrinol Metab 1992;75:234–238.
11. Schoenle E, Zapf J, Hauri C, Steiner T, Froesch ER. Acta Endocrinol (Copenh) 1985;108:167–174.
12. Guler HP, Zapf J. Scheiwiller E, Froesch ER. Proc Natl Acad Sci USA 1988;85:4889–4893.
13. Young SCJ, Underwood LE, Celniker A, Clemmons DR. J Clin Endocrinol Metab 1992;75:603–608.
14. Baxter RC, Martin JL. Prog Growth Fact Res 1989;1:49–68.
15. Kupfer SK, Underwood LE, Baxter RC, Clemmons DR. J Clin Invest 1993;91:391–396.
16. Stein PT. J Parenteral Enteral Nutr 1982;6:444–452.
17. Cohn SH, Vartsky D, Yasumra A, Sawitsky A, Zanzi I, Vaswani A, Ellis KJ. Am J Physiol 1980;239:E524–530.
18. Lieberman SA, Butterfield GE, Harrison D, Hoffman AR. 75th Annual Meeting of the Endocrine Society, Las Vegas, NV, June 1993; abstract no. 1664.
19. Chen SA, Bukar JG, Mohler MA, Cook J, Lewis D, Hatton J, Young AB, Rapp RP, Kudsk KA, Gesundheit N. 75th Annual Meeting of the Endocrine Society, Las Vegas, NV, June 1993; abstract No. 1596.
20. Johansson AG, Lindh E, Ljunghall S. Lancet 1992;339:1619.
21. Canalis E. J Clin Invest 1980;66:709–719.
22. Hock JM, Centrella M, Canalis E. Endocrinology 1988;122:254–260.
23. Schmid C, Guler H-P, Rowe D, Froesch ER. Endocrinology 1989;125:1575–1580.
24. Eberling PR, Jones JD, O'Fallon WM, Janes CH, Riggs BL. J Clin Endocrinol Metab 1993;77:1384–1387.

457

IGF-I treatment of syndromes of growth hormone insensitivity

Ron G. Rosenfeld[1], Jaime Guevara-Aguirre[2], Sharron E. Gargosky[1] and Arlan L. Rosenbloom[3]

[1]*Department of Pediatrics, Oregon Health Sciences University, Oregon, USA;* [2]*IEMIR, Quito, Ecuador;* [3]*Department of Pediatrics, University of Florida, Florida, USA*

Syndromes of GH insensitivity

The report in 1966 by Laron, Pertzelan and Mannheimer [1] of the clinical phenotype of GH deficiency combined with elevated serum levels of GH, provides the first documentation of "classical" growth hormone insensitivity (GHI). Subsequent studies demonstrated that increased GH secretion in such patients was the consequence of GH resistance at the level of the target tissue, typically resulting from abnormalities of the GH receptor gene [2]. It is now apparent that Laron syndrome, or GH receptor deficiency, encompasses both quantitative and qualitative defects in the GH receptor. Furthermore, pure Laron syndrome constitutes part of a spectrum of disorders of GH responsiveness (GH insensitivity) that also includes abnormalities of GH signal transduction, primary defects in synthesis of IGF-I, GH insensitivity resulting from antibodies to GH or its receptor and GH insensitivity resulting from malnutrition, liver disease or related disorders [3]. While it seems likely that the clinical response of patients with GHRD (Laron syndrome) to IGF-I treatment will be predictive of the response of other forms of GHI, this remains to be documented.

The elucidation of the molecular pathophysiology of GH insensitivity has provided an ideal source of subjects for clinical trials of recombinant DNA-derived IGF-I [2]. Such patients manifest gross abnormalities in growth and body composition and are, by definition, unresponsive to GH therapy. Consequently, much of the early clinical experience with IGF-I therapy has been in this group of patients.

The preliminary results of these investigations, detailed below, have proven to be of importance in our understanding of the physiology of the IGF axis. The prototypic patient with GH insensitivity (e.g., GHRD) behaves as if he were "functionally" GH deficient. He can, thus, be compared physiologically to a patient with classical GH deficiency, thereby providing an excellent opportunity to see how much of the anabolic actions of GH can be mimicked by IGF-I. Similarly, administration of IGF-I to such patients allows investigation of the regulation of IGFBPs by the IGF peptides themselves and the ability of IGF-I to modulate serum IGFBP-3 concentrations, in both its binary and ternary forms, can be documented. Finally, the physiological response of the patient to systemic IGF-I administration permits evaluation of the "endocrine," vs. "autocrine-paracrine" actions of IGF peptides.

IGF-I administration to normal men

The development of clinical trials of IGF-I therapy in patients with GHRD was based upon the demonstration of bioactivity and safety, following administration to normal volunteers. The initial reports of IGF-I administration to normal men was as a single intravenous injection of 100 µg/kg to eight healthy volunteers [4]. Hypoglycemia was noted within 15 min following rapid intravenous administration, with a nadir at 30 min to approximately 50% of baseline glucose and a return to normal glucose levels by 120 min. When compared with insulin, IGF-I was shown to have 6% of insulin's potency on an equimolar basis. Hypoglycemia is most likely attributable to an increase of free IGF-I from 19% of total serum IGF-I at baseline to 80% of total serum concentrations by 15 min postinjection, and a return to baseline proportions by 7 h after administration. Although calculations of "free" IGF-I in serum are still suspect, it seems reasonable to assume that rapid intravenous administration results in an increase in the free:bound ratio in serum, for at least some period of time before the "free" peptide is bound by the various IGFBPs. Subsequently, longer-term studies were carried out with 6-day infusion in two normal adult males at a rate of 20 µg/kg/h, which raised serum IGF-I concentrations from 150 to 700 ng/ml, but without producing clinically significant hypoglycemia [5]. Bioactivity of the administered IGF-I was supported by the observations that serum GH levels were suppressed, creatinine clearance was increased by 30%, and plasma urea decreased, without any change in urinary excretion of urea, thereby indicating increased protein synthesis. The short-term half-life of IGF-I bound to the 50K binding protein was 20–30 min, with a prolonged half-life of 12–15 h for IGF-I bound to the 150–200 K ternary complex, made up of IGFBP-3 and the acid-labile subunit. Following subcutaneous injection, the half-lives of free IGF-I and -II were estimated to be 10–12 min and their production rates 10–13 mg/day [6]. Increases in serum IGF-I were accompanied by reciprocal falls in serum IGF-II levels, presumably representing displacement of IGF-II from IGFBPs. IGF-I disappeared from serum within 14–18 h following subcutaneous administration. This relatively long half-life for IGF peptides demonstrates the importance of IGFBPs as reservoirs for both IGF-I and -II.

Subsequently, six normal subjects and two patients with GH deficiency were given 100 µg/kg IGF-I by daily subcutaneous injection for 7 consecutive days [7]. Normal subjects had a 250% increase in serum IGF-I levels following the initial administration, with a depression of blood glucose levels 4 h postinjection, but not to abnormally low levels. Similar results were seen in the GH deficient subjects, but with lower serum IGF-I levels at all time points evaluated. This latter observation presumably reflects the deficiency in serum IGFBP levels in GH deficient or resistant individuals, and is an important factor in the pharmacokinetics of IGF-I administration to such patients (see below). During the course of this brief trial no significant changes were seen in the excretion of urea nitrogen, creatine, creatinine, sodium, potassium, calcium or insulin C-peptide during the 7 days of IGF-I administration. Following single subcutaneous injection of 40 or 80 µg/kg IGF-I in healthy volunteers, Wilton et al [8] found mean serum IGF-I concentrations to increase by

150 and 254 ng/ml, respectively. Repeated daily injections of 40 µg/kg produced a steady state serum IGF-I level of 150 ng/ml above baseline. The only pharmacokinetic index that changed between single and repeated injections was the T-max, which decreased from 6.9 h following a single injection to 3.5 h after a week of administration. There were no hypoglycemic symptoms, no suppression of endogenous IGF-I production and no suppression of fasting insulin levels. Postprandial insulin concentrations, however, were lowered by IGF-I, when compared with placebo injection.

Short-term treatment of GHRD with IGF-I

As GHRD individuals are markedly deficient in IGFBP-3, as well as IGF-I, concern existed that they might attain higher concentrations of free IGF-I for an extended period of time following IGF-I administration and might be more susceptible to IGF-I-induced hypoglycemia. There was also concern that the therapeutic response to IGF-I might, at least in part, be dependent upon adequate serum levels of IGFBP-3, presumably necessary to sustain a circulating pool of IGF-I for delivery to IGF receptors. Previous reports of IGF-I administration to rodents had indicated a rise in serum levels of IGFBP-3 [9—11], suggesting that treatment of GHRD patients with IGF-I would stimulate an accompanying rise in serum IGFBP-3 levels, thereby "normalizing" IGF-I pharmacokinetics.

In the initial report of administration of recombinant IGF-I to patients with GHRD, acute symptomatic hypoglycemia was induced by an intravenous bolus of 75 µg/kg in nine individuals, between 11—33 years of age, who were in a prolonged fasting state [12]. Serum glucose levels dropped to an average of 45% of baseline 30 min following injection and hypoglycemia persisted until a meal was given at 2 h. A paradoxical rise in serum GH levels was noted, presumably reflecting the IGF-I-induced hypoglycemia. Of note, however, is that in patients with defects of the GHR, the counter-regulatory effects of GH on glucose levels cannot be expected to normalize serum glucose levels.

Subcutaneously administered IGF-I to eight GHRD patients, including three children, at a dosage of 150 µg/kg/day for 7 days, in contrast to the experience with i.v. drug in the fasting state, did not produce symptomatic hypoglycemia [13]. Walker et al [14] administered IGF-I intravenously for up to 11 days to a 9-year-old child with GHRD. Significant anabolic effects were noted, including a decrease in serum urea nitrogen, increase in urinary calcium excretion and decrease in urinary phosphate and sodium excretion. Asymptomatic hypoglycemia, as well as hyperglycemia and ketonemia were observed, as was suppression of IGF-II levels.

The effects of giving subcutaneous IGF-I at a dose of 40 µg/kg q12 h over 7 days in 6 Ecuadorian adults with GHRD were studied by Vaccarello et al [15]. This frequency of administration was employed in an effort to overcome the deficiency in serum IGFBP-3 levels and allow for "sustained" increases in serum IGF-I levels. With regular feeding, no hypoglycemia was observed, although there was suppression of 2 h postprandial insulin levels. Urinary calcium excretion increased 2-fold without an accompanying change in serum calcium levels. Mean integrated 24-h GH levels were significantly suppressed, as were the number of peaks, area under the curve and clonidine-stimulated GH release, demonstrating that administered IGF-I was capable of feedback inhibition at the pituitary and/or hypothalamic level. At this dosage of IGF-I, a mean peak serum IGF-I level of 253 ± 11 ng/ml was achieved between 2–6 h after injection, with a mean trough level of 137 ± 8 ng/ml. These peak and trough serum IGF-I levels are not significantly different from IGF-I levels seen in normal adult Ecuadorian controls. As previously reported [14], serum IGF-II levels were suppressed, although the total serum IGF levels (IGF-I + IGF-II) did not change significantly. Surprisingly, serum IGFBP-3 levels did not increase with IGF-I administration, although IGFBP-2 levels did rise. The failure to demonstrate an IGF-induced rise in serum IGFBP-3 concentrations differed from previous reports of IGF-I administration to rats (see above).

Long-term treatment of GHRD with IGF-I

Although the short-term studies cited above demonstrated the bioactivity of exogenous IGF-I, it was still not clear that administered IGF-I could function as an "endocrine" hormone and stimulate skeletal growth. Subsequently, growth acceleration comparable to that seen with GH treatment of GH deficiency was reported in five children treated for 3–10 months with recombinant IGF-I at an initial daily dosage of 150 µg/kg given as a single daily injection [16]. Growth velocity on therapy ranged from 8.8–13.6 cm/year. Similarly, the patient previously reported by Walker et al [14] demonstrated sustained growth on twice daily injections of 120 µg/kg/dose, with an acceleration of growth from 6.5 to 11.4 cm/year during 9 months of treatment [17]. Serum and urinary urea nitrogen decreased; urinary calcium increased, as did creatinine clearance and urine volume. Fasting and postprandial glucose concentrations were normal and clinical hypoglycemia was not a problem.

To date, the largest experience with treatment of GHRD (and GHD-IA) children with IGF-I is that reported by Wilton et al [18] in a study group of 30 patients from Europe and Australia, ages between 3–23 years. Five patients responded with growth acceleration to 40 µg/kg b.i.d. for 6–12 months; other patients were either increased progressively to 120 µg/kg b.i.d., often because of a marginal response on the lower dosage or were started on the higher dosages. All, but the oldest (20 and 23 years old), responded with a growth rate increase in excess of 2 cm/year, compared to pretreatment. Hypoglycemia, defined as a blood glucose level <3 mmol/l, with or without symptoms, occurred in 17 patients, and in two of these was severe with convulsions. Twelve patients reported mild to moderate headache, which in one case was severe and was accompanied by vomiting and bilateral papilledema that resolved after cessation of treatment. One child had hypotension, a modest decrease in serum potassium and fatigue following each injection, so treatment was stopped. Partial peripheral paresis of the right facial nerve was seen in one child after 10 days of therapy and resolved within 14 days. Savage et al [19] have recently updated these results. Five subjects treated for 9 months with 40 µg/kg b.i.d. had a mean annual growth rate of 7.8 cm; seven subjects treated for 9 months with 40 µg/kg b.i.d., increasing to 120 µg/kg b.i.d., had a mean annual growth rate of 7.1 cm. Nine subjects treated for 9 months with 120 µg/kg b.i.d. had a mean annual growth rate of 11.0 cm.

Two pubertal Ecuadorian GHRD patients treated with long-acting GnRH analog and IGF-I (120 µg/kg b.i.d.), have also demonstrated a sustained growth response during 9 months of therapy. The large number of recently identified cases of GHRD in southern Ecuador (now more than 70) offers an unique opportunity for clinical testing of the efficacy of IGF-I therapy without the potential confounding effects of altered nutritional or health status. Furthermore, since these patients share a common point mutation in exon 6 of the extracellular domain of the receptor, considerable clinical homogeneity exists among the subjects. A randomized, placebo-controlled study of recombinant IGF-I in prepubertal children from this population is underway, with completion of the 1st year scheduled for early 1994.

Remaining treatment issues

Clinical trials of recombinant IGF-I in syndromes of GH insensitivity are still in their early stages. While IGF-I therapy has been shown to stimulate growth acceleration (short-term, at least), we know little about optimal dose or frequency of administration. The dosages of IGF-I employed in the early clinical trials were based in part on safety issues (e.g., hypoglycemia) and the twice daily frequency result from concern about a short half-life in patients who were IGFBP-3 deficient. The failure of serum IGFBP-3 levels to rise has been unexpected and it is all the more remarkable that growth acceleration has occurred in the absence of any rise in serum IGFBP-3 levels or major change in the pharmacokinetics of IGF-I. In this regard, it is of note that Laron and colleagues [20] have reported that two patients with GHRD treated with IGF-I for 12 weeks showed increases in IGFBP-3 levels, measured by western ligand blot. This is in contrast to the observation by Gargosky et al [21] that 1-week treatment with IGF-I did not alter serum IGFBP-3, ALS, or the distribution of the IGF peptides among binary and ternary forms of IGFBP-3. Longer-term studies in Ecuador have failed to demonstrate IGF-I induced increases in serum IGFBP-3, measured by either RIA or western ligand blot (data not shown).

It is now clear that IGF-I, long-thought to be important as an autocrine or paracrine growth factor, is fully capable of acting as an endocrine hormone. In GHRD, the bioavailability of administered IGF-I may be enhanced by the failure of serum IGFBP-3 levels to rise. The growth response to exogenous IGF-I also discredits the "dual effector" hypothesis which states that growth results from the dual effects of GH, involved in differentiation of precursor cells in the epiphyseal plate and IGF-I, involved in stimulating cell replication. IGF-I, by itself, is fully capable of stimulating skeletal growth. Whether the growth response to IGF-I will be sustained and free of toxicity remains to be established.

The finding of diminished bone density and relative obesity in adults with GHRD suggests the possibility of IGF-I replacement therapy in affected adults [22]. IGF-I stimulates osteoblastic activity in vitro and in vivo in mature rat bone, while decreasing osteoblastic activity, resulting in a net anabolic effect on bone mineral. This can be accomplished in the absence of GH, as demonstrated by IGF-I treatment of hypophysectomized rat [23]. Bone density is also increased in hormonally normal sheep given 50 µg/kg/day of IGF-I, suggesting potential efficacy of IGF therapy of osteoporosis in GH/IGF replete normal aging individuals [24].

At this point, it appears clear that systemic administration of IGF-I is capable of stimulating both short-term anabolic effects and growth [25,26]. On the other hand, preliminary data suggest that the growth response observed in GHRD patients given IGF-I once or twice a day does not quite equal that observed in naive GH deficient children treated with daily GH. This apparent limitation in the growth response may indicate:

1. IGF-I needs to be administered at a higher dosage;
2. IGF-I needs to be administered more frequently, especially in light of the low serum IGFBP-3 concentrations;
3. IGF-I should be administered together with IGFBPs; and
4. GH has an added differentiative or mitogenic action which makes it superior to IGF-I.

This action may be as simple as the induction of IGFBP-3 gene transcription.

Acknowledgements

Supported in part by grants from the National Organization for Rare Disorders, Inc. (RGR), Grant DK45830 from the NIH (RGR, JGA, ALR), the FDA (RGR, JGA, ALR), and Pharmacia (RGR, JGA, ALR).

Note

Portions of this manuscript were derived from reviews listed as references 25 and 26.

References

1. Laron Z, Pertzelan A, Mannheimer S. Isr J Med Sci 1966;2:152–155.
2. Rosenfeld R, Rosenbloom AL, Guevara-Aguirre J. Growth hormone insensitivity due to growth hormone receptor deficiency. Endocrinol Rev 1994 (in press).
3. Laron Z, Blum W, Chatelain P et al. J Pediatr 1993;122:241.
4. Guler HP, Zapf J, Froesch ER. N Engl J Med 1987;317:137–140.
5. Guler HP, Schmid C, Zapf J, Froesch ER. Proc Natl Acad Sci USA 1989;86:2868–2872.
6. Guler HP, Zapf J, Schmid C, Froesch ER. Acta Endocrinol (Copenhagen) 1989;121:753–757.
7. Takano K, Hizuka N, Shizume K, Asakawa K, Fukuda I, Demura H. Growth Reg 1991;1:23–28.

8. Wilton P, Sietnicks A, Gunnarsson R, Berger L, Grahnen A. Acta Paediatr Scand 1991;377(suppl): 111–114.

9. Zapf J, Hauri C, Waldvogel M et al. Proc Natl Acad Sci USA 1989;86:3813–3817.

10. Clemmons DR, Thissen JP, Maes M, Ketelslegers JM, Underwood LE. Endocrinology 1989;125: 2967–2972.

11. Glasscock GF, Hein AN, Miller JA, Hintz RL, Rosenfeld RG. Endocrinology 1992;130:203–210.

12. Laron Z, Erster B, Klinger B, Anin S. Lancet 1988;2:1170–1172.

13. Laron Z, Klinger B, Jensen JT, Erster B. Clin Endocrinol 1991;35:145–150.

14. Walker JL, Ginalska-Malinowska M, Romer TE, Pucilowska JB, Underwood LE. N Engl J Med 1991;324:1483–1488.

15. Vaccarello MA, Diamond Jr FB, Guevara-Aguirre J et al. J Clin Endocrinol Metab 1993;77:273–280.

16. Laron Z, Anin S, Klipper-Auerbach Y, Klinger B. Lancet 1992;339:1258–1261.

17. Walker J, Van Wyk JJ, Underwood LE. J Pediatr 1992;121:641–646.

18. Wilton P (on behalf of the Kabi Pharmacia Study Group). Treatment with recombinant insulin-like growth factor-I of children with growth hormone receptor deficiency (Laron syndrome). Acta Paediatr Scand 1992;282(suppl):137–141.

19. Savage MO, Wilton P, Ranke MB et al. Pediatr Res 1993;3:S5 (abstract 17).

20. Kanety H, Karasik A, Klinger B, Silbergeld A, Laron Z. Acta Endocrinol 1993;128:144.

21. Gargosky SE, Wilson KF, Fielder PJ et al. J Clin Endocrinol Metab 1993;77:1683.

22. Guevara–Aguirre J, De la Torre W, Rosenbloom AL, Acosta M, Rosenfeld RG. Proceedings of the 73rd Annual Meeting of the Endocrine Society 1991;385 (abstract 1417).

23. Guler HP, Zapf J, Schweiwiller E, Froesch ER. Proc Natl Acad Sci USA 1988;85:4889–4893.

24. Cottam YH, Blair WT, Gallaher BW et al. Endocrinology 1992;130:2924–2930.

25. Rosenfeld RG, Rosenbloom AL, Guevara-Aguirre J. Growth hormone insensitivity due to growth hormone receptor deficiency. Endocrinol Rev (in press).

26. Rosenfeld RG, Rosenbloom AL, Guevara-Aguirre J. In: Blackman M, Harman SM, Roth J, Shapiro J (eds) GHRH, GH and IGF-I: Basic and Clinical Advances. Serono Symposia (in press).

Index of authors

Scheper, W. 43
Schwander, J. 151
Schwartz, J. 3
Segovia, B. 217
Shimasaki, S. 193
Siddle, K. 95
Silverman, L.A. 275
Silvian-Drachsler, I. 329
Skottner, A. 329, 401
Soos, M.A. 95
Steeb, C.-B. 409
Stepaniuk, O. 263
Stephenson, E. 3
Straus, D.S. 33
Streck, R. 253
Strong, D.D. 205
Suh, D.-S. 163
Sumitomo, S. 193
Sussenbach, J.S. 43
Suwanichkul, A. 141

Tanahashi, H. 193
Taylor, A.M. 437
Thomas, M.J. 13
Tomas, F.M. 131
Trivedi, B. 77

Underwood, L.E. 449

Vu, T.H. 351

Wallace, J.C. 57
Walton, P.E. 131
Warburton, C. 247
Werner, H. 107
Werther, G.A. 291
Williams, C.E. 427
Wissink, S. 175
Wood, T. 253

Zapf, J. 381

Subject index

474